Choosing Cesarean

Choosing Cesarean

A NATURAL BIRTH PLAN

Magnus Murphy, MD, and
Pauline McDonagh Hull

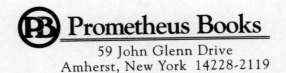

Prometheus Books

59 John Glenn Drive
Amherst, New York 14228-2119

Published 2012 by Prometheus Books

Cover image © 2012 Media Bakery
Cover design by Nicole Sommer-Lecht

Inquiries should be addressed to
Prometheus Books
59 John Glenn Drive
Amherst, New York 14228–2119
VOICE: 716–691–0133
FAX: 716–691–0137
WWW.PROMETHEUSBOOKS.COM

16 15 14 13 12   5 4 3 2 1

Library of Congress Cataloging-in-Publication Data

Murphy, Magnus, 1963–
    Choosing cesarean : a natural birth plan / by Magnus Murphy and Pauline
McDonagh Hull.
        p. ; cm.
    Includes bibliographical references and index.
    ISBN 978–1–61614–511–8 (pbk.)
    ISBN 978–1–61614–512–5 (ebook)
    I. Hull, Pauline McDonagh, 1973– II. Title.
    [DNLM: 1. Cesarean Section. WQ 430]

618.8'6—dc23

2011037521

Printed in the United States of America

Disclaimer

1. NOT MEDICAL ADVICE

Information contained in *Choosing Cesarean: A Natural Birth Plan* is intended for educational and informational purposes only and is not professional medical advice, diagnosis, treatment, or care, nor is it intended to be a substitute thereof. Always seek the advice of a physician or other qualified health provider duly licensed to practice in your jurisdiction. Never disregard professional medical advice or delay in seeking advice because of something you have read in *Choosing Cesarean: A Natural Birth Plan*. Always consult with your physician or other qualified healthcare provider before embarking on a new treatment plan. Information contained in *Choosing Cesarean: A Natural Birth Plan* is not exhaustive and does not cover all contingencies.

2. NO PHYSICIAN-PATIENT RELATIONSHIP

The information contained in *Choosing Cesarean: A Natural Birth Plan* does not establish a physician-patient or professional relationship between the reader and the authors of *Choosing Cesarean: A Natural Birth Plan*, nor is it intended as a solicitation of individuals to become patients or clients of the authors.

3. DISCLAIMER OF WARRANTIES

The authors and publisher of *Choosing Cesarean: A Natural Birth Plan* disclaim any warranty concerning the application of the information contained therein to your specific circumstances. Always seek the advice of a physician or other qualified health provider duly licensed to practice in your jurisdiction.

4. LIMITATION OF LIABILITY

In no event shall the authors and publisher of *Choosing Cesarean: A Natural Birth Plan* and their respective successors be liable for damages of any kind, including and without limitation any direct or indirect, special, punitive, incidental, or consequential damages including and without limitation any loss or damages in the nature of, or relating to, lost business, medical injury, personal injury, wrongful death, improper diagnosis, inaccurate information, improper treatment, or any other loss incurred in connection with the information contained in *Choosing Cesarean: A Natural Birth Plan*, regardless of the cause.

Contents

Acknowledgments

If you are facing in the right direction, all you need to do is keep on walking.

—Buddhist proverb

Pauline McDonagh Hull

With thanks to all the people in my life who have helped me to keep on walking.

The many doctors, medical professionals, and fellow advocates who have encouraged me to campaign confidently for clarity and real choice. I set out on this journey alone, as a journalist and woman determined to set the record straight on cesarean birth, and I've been lucky to make so many wonderful allies along the way. Thank you all.

Visitors to my website and blog, thank you for all your motivating comments and shared stories. On tired days, in defeated moments, or when my resolution has wavered, with uncanny timing someone has written to me with personal gratitude or a request for help, reminding me all over again why I must persevere.

My brother Steve, thank you for always being there for me; and my parents, Theresa and Steve, thank you for nurturing my love of books and instilling in me the courage to stand up for what I believe in. Mum, I still carry your silver typewriter bracelet charm.

My obstetrician, Dr. Patricia Dreyfuss, thank you for bringing our children into the world safely, and for giving me the best care and support imaginable.

My coauthor, Dr. Magnus Murphy, with whom I have experienced this most unique and enjoyable writing partnership, thank you for your shared passion and conviction, and not least, for your incredible patience with my inclusion of ever more references! I look forward to finally meeting you.

And most of all, my family—Richard, thank you for your unwavering support, understanding, and love, and for being my long-suffering cesarean sounding board. Charlotte and Jack, for making my heart swell so much it hurts, every single day. And Balto, for the canine company and screen breaks you continue to provide me with throughout many a late night working. I love you all.

Magnus Murphy, MD

For me, this book is the culmination of a very long road of professional development, academic growth, and changed beliefs. My work as an obstetrician and gynecologist and latterly as a urogynecologist has been profoundly influenced by my thoughts and conclusions regarding the subject matter of this book.

My development has also been influenced by too many past and present colleagues and mentors throughout the years to mention individually, but to all of them I am grateful, especially my first teachers—my wonderful parents, who taught me to think independently and never take anything at face value. I also specifically want to thank my teachers and professors at my alma mater, Stellenbosch University Medical School in South Africa, for a medical education that was second to none.

This joint project was first conceived within hours of my "meeting" Pauline online and discovering a shared interest, and more than that, the shared desire to bring this topic to the attention of women everywhere. Without Pauline as my partner, this would not have been possible. To Pauline, thank you.

To my family—Ronel, Michele, and Meghan. Thank you for your love, encouragement, and putting up with all the hours I've spent over the years, on weekends and in evenings, researching, writing, and on Skype™.

Finally, to my patients, you have shaped my thinking more than all the knowledge I've gained in books and journals. Your stories have inspired me to do better. Your courage has forced me to rethink old paradigms. Together with Pauline, our individual roads of discovery merged into the process that has culminated in this book.

Preface

*In fact the a priori reasoning is so entirely satisfactory to me
that if the facts won't fit in, why so much the worse for the
facts is my feeling.*
   —Erasmus A. Darwin, in a letter to his brother Charles,
       after reading *The Origin of Species*
     (in *The Life of Charles Darwin*, Francis Darwin, 1902)

This book will have its critics, which we completely expect and even understand, given the magnitude of the emotions that are associated with birth. At a time when it seems like the loudest rallying cries are from women with a desire to return to less "medicalized" and more natural birthing methods, it may be disconcerting to some readers that the opposite is also true—there are many women who prefer surgery and *choose* a cesarean birth, and there are many doctors and other medical professionals who completely support this choice. And although this choice still represents a relatively small minority of women, we believe that as more and more women learn the truth about different birth risks and benefits, the numbers requesting surgery are very likely to increase and will continue to have an impact on cesarean rates in the future.

That said, it is *not* the authors' intention to advocate cesarean birth for *all* women, and our alluding to the inevitability of increasing cesarean rates should not be interpreted as any ideological desire on our part for more women to have cesareans. In fact, we are firmly of the opinion that some women are not suitable candidates for surgery, and our support of maternal request is certainly not synonymous with a policy of cesarean on demand for everyone.

Primarily, the premise of this book is to defend the legitimacy of a planned cesarean on maternal request, and by doing so, to highlight the problem that has existed in cesarean research for decades—that is, *mixed data*. Unfortunately, the majority of birth research to date has not compared apples with apples, and this has led to widespread criticism, ignorance, and misrepresentation of planned cesareans. At best, the information that is

19

available on maternal request cesareans can be difficult to navigate and is reliant on *most probable* approximations of risks and benefits; at worst, it can be irrelevant or even disingenuous. This, in turn, has led to inaccurate and sometimes biased interpretations of the facts, which are then presented to the news media for public consumption.

For example, the outcomes of *all* cesareans (emergency and planned) have often been compared with successful, spontaneous vaginal birth outcomes only—ignoring the fact that emergency surgery, with its associated risks, is more likely to occur with a vaginal birth plan than a cesarean birth plan. And even studies that acknowledge the need to separate planned and emergency caesarean births do not always take the next logical step of assigning the relevant emergency outcomes to the group with planned vaginal births. Similarly, planned cesarean births are often a combination of primary and repeat surgeries, and the different indications for the surgery are rarely separated (for example, medical indication, obstetrical indication, and maternal request with no indication). As a consequence, cesarean births with inherently higher risks are pooled with lower-risk surgeries and used to inform women of risks that may not actually apply to them. In effect, the risks of a planned cesarean are frequently overestimated, while the risks of a planned vaginal birth are understated.

Of course, in presenting our arguments in this book, we have had to navigate this very same pool of research to produce sufficient evidence to support our case, so it's understandable that some readers might question the quality of our evidence. However, we assure you that by taking a worldwide view of the research into planned cesarean outcomes, by unearthing facts and data that are not commonly publicized or juxtaposed, and by separating high-quality evidence from anecdotal or personal contributions, we are confident that our portrayal of maternal request as a legitimate birth choice is sound, and furthermore, that our position is supported by a number of professional bodies in the United States and other countries. We make properly referenced arguments and statements using all levels of scientific evidence, including the highest, level 1 and 2, wherever possible, but we also incorporate the personal experience of medical professionals and women who have had various types of births. And although we realize that personal evidence is not the equivalent of well-designed, randomized controlled studies, we feel that in the absence of such studies, these voices demand attention.

What *may* be challenging at times—and indeed has sometimes been a challenge for us as authors—is that because the research and examples we cite are taken from a wide variety of countries, there are statements in the book that are not necessarily relevant to every single reader's country of residence or place of work. You might not always recognize certain trends, problems, or arguments as part of your reality, and therefore we ask you to bear this in mind when reading.

We would also like to preempt some of the criticism we will inevitably receive and to urge readers to be mindful that the quality of different criticism can vary. As we've said, a book such as this can be expected to elicit strong reaction, since the topic is emotive and personal and goes against ingrained paradigms. As such, while constructive criticism is useful, and indeed evidence-based criticism opens up a platform for healthy debate (which is precisely what this subject needs), where criticism is purely an unsubstantiated, emotional, or ideological reaction, it is not only unhelpful for the debate itself but is likely elicited by those who have no knowledge of much of the research quoted in this book.

Finally, lest we are presented as irresponsible, scalpel-happy advocates of all things surgical, we would like to stress that our motivation for writing this book comes from a deep-rooted desire to improve the health outcomes of mothers and babies. We are genuinely concerned about the physical and psychological well-being of women whose maternal request is ignored or refused, but also about the wider population of women who may be coerced into making birth choices without being fully informed of the potential risks. The obsession in many countries with reducing cesarean rates seems to be *at any cost*—all that matters is getting that magic number down. And meanwhile, women and babies die in droves or endure devastating injuries in the developing world, largely because they lack access to the lifesaving benefit that is cesarean surgery.

We don't claim to know what every woman wants or needs, but we are confident that despite the ideological rhetoric that abounds, very few contemporary women want the equivalent of a natural birth from centuries ago, when death and injury rates for babies and mothers were horrifically high. It's easy to forget sometimes that pregnancy and childbirth are inherently risky events, and while some women look forward to their experience being a wonderful rite of passage or an empowering personal journey with as few medical interventions as possible, this is neither the desire nor the reality of others. We strongly object to the idea that *every* pregnant woman would or should want to take this approach.

It is our wish that women would be fully educated, counseled, and supported by medical professionals regarding their birthing choices, and we believe that for most women, planned cesarean birth should be included in the range of choices available to them.

Introduction

Normal women come to us demanding a cesarean delivery to
avoid the agonies of childbirth. While none would grant them
this request, it is well to remember that what is a fantasy today
may be a fact tomorrow.

—O. Paul Humpstone, MD, FACS,
in the published proceedings
of a 1920 symposium titled
"Cesarean Section vs. Spontaneous Delivery"

In the very first volume of its production, the *American Journal of Obstetrics and Gynecology* published an article by a doctor who was eminently ahead of his time, and whose words this book echoes almost a century later. In 1920, Dr. O. Paul Humpstone wrote the prophetic words above and also these statements:

> Hysterotomy (cesarean) [is] the easiest way for any primiparous woman to have her baby; and it is the surest way of having a live baby. It is the only painless childbirth that occurs today.
>
> The old idea that childbirth is limited to a process of expulsion or extraction of a child from a uterus in a woman's abdomen by way of the narrow tortuous canal of the human pelvis; by the forces of nature alone, or with the aid of a man stretching or tearing or cutting the soft parts or even severing the pelvis itself, has passed away in the light of aseptic abdominal surgery.[1]

Unfortunately, we are not privy to the reaction Dr. Humpstone received from his professional peer group at the time or indeed the reaction (if there was any) from the news media. But what we do know is that the twentieth century was almost over before the subject of maternal request cesareans was being seriously considered by doctors again. Up until then, surgery was considered too dangerous, with too high a risk of death, for cesareans to be allowed to develop into a "method of choice."[2]

Nevertheless, as we enter the second decade of the twenty-first century, and despite agreement from groups such as the American College of Obstetricians and Gynecologists (ACOG) and the National Institutes of Health (NIH) that in certain situations, maternal request is a valid birth choice, this position is not universally accepted. The International Federation of Gynecology and Obstetrics (FIGO), for example, has not wavered from its 1998 position, and maintains, "Physicians have the responsibility to inform and counsel women in this matter. At present, because hard evidence of net benefit does not exist, performing caesarean section for non-medical reasons is ethically not justified."[3]

One of the main problems, aside from an often instinctive negative reaction to the idea that surgical means might be a legitimate alternative to a natural process, is the issue with mixed cesarean research and data that we discussed in the preface. With so much evidence demonstrating greater risks with cesarean birth (regardless of the reason for, type of, or timing of each surgery), the perception often is that this birth choice is both irresponsible and dangerous. Yet in 2003, when Australian doctors Stephen Robson and David Ellwood discussed the possibility of conducting a study of cephalic (head-down) births to measure the "intent to treat" outcomes of planned vaginal births versus planned cesarean births, they acknowledged a seldom recognized but extremely telling fear that exists: "What a disaster it would be if it was found elective cesarean was safer than vaginal birth."[4]

And to a certain extent, we can sympathize with this fear; after all, many hospitals in the United States drastically reduced their VBAC (vaginal birth after cesarean) rates following research in which repeat cesarean delivery was shown to be safer than a trial of labor. It therefore follows that some groups might fear the impact that positive data from primary planned cesarean research might have on first-time vaginal births as well. Nevertheless, we believe in the autonomy of *all* birth choices and don't feel it's ethical that the benefits of one birth choice be subdued lest the risks of another birth choice are revealed. Women should be fully informed and (if they choose to be) personally involved in the decision-making process.

Interestingly, in the same year that Robson and Ellwood's deliberations were published, the American College of Obstetricians and Gynecologists addressed the lack of evidence surrounding cesarean versus vaginal birth as well and concluded, "With better data, there may be a shift in clinical practice."[5] And so we are left with a paradoxical state of affairs in which increasing numbers of medical professionals agree that the benefits of a planned cesarean birth, for both the baby and the mother, may indeed outweigh those of a planned vaginal birth—or at least, the two types of birth are so balanced that neither can be considered categorically safer—yet vehement opposition from other medical professionals prevents them from conducting the studies that would help prove it one way or another.

So in the absence of such level 1 evidence (i.e., properly designed randomized trials), and the very low likelihood of such evidence becoming available in the immediate future, what remains is extrapolated data from a vast amount of research that has often been done for other reasons. In this book, we have attempted to mine the available evidence to demonstrate that a planned, elective cesarean is not only a legitimate choice but in many respects is safer than a planned vaginal birth. Clearly, our presentation of this viewpoint deals with statistics and generalities, not an individual woman's health risks or prognosis, and therefore, a personalized consultation is essential. However, as the authors of the first-ever book to set out such an ambitious mandate on cesarean birth, we are pleased to present it in an accessible form.

The cesarean has been undeservedly associated with negative connotations in most discourses on birth, but in our opinion, if there was ever a procedure in medicine that deserved the honor of celebration for its services to saving lives and protecting quality of lives, this is surely it. In fact, we'd like to suggest an International Cesarean Celebration Day!

Chapter 1

A Cut above the Rest: My Own Informed Decision

By Pauline M. Hull

First they ignore you, then they ridicule you, then they fight you and then you win.
— Attributed to Mahatma Gandhi (1869–1948)

P robably the most frequent question that I am asked by journalists, and also by friends and family, is "Why did you *choose* to have a cesarean?" So here, for the record, is my answer.

IT WAS IN MY NATURE

The onset of puberty spurred some of my earliest conflicts with Mother Nature and all things natural, and funnily enough (depending on your sense of humor), a sharp-edged blade was involved in one of these too. The first example was when I made the apparently contentious decision to introduce the hair on my legs to a nice sharp razor, against the sternest advice from an aunt.

"Don't!" she warned. "Your hair will grow back twice as thick as it is now, and you'll regret it forever."

Needless to say, I haven't regretted my decision to live with fuzz-free shins since that day forward (although I did wait a few weeks before shaving my *whole* leg, just in case), and indeed, other areas of depilatory care were to follow without further ado. Next up was my desire to buy a bra. The natural look just wasn't cutting it anymore inside the thin white cotton shirt of my school uniform, so I decided to intervene.

"You don't need to measure me," I insisted in the shop. "I can tell just by looking at all the bras which size I'll need." But as it turned out, I couldn't. My youthful impatience and ignorance of this new set of ABCs created such angry red marks around my chest and back that barely a week later I had to make a rather sheepish return to the store for a proper fitting. What's the point of these childhood anecdotes?

First, they illustrate that from a very early age, so much of what women choose to do with their bodies is *not* natural. In our attempts to make our-selves prettier, smarter, younger, thinner, happier, or whatever it may be (you name it, there's an artificial method available), we often employ un-natural means to facilitate our own perceived satisfaction. Yet while we're busy trying to make these choices, there are external influences telling us what choices we *should* or *shouldn't* make and putting constant pressure on us to rethink our natural instincts or desires. And perhaps nowhere is this more prevalent than when it comes to having children. For example:

- Birth control (pills, condoms, injections, diaphragms, coils, etc.) helps us manipulate when or if we get pregnant, which for increasing numbers of women means delaying motherhood long after the alarm on their naturally ticking clock has gone off. We simply hit the snooze button to buy ourselves a little more time, and then another month or even year passes before the alarm bells begin to ring once more.
- Abortion offers us an alternative to carrying our babies to term, and whether it's legal, ethical, moral, or otherwise, the fact remains that it is medically possible and widely available.
- In vitro fertilization (IVF) and surrogacy provide us with an alter-native means of starting a family (or the chance of having one, at least) if we, or our partners, are infertile or struggling to conceive.
- Ultrasound technology, blood tests, urine samples, and other regular medical monitoring (some or all of which are employed throughout pregnancy) give us a special preview of life formation and alert us to potential problems at a level that is just not available naturally.

My childhood anecdotes also highlight the importance of making an informed decision. For example, my decision to wear a bra was one born of personal size, comfort, and timing more than it was a symbolic step into

womanhood, but even so, in choosing to strap a (wo-)manmade contrap-
tion to my body, I should have done my homework first.

And so this is precisely what I did when it came to my birth plan. I
realized that some women feel a natural pull toward vaginal birth and that
others feel entirely ambivalent about delivery type, and I also knew that I
felt differently. For me, there *was* a choice to be made, and again, initially
at least, this choice was purely instinctive.

But with more than just a few red bra strap marks at stake this time, I
made sure that my decision about which birth plan would fit me best was
an informed one, and after careful consideration, research, and planning,
I chose a cesarean, and these are my reasons why.

MY PERSONAL RISK-BENEFIT ANALYSIS

Truthfully, ever since I understood that it was a possibility, I knew I
wanted a cesarean. Even as a young woman, it seemed a perfectly logical
and natural choice to me: a planned, controlled birth with the aid of a com-
petent surgeon in favor of an unpredictable, potentially painful birth plan
dependent on the vagaries of Mother Nature. I never felt an urge or desire
to pursue the physical rite of passage into motherhood that I'd heard other
women describing, and indeed, I felt the exact opposite of eagerness when
they would talk excitedly about the drama of waters breaking; contractions starting; Hollywood-style car races to the hospital; and the number
of hours, days, and perineal stitches they could chalk up to their children's
births. To my ears, it all sounded like the most barbaric initiation cere-
mony for membership into a paradoxically competitive club that I had no
intention of joining. I might want a baby, but I certainly didn't want one
the traditional way.

That said, by the time I began thinking seriously about becoming
pregnant in my early thirties, there was much more involved than an
instinctive desire to avoid pain and trauma for myself. I'd done a great deal
of research and decided that without doubt, my baby would be safer if I
took a planned surgical route rather than a trial of labor. Ironically, after
everything I'd read, I now had some fears about a cesarean birth in terms
of my own risk and discomfort, but not my baby's. For example, I hated

the idea of spinal anesthesia (which is partly why promises of an epidural did nothing to entice me toward a trial of labor—I was worried enough about someone sticking a needle into my spine without adding the force of a labor contraction into the mix), and I wondered how difficult the recovery might be as a new mom. But these were things I decided I could tolerate because to my mind, I was 100 percent convinced that the least traumatic outcome for my baby would be cesarean delivery at thirty-nine-plus weeks into my pregnancy.

And how did I reach this controversial conclusion? Due to the nature of my website, which I began work on back in 2004 while still working as a BBC journalist, I had knowledge of numerous medical studies from around the world that demonstrated very positive outcomes with planned cesarean birth that had never really received the wider attention they deserved, in news media, mainstream books, and websites, or by medical professionals providing prenatal information. After reading these and essentially conducting a personal risk-benefit analysis that culminated in a supportive and individualized consultation with my obstetrician (a process every woman is advised to carry out, whatever her birth preference), I felt confident I was able to make a truly informed decision about how to give birth.

THE SAFE ARRIVAL OF OUR BABY

It is true that the majority of babies born vaginally arrive safe and healthy, but it is also true that natural birth is fraught with complications and trauma that can lead to moderate or severe injuries and even death. And while many experts point to various statistics and data to demonstrate that these frightening incidences are relatively rare in the developed world or that the percentage of babies actually affected is relatively low, I would always think of the words of a doctor I'd heard speak at a birth conference. The gist of what he said was exactly how I had always felt about risk: "Whatever the statistics say, when it's *your* birth, and *your* baby, the only number that matters to you in the end is 'number one' [you], and if anything bad does happen, it's happening to you and your baby 100 percent."

MY TOLERANCE OF PAIN

When I asked myself which type of birth pain I could tolerate best, the answer was simple. I had read the evidence on postpartum pain, injury, and discomfort in women following both vaginal births and cesarean births, and I concluded I would be better able to tolerate and live with those described by women in the latter group. Obviously, I was aware of examples of women with spontaneous vaginal births who had escaped any perineal laceration or episiotomy, but with around half of all mothers experiencing at least one of these, I didn't see this as an insignificant risk. As for the cesarean, I understood that there would be a surgical incision and multiple layers of bruised and torn internal tissue to contend with, but I still felt confident that I'd be able to manage this pain.

AN ORGASMIC POST-BIRTH

We've dedicated a whole chapter to this very controversial reason for choosing a planned cesarean ("Cesarean for Sex: The Ultimate Birth Taboo?"), and I must admit that it was a factor I considered. Quite simply, I valued my sex life and didn't want to take any unnecessary risks with the birth of my child that might endanger it. Does that make me a bad mother? I don't believe so. Again, it seemed to me to be a question of tolerance. I knew a number of women who'd had stitches following their vaginal births, and the lucky ones completely accepted any changes in their perineal area as normal; some even joked about receiving an "extra stitch" for their husband (also known as "the husband's knot") or described to me through laughter the new harmless "knobbly bits" they could feel that weren't there before. But others described how their sex life was altered due to ongoing pain and discomfort in and around their vagina. Meanwhile, what I found incredible when discussing and researching this particular risk was that while I wasn't really supposed to be thinking about post-birth sex, the possibility of women experiencing an orgasm *during* vaginal birth seemed far more acceptable. And I remember thinking, "It's a funny old world."

PLANNED VERSUS UNPREDICTABLE

When I became pregnant, my husband and I agreed that whatever could be known, we wanted to know. For example, when my fetal nuchal translucency and blood tests showed our baby to be at high risk of a chromosomal condition (such as Down syndrome), we chose to have an amniocentesis and find out for sure. And when we were asked whether we wanted to know the sex of our child, we replied with an emphatic yes in both pregnancies. For the birth itself, we liked the fact that with a cesarean, the baby would be delivered very quickly and taken away for a thorough health check while I was being stitched back up. No waiting around for contractions to start, no lottery ticket as to who would be taking care of me when I arrived at the hospital. No debate among the medical team halfway through about what to do or when to do it, or even whether the necessary staff and resources would be available. That's not to say I didn't appreciate that a cesarean plan could be unpredictable too (quite naturally, I imagined all sorts of worst-case scenarios); I just felt that it was *more* predictable than labor. And should anything go wrong, I couldn't think of a better place to be than in the operating room with my trusted doctor and her team. Also, on a purely practical level, it was beneficial being able to plan the time and date of my births, particularly for arranging the care of our daughter during our son's birth and managing packers for our house moves. However, I would stress that our schedule did not dictate our birth choice; rather, our birth choice facilitated our schedule.

BIRTH SATISFACTION

I was very satisfied with each of my cesarean birth experiences (and I say this gratefully, not smugly). I came home with two healthy babies, my obstetrician was wonderful, I recovered well, and I have never suffered flashbacks or any other psychological trauma related to the births. My husband was happy with how the births went, too, and I mention this because sometimes the birth experience of men is downplayed or forgotten. Interestingly, my husband had no notion of birth preferences at all when we discussed having children. He says that back then, he would have gone along with whatever I wanted, natural or surgical. But now, after years of hearing stories from his peers about their more traditional birth events, my husband says he appreciates how different his more relaxed experience was from many of their realities: for example, one colleague's hour-long emergency transfer from a birthing center thinking he was going to miss the birth because he wasn't allowed to go with his wife when she was sent ahead in an ambulance, another whose wife has just had a second surgery for prolapse in her early forties, and a friend's etched memory of blood on the labor ward floor and a doctor's stark warning to prepare himself because his wife might not make it.

MOTHERING THE FUTURE'S MOTHERS

Finally, I feel that motherhood is a very personal journey for every woman right from the start. We each have a unique perspective and approach, and we all feel differently about raising our children—just as we do about birth. I viewed birth merely as a means to an end and had no expectation or desire that it should be personally fulfilling or special in itself. In fact, I'd probably never have thought much of it again except for the nature of my work, and I have sometimes wondered whether this could be one of the reasons maternal request has earned itself an almost mythical reputation. Perhaps women choosing cesareans just don't consider their birth experience as something worth talking, writing, or shouting about once it's over, and consequently, their silence is misconstrued as nonexistence. But even though their birth stories are not necessarily being heard in a public forum, it's highly likely that they are being heard by a very large audience indeed: their daughters, the next generation of mothers. And if I'm right, and this *is* the case, surely the time has finally come to stop denying that women like me exist, and as a society, to accept that the phenomenon of maternal request cesareans is not going away anytime soon. On the contrary, if our daughters have anything to do with it it's simply an inevitable feature of our birthing future.

Chapter 2

How Two Cesareans Shaped a Life's Work

By Dr. Magnus Murphy

A moment's insight is sometimes worth a life's experience.
—Oliver Wendell Holmes,
The Professor at the Breakfast Table, 1860

My first realization that the birthing experience is to a large degree a cultural experience happened during my fourth year as a medical student, when I spent an elective month in a missionary hospital in northern South Africa. The hospital served a population made up mainly of two tribes, and during the course of my time there, I made a remarkable discovery. It was not obvious at first blush, but the labor ward was clearly divided—not by any physical separation, but by a sound barrier so distinct that walking from one side to the other brought about a decibel variation that could only be described as deafening. On one side, there was the auditory assault of screaming women, while on the other, a silence that permeated the air, broken only by whispered instructions or the odd machine noise.

Upon inquiring, I found that one tribe had a social taboo against making noise and showing any fear or pain in the face of childbirth. Expressing such emotion during the arrival of their baby brought shame and contempt upon these women. On the other hand, the second tribe's women could give free rein to their real and embellished distress in the knowledge that the customary gift they would receive after the baby was born would depend on how hard they had to work to bring their husband's child into the world. In both instances, the underlying chauvinism was neither expressed nor probably even realized, and at the time I didn't make much of it. Only later did I contemplate the tribal cultural prison all these women were in. They had no freedom to make *any* birth choices — not even the simplest choice about how much or how hard they could cry.

MY PERSONAL EXPERIENCE

Many years later, my own journey into parenthood started off pretty routinely. My wife had a normal pregnancy with our first daughter; we were not expecting the biggest of babies since neither of us can be described as "tall" or "big." In fact, we were quite relaxed about the whole thing. A maternal request planned cesarean had never even come up as a thought in our minds. I was an obstetrical resident at the time, busy with training to be a specialist obstetrician and gynecologist, and I was learning all the tricks of the trade skills of vaginal delivery (by hook or by crook with forceps or vacuum), as well as cesarean delivery for medical or obstetrical indications. When my wife had reached forty-one weeks' gestation, both she and I became a bit uncomfortable with the lack of change in her cervix and the obvious dilemma that this situation caused for our plan (or non-plan) of a normal conclusion to the whole pregnancy and birth. We had no intention to be alternative, to rock the boat, or to go against the established knowledge. However, induction of labor became increasingly likely to fail, since her cervix showed absolutely no intention of being cooperative. If she didn't go into spontaneous labor soon and induction failed, it would lead to an emergency cesarean. And so when finally, at forty-two weeks, an ultrasound discovered there was absolutely no amniotic fluid present, and a fetal heart monitor trace showed the first ominous signs of trouble, a cesarean delivery was immediately arranged.

This is where our normal pregnancy quickly came off the rails, and our daughter ended up in a neonatal intensive care unit (NICU) for five days. I know for a fact that any attempt at induction at that time or natural vaginal birth would likely have ended in tragedy. As it was, the cesarean was unplanned, traumatic, and although ultimately necessary, not something we had given much thought to prior to its sudden inevitability. Conversely, every thought we'd had about how things might go had to be thrown out and a new reality accepted. Fortunately, today, our daughter is a beautiful, healthy, and normal teenager who thinks her parents are just a little bit weird, know nothing at all, and are very old.

About two years after this, we emigrated from our native South Africa to Canada, where I began work as an obstetrician in a small town, and we quickly managed to increase the population of Canada by one more female. This time, my wife decided as soon as she knew she was pregnant that she would be planning a cesarean birth and nothing else. My answer? "Yes, dear."

The difference in our second daughter's birth experience cannot be overstated. We were much more relaxed, and we knew to within a few minutes when our baby would arrive. The procedure took all of fifteen minutes before my wife had our baby in her hands and on her chest. Although she had pain for about twenty-four hours, it started only after about eighteen hours (once the spinal anesthesia had worn off), and thus she had a good night's sleep that first night. OK, I'll admit, my wife might remember that first night slightly differently, but the fact is that the pain was not a great problem, and she was certainly able to move around and eat immediately afterward. After two days, she and our baby were home, and the rest is history. Unfortunately, this daughter also thinks her parents are a little weird, know nothing at all, and are, oh, yes—very old.

This experience of entering fatherhood, with my very different experiences of two birth choices, has had a profound impact on me, personally as well as professionally. It has made me considerably more likely to listen to women's fears about vaginal birth and to accept requests for planned cesareans, provided there are no obvious reasons not to do so. Also, I am mindful of quite a few cases during my career as an obstetrician in which I had to break the news to a couple that their full-term baby had died in the womb for no immediately apparent reason. A fetus that was perhaps completely healthy only one day earlier, and who could have become a newborn child at anytime, had suddenly morphed into a lifetime's worth of suffocating anguish and grief. And each time, I was reminded of the realization that my wife and I had come terrifyingly close to having something in common with these couples.

I thus freely admit that I come to this project with no claims of a purity of innocence and completely objective lack of bias.

Yes, I've said it: I am biased . . .

. . . toward a woman's right to choose a planned cesarean birth, to make up her own mind, and to use her own intellect to break free from the cultural shackles that are based on myth, tradition, or simply inertia. At the very least, a woman has the right to be respected enough to be taken seriously if she raises the issue. And if it is believed that a planned cesarean is genuinely not in her best interest, a woman has the right to be persuaded with solid arguments and evidence—as opposed to platitudes or insulting generalizations.

MY PROFESSIONAL EXPERIENCE

My professional life has taken some interesting turns. As a recently immigrated general obstetrician and gynecologist, I initially had to struggle for recognition in a foreign country with a relatively closed—but at the same time, encouraging—professional corps in my field. Since I graduated in South Africa with some potential and interest in an academic career, I slowly but doggedly worked my way up, against all odds, to where I one day found myself as Division Chief and Fellowship Director for Urogynecology in Calgary, the biggest city in Alberta, home of the Calgary Flames Hockey and the Calgary Stampede. My interest in urogynecology started about ten years prior to this, when I realized that the problem of pelvic floor disorders is the orphan child of gynecology, but with tremendous prevalence. It was reinforced by my many experiences of seeing and feeling with my own eyes and hands the absolutely obvious sensation of a pregnant woman's internal pelvic tissue tearing or giving way the moment before the baby would suddenly descend. This sensation, and the knowledge that this woman was likely to enter the world of the pelvic floor "disabled," was partly to blame for my eventually giving up obstetrical practice and focusing my life's work on the management and treatment of women with pelvic floor problems, often a direct result of vaginal birth.

Today, I work as a clinical professor in urogynecology at the University of Calgary. A urogynecologist is someone who deals with all manner of pelvic floor disorders, including prolapse and incontinence of urine and fecal matter, as well as pelvic and bladder pain problems. The main issue with the specialty is that no one outside those who suffer with these problems seems to have heard of it. Furthermore, many of the caregivers who look after pregnant women don't ever see these problems except in their most severe and immediate form, since most appear long after the birth (and certainly longer than the standard six weeks' postpartum care). As a result, they more often than not downplay the risks of vaginal birth while giving full attention to the risks of a cesarean birth.

I am constantly amazed at how often I hear the following from women: "Until it happened to me, I didn't even know this was possible," or: "It all started after my [*fill in number*] vaginal birth." Every time I meet a new young patient with severe pelvic floor problems related to vaginal birth, I wonder to myself whether, knowing what she knows now, she would still choose a vaginal birth if she had her time again. Such interesting but ultimately pointless speculation is, however, not helpful in a busy clinical practice. We are far too busy diagnosing and operating (and trying to stay ahead of the deluge of patients) to entertain esoteric what-ifs.

If only I had unrestricted and unlimited research funds to do with what I want!

But I don't. So I decided to join forces with Pauline, who was also writing a book on the benefits of cesarean birth, so that future pregnant women might answer for themselves which type of birth they want without being deafened by a bombardment of shrill generalizations, or worse, the silence of a lack of knowledge.

Chapter 3

The Safest Birth Choice for Your Baby: Planned Cesarean

We cannot sit back and let nature overcome our babies.
—Professor Kypros Nicolaides,
Fetal Medicine Foundation, 2010

W hat we have to say in this chapter may seem hugely controversial to many readers. We know there may be a flood of criticism in response to it. Nevertheless, it is our unwavering position that in
a healthy pregnancy, the safest way for a baby to be born is via planned
cesarean delivery at thirty-nine-plus weeks' gestation.

That's not to say there are *no* risks involved for the cesarean-born
baby. Of course there are, and we discuss these in chapter 13, "The Risks
of Planning a Cesarean." But it is our belief that a planned cesarean in a
healthy pregnancy involves fewer and *less serious* risks than those associated
with a planned vaginal birth. How can this be? In a nutshell, it's because
with doctors delivering your baby surgically, you're in considerably more
reliable and safer hands than those of the unpredictable Mother Nature
could ever be. And you don't need to take our word for it, either. Research
studies and the information contained in national birth data have demonstrated this too. It's just that, unfortunately, women are not always told
about these facts in prenatal appointments or classes, and they don't come
across them more generally because (as we describe in chapter 9, "The
Politics of Birth") positive cesarean news does not always receive the
media attention it deserves. And so we present here some of the missing
pieces of a birth puzzle that, when completed, paints a very different picture of birth safety than the natural one that is traditionally portrayed.

DEATH

Statistically, the risk of a baby dying is reduced if it is delivered at thirty-nine to forty weeks' gestation, so this is an important benefit of planned cesarean birth, which is normally scheduled for thirty-nine-plus weeks' gestation. Births at an earlier or later gestation than this have been shown to have more complications for the baby, and while labor or an earlier cesarean birth scheduled for medical reasons (e.g., preeclampsia) are sometimes unavoidable, the risks associated with later gestational ages, while very small, can be avoided through surgery.

And yet this is not always recognized in the public discourse, partly because the number of full-term babies that die at or before birth is still relatively low in the developed world, and their deaths are often explained as a distressing but unfortunately natural occurrence. The fact that some of these deaths might have been avoided with a planned cesarean is rarely discussed, and, understandably, to suggest that all babies be delivered at that gestation would be highly controversial. Currently, women are usually induced at forty-one weeks to avoid risks including stillbirth, but this is something that many natural-birth advocates vehemently disagree with, and so you can imagine how the idea of bringing this date even further forward would be unacceptable to many. And to be fair, of course, gestational age estimates are not infallible (even the best estimates rely on very early scans and accuracy of menstruation dates), but the point here is that the gestational pattern of risk evidence is inescapable. What a woman does with this information is for her to decide.

A nationwide investigation into ten years of intrauterine fetal demise (when a baby dies in the womb) in the United States found a significant increase in the stillbirth rate after thirty-nine weeks' gestation. As a result, the researchers calculated that by delivering all babies at this stage in pregnancy, two deaths in every one thousand living fetuses could be prevented, which is equivalent to averting as many as six thousand intrauterine fetal deaths in the United States each year. Dr. Gary Hankins and his coauthors called this "an impact that far exceeds any other strategy implemented for stillbirth reduction thus far."[1] Similarly, of almost two million babies in California born alive between 1999 and 2003, singleton babies born later than forty-one weeks were shown to have greater neonatal mortality than those born between thirty-eight and forty-one weeks.[2] And despite persistent criticism of the current over-medicalization of birth, a large review of 540,834 live births and stillbirths in more than sixty maternity units in Britain found that a "higher intervention score and higher number of consultant obstetricians per one thousand births were both independently and significantly associated with lower stillbirth rates."[3]

Further afield, in a study of twenty thousand births at hospitals in nine Asian countries, the neonatal mortality rate (NMR) was seven per one thousand live births with vaginal birth, 2.2 with planned cesareans, and 12.4 with emergency cesareans. Vaginal birth also had higher rates of severe asphyxia (oxygen deprivation) and palsy than did planned cesarean birth, and—another benefit for babies—fewer mothers died with a planned cesarean.[4] There may be differences in hospital practice in some of these hospitals compared with the United States or Europe, but even so, there is no escaping the fact that planned cesareans had *considerably* safer outcomes for babies.

SERIOUS BIRTH INJURY

Babies delivered by cesarean are at risk for different types of birth trauma and injury than babies delivered vaginally. Unfortunately, most of the research carried out to date has compared just two groups: all cesarean births and all vaginal births, a comparison method we now know is fundamentally flawed. Newer studies, however, with improved methodologies (for example, attributing infant injuries that occur during an emergency cesarean to "risks associated with planned vaginal birth," not automatically grouping them with "planned cesarean birth risks" instead) are beginning to shed light on the truth.

For example, in 2009, Canadian researchers examined almost forty thousand term deliveries of healthy, first-time mothers between 1994 and 2002 by comparing the outcomes of "planned cesarean delivery for breech presentation" with "spontaneous labor with anticipated vaginal delivery at term in pregnancies with a cephalic-presenting singleton." In other words, babies lying in the wrong position with a cesarean birth plan were compared with correct (head-down) position babies with a vaginal birth plan. Dr. Leanne S. Dahlgren and her team found that life-threatening injuries to the mothers were similar in both groups, but that life-threatening injuries to babies were decreased in the cesarean group.[5] Importantly, more detailed analysis of the planned vaginal birth group demonstrated that the increased risk for babies was associated with operative vaginal births (forceps- and vacuum-assisted deliveries) and emergency cesareans, but not with spontaneous vaginal births. And since 63 percent of the mothers who *planned* a vaginal birth actually *had* a spontaneous vaginal birth, the study authors note that these women would not have benefited from a planned cesarean birth. Rather than advocate planned cesarean delivery as the safest birth plan, they suggest that more research into which women are more likely to have assisted births is needed.

However, while we agree that a study like this is not a reason to suggest planned cesareans for all mothers, we are resolute in our opinion that pregnant women should be made aware of the facts found (especially when you consider that the cesarean surgeries were breech births, not the more straightforward cephalic births of the vaginal group) and that they should be fully involved in deciding whether to take a 37 percent risk (in this case) of worse outcomes for their baby. In the absence of concrete data about the possible chances of achieving a spontaneous vaginal birth, do pregnant women feel confident about their chances?

The other good thing about this study is that it helps explain away the long-held myth that planned cesarean births are more dangerous for babies. Remember, the vast majority of previous studies not only used "successful spontaneous vaginal birth outcomes only" as one comparison group; they then used "all cesarean birth outcomes" as the other group. Therefore, it is clear from the Canadian outcomes above that the serious injuries that occur during assisted vaginal birth and emergency cesarean birth have most often been separated from their true origin (planned vaginal birth) and some then erroneously attached to lists of planned cesarean birth risks. It's taken a long time and a great deal of pressure from planned-cesarean advocates like ourselves to get this situation recognized and resolved, but we think the truth is finally (albeit slowly) becoming known, and that once it is known more widely, then more women, more journalists, and indeed more medical professionals will be able to look back at some of the established "evidence-based" literature on negative cesarean birth outcomes and see it from a fresh perspective.

New approaches in research are useful for this purpose as well. Take, for example, the US analysis of the approximately 2.6 percent live single-ton births (out of eight million) in 2004 and 2005 that were complicated by some type of birth trauma. The researchers found that even when comparing vaginal birth outcomes alone (spontaneous and assisted) with all cesarean outcomes (emergency and planned), cesarean birth was still consistently associated with reduced odds of birth trauma—across all birth weight subgroups, whether or not fetal distress was present.[6] Moreover, the researchers demonstrated how the very opposite conclusion—greater risk for birth trauma with cesareans—had been mistakenly reported prior to this. By not including all scalp injuries, which accounted for 78.24 percent of all birth trauma, vaginal birth was inadvertently favored in the standard measure of birth trauma.

Finally, should further evidence be needed, Dr. Hankins's analysis, cited in the evidence on stillbirths above, also concluded that overall, "the frequency of significant fetal injury is significantly greater with vaginal delivery, especially operative vaginal delivery, than with cesarean section at 39 weeks."[7] More specifically, babies born by planned cesarean had a significant reduction in the occurrence of moderate or severe encephalopathy (a condition of abnormal brain functioning as a result of some insult, like an infection or lack of oxygen) and brachial plexus palsy (paralysis of the arm due to an injury to the brachial plexus).[8]

SHOULDER DYSTOCIA AND ITS CONSEQUENCES

Shoulder dystocia, which is when a baby's shoulder gets stuck or lodged inside the pelvis of its mother during a vaginal delivery, occurs only in around 1 to 2 percent of vaginal births, although it occurs much more frequently in a subsequent pregnancy if it's happened once already (about ten times higher than in the general population).[9] And the repercussions when it does happen can be very serious: for example, brachial plexus injury (which is almost entirely unpredictable),[10] asphyxiation, or even death.[11] Large babies are particularly at risk for shoulder dystocia, and some researchers have warned that the current fetal weight guidelines for recommending a planned cesarean are too high and may expose these babies to a high risk of permanent neurological damage.[12] However, it is also the case that brachial plexus injuries can occur in otherwise normal vaginal births without shoulder dystocia; although shoulder dystocia increases the risk for brachial plexus injury one hundredfold, it is estimated that up to half of cases are associated with factors like compression during labor contractions, or simply injuries in the uterus during development. As a result of this, although brachial plexus injury is much less likely with a planned cesarean, it is not a risk that can be completely ruled out.[13]

HEAD AND SCALP INJURIES

Cranial traumatic injury is almost always associated with physical difficulty during attempted vaginal birth and the use of instruments, with "poorly judged persistence with attempts at vaginal delivery in the presence of failure to progress or signs of fetal compromise [being] the main contributory factor."[14] All types of scalp injuries as well as intracranial hemorrhage have been shown to be more common with vacuum- or forceps-assisted delivery than with spontaneous vaginal deliveries.[15] And although scalp injuries caused by a blade cutting the baby's head mostly occur with cesarean birth and are thus often cited as a risk of planned cesareans, such injuries are predominantly associated with *emergency* surgery and, therefore, with planned vaginal birth. This is discussed in more detail in chapter 13, "The Risks of Planning a Cesarean."

INFANT HEMORRHAGE

Research has shown that intracranial hemorrhage is significantly associated with vaginal birth, and in particular, assisted vaginal birth or emergency cesarean.[16] In one small but in-depth US study using magnetic resonance imaging, the only cases of hemorrhage occurred with vaginal births, and in fact, 26 percent of all vaginally born babies in the study were shown to have noticeable brain bleeds.[17]

There has also been research into which type of assistance in vaginal births—vacuum or forceps—is more likely to cause injuries to the baby. And although vacuum delivery causes fewer injuries to the mother than do forceps, it is not necessarily superior to forceps delivery as far as the baby is concerned. The risks are just different,[18] and whereas intracranial bleeding with forceps deliveries is more often associated with skull fractures, the overall incidence of brain and scalp hemorrhage is similar. In fact, two potentially serious types of hemorrhage, cephalhematoma (hemorrhage between the skull bone and its covering membrane) and subgaleal hematoma (bleeding into a potential space underneath the galeal aponeurosis, which is part of the scalp), have been found to be more commonly associated with vacuum delivery. The subgaleal type of bleeding is potentially more serious, since this particular space (in contrast to the space where cephalhematoma occurs) is not limited by membranes attached to the skull bones and thus can accommodate a significant volume of blood, even to the point of compromising the newborn's circulation.[19]

MECONIUM ASPIRATION

This is when a baby inhales its own meconium: its first greenish, sticky, but completely sterile poop. Although this is possible during a planned cesarean birth, it is far more likely to happen during a planned vaginal birth.[20] It's dangerous because the meconium can cause respiratory distress or failure and collapsed lungs, sometimes leading to severely ill babies requiring oxygen, mechanical ventilation, NICU admission and even artificial lung treatment. Although such severe repercussions of meconium aspiration are not very likely, its occurrence is by no means rare.

EMERGENCY TRAUMA

Have you ever thought about what actually happens to a baby during a vaginal birth that ends up in difficulty? How it actually makes its way out in an emergency situation? For example, sometimes the baby's head has crowned but is not going any farther, and doctors may have tried pulling it out with their hands, with forceps, and with vacuum, but to no avail. The only option is to do an emergency cesarean. Even then, trying to deliver the baby from above is difficult and hazardous for both the baby and the mother. Usually, someone has to push the baby's head up forcefully from below after the incision has been made in the uterus. The force required may even cause skull injuries. The doctor doing the surgery and the assistant pushing from below have to work in tandem so that as soon as the head is pushed up, the doctor can slip a hand below it to continue to lift it up. Unfortunately, such considerable force is often required that this process, in combination with the considerable thinning out of the lower segment of the mother's uterus because of all the contractions, often leads to tearing of the lower uterus. These tears might extend into the bladder or larger blood vessels and cause considerable further risk as a result. In short, obstructed labor is a dangerous and unpredictable situation for the baby, as well as its mother, and the birth canal is a hazardous route. And even though these risks are not 100 percent exclusive to cesarean after obstructed labor, they are significantly increased in such cases. Planned cesarean birth avoids this situation in the majority of women.

HUMAN ERROR

This risk factor is rarely included in comparative studies, but it is unquestionably important. Think back to news stories you may have heard or read where a cesarean is dangerously delayed and, in the end, not done in time to preserve the baby's well-being (or not done at all). In the aftermath, it usually comes to light that there was some disagreement by staff regarding the management of the vaginal birth attempt, or that staff did not notice or ignored the warning signs of fetal distress, or just that the signs of distress were so subtle that they were observed only with careful hindsight after a bad outcome. Remember, a planned vaginal birth can take place over a prolonged period of time, with numerous medical staff (all of whom have varying levels of training and experience and different attitudes to birth risks), plus reliance on the twenty-four-hour availability and quality of emergency care, all of which can introduce the possibility of human error.

Obviously, human error is a possibility with planned cesarean births too, but a quick review of any historical litigation cases will demonstrate that the overwhelming majority of incidents are associated with planned vaginal births. Lawsuits regarding labor and delivery management almost universally claim that a cesarean was not done early enough. The reverse is almost unheard of. And that's not to say that all successfully litigated cases necessarily indicate willful neglect or incompetence — sometimes technology simply cannot predict or isn't clear — but the association with birth type remains.

Here are just some examples of horrific birth outcomes described in news reports, and regrettably, we're confident that you will have read about similar cases elsewhere:

Baby A survived four hours after his skull was fractured in a desperate bid to free him with a pair of forceps during a delayed emergency cesarean; an inquest heard that his death could have been avoided.[21]

Baby B died at less than two days old after an attempted forceps and vacuum delivery left him brain damaged and with two types of hemorrhage: one caused by the vacuum and another akin to that suffered by someone in a traffic accident.[22]

Baby C was awarded undisclosed financial compensation for her injury, which occurred during vaginal birth with a shoulder dystocia complication; she has Erb's palsy, and her arm is paralyzed.[23]

Baby D died at just a few days old after his head got stuck during vaginal birth and a vacuum was used to deliver him; his parents said they'd have chosen an emergency cesarean had they known the risks. The compensation awarded included an amount for the pain and suffering the baby would have felt during and after the birth.[24]

Baby E, at thirteen months of age, has already had one operation to reposition his shoulder and undergoes numerous daily physiotherapy sessions, and although further surgery and grafts are planned, they bring no guarantees that the damage will be repaired; following shoulder dystocia during his vaginal delivery, he has Erb's palsy and limited use of his arm.[25]

Baby F was delivered so violently with forceps that he not only suffered a fractured skull and bleeding on the brain (with likely brain damage), but one of his eyeballs came out of its socket. During the procedure, his mother was actually dragged down the bed by the force employed. The father was so distressed by the baby's appearance that he couldn't hold his son for months, and the baby now faces further surgeries in addition to the three he has already had in his ten months of life.[26]

Baby G was three days old when she died on life support after a Kielland's forceps delivery caused a severe spinal injury. She had been stuck with her head sideways, and the delivery resulted in her head being twisted around without her body. Her mother had repeatedly appealed for a cesarean during the labor, but her request was not granted.[27]

THE COUNTERARGUMENT: "Vaginal birth has more benefits, and cesarean birth has more risks"

Even given the evidence-based argument we have presented in this chapter, the debate over which type of birth is safest for healthy babies is essentially one of perspective. Your perspective of pregnancy and the birth process itself (for example, do you view it as inherently safe, with medical intervention only necessary in emergency situations, or as inherently risky, with medical intervention an essential and valuable support throughout?), and your perspective of the different risks and benefits (for example, are you more concerned about the possibility of shoulder dystocia and fetal distress or of impaired bonding and respiratory distress?) will come into play, and they will be different for each person.

That said, there is strong opposition to the idea that a planned cesarean could offer more benefits to the unborn baby than a natural, vaginal birth, and so we will address this opposition now.

Breathing Problems

Risk: Babies born by planned cesarean delivery are more likely to have breathing difficulties.

Few people realize the dramatic physiological changes that occur in the body of a newborn baby, or that other than death, the moment of birth represents the singular most rapid and profound physiological stress and change ever to be experienced during life.[28] In fact, the transition from fetus to neonate, or newborn baby, is remarkable, and nowhere is this more dramatically illustrated than in the ability of the fetus to resuscitate itself by clearing its lungs of fluid at birth. Up until then, it has been completely submerged and effectively breathing fluid in and out of its lungs. Not only do the lungs have to be cleared, but the whole blood circulation system has to change by shunting blood away from a placental circulation and through the lungs instead. This ability to biologically adjust, and the fact that the overwhelming majority of babies do so successfully, is almost miraculous.

When discussing with laypeople the process of clearing fluid from the lungs, medical professionals often credit the squeezing of the baby's chest during vaginal birth, a simplistic mechanism that is easy to explain and understand. However, this squeezing is only responsible for a very small amount of fluid clearing,[29] and the exact mechanisms of fluid clearance are not completely understood. It is a complicated process involving the active transportation of fluid into circulation by the lung alveolar epithelial (lining) cells.[30] The ability of these cells to perform this feat depends on numerous metabolic pathways, gene effects, and steroid hormones.

There are some studies that suggest that babies born by planned cesarean are more likely to have breathing difficulties than those born vaginally. However, most respiratory problems occur in infants delivered before thirty-nine weeks' gestation, as we discuss in our chapter on risks. Even the difference of one week can make a significant difference to a baby's respiratory health. Therefore, the recommended gestational age for a planned cesarean delivery on maternal request is thirty-nine-plus weeks, and this is essential to understand when reading studies on birth type comparisons.[31]

It is also essential to understand the *size* of a particular risk, as Pauline highlighted during a BBC radio interview in 2007 following the publication of Danish research on respiratory morbidity. The study found that babies born by planned cesarean at thirty-nine weeks' gestation had a "doubled risk" of breathing difficulties compared with babies born vaginally, and this news received considerable media attention at the time. In fact, the actual percentage risk was very small: 2.1 percent versus 1.1 percent respiratory morbidity, and 0.2 percent versus 0.1 percent serious respiratory morbidity.[32] Besides, doctors are now extremely conscious of the importance of gestational age at birth, and, increasingly, so are women. In fact, there have been so many studies emphasizing the importance of gestational age in recent years that many hospitals have introduced strategies to reduce premature late-term births (thirty-six to thirty-eight weeks' gestation) and have reported reductions in their rates of neonatal respiratory morbidity as a result.[33]

Of course, some babies will always need to be delivered earlier than thirty-nine weeks' gestation, and researchers are always working to develop ways to reduce the respiratory morbidity for these babies whose lungs have not fully matured. For example, the use of steroids has been found to help with lung maturity in some babies.[34] And while the idea of breathing difficulties sounds very scary for mothers whose medical conditions or those of their babies warrant early delivery, it's worth remembering that the vast majority of difficulties are transient and successfully treated, and that the alternative would likely be far worse.

Gestational Age

Risk: It's almost impossible to know for sure what a baby's true gestational age is.

Estimating a baby's true gestational age is challenging, and the correct assessment of gestational age and fetal growth is essential for optimal obstetric management.[35] Fortunately, improvements in measuring gestational age and the evaluation of lung maturity continue to be made, and what we do know is that the earlier a woman has an ultrasound assessment in pregnancy, preferably between ten and twelve weeks, the better the estimate of gestational age.[36] Obviously, it is a good idea to also keep a diary of your menstruation dates while you are trying to conceive, or even if you're not (accidents and surprises can happen!), but you should have an early ultrasound assessment as well to reduce the risk of getting it wrong.

Vaginal Passage

Risk: Cesarean-born babies miss out on exposure to the essential bacteria in the mother's vagina.

There are absolutely some differences between babies born vaginally and babies born surgically, but the long-term effect of many of these differences is still unknown. For example, prophylactic antibiotics are a standard duty of care for most cesarean surgeries, and these may be passed on to cesarean babies before birth or through breast milk, although babies born both vaginally and surgically have been reported to develop the yeast infection known as oral thrush. We also know that vaginally delivered babies acquire bacterial communities resembling their own mother's vaginal and bowel microbiota, while cesarean-delivered babies have bacterial communities similar to those found on the skin surface.[37] But what does this mean? It isn't known for certain. There have been attempts to make a link between cesarean births and increasing rates of allergies in children, but researchers have been unable to isolate birth type as an absolute risk factor. For example, pollution, cleaning products that reduce human contact with dirt and germs, and changes in our diet and environment may all play a part. Also, it's been suggested that regardless of birth type, breastfeeding provides an alternative source of healthy bacteria for babies to ingest, if this is something a woman wants to do.

Bonding

Risk: *Cesarean delivery impedes the natural bonding process between mother and child.*

There is actually very little evidence that either vaginal squeezing or hormones secreted mostly during labor (for instance, oxytocin) are essential contributors to the process of a baby's bonding, or to its development or safety, other than through their effects on the process of labor itself. In fact, it's difficult to prove that so-called love hormones have any additional effect at all, but equally, it's difficult to prove that they don't. Interestingly, however, whether a woman has a vaginal or a cesarean birth, she is given a synthetic dose of oxytocin immediately afterward, as this has been shown to significantly reduce the chances of her hemorrhaging.

Overall, we tend to navigate toward research that measures women's own assessment of whether they've bonded with their baby, and we are satisfied that the level of bonding enjoyed by mothers and babies has more to do with a woman's personal health and satisfaction following the birth—and, of course, with her personal nature and circumstances—than with what type of birth she had. We discuss this in more detail in chapter 4, but essentially, there are too many women who have cesarean births prior to labor ever starting, and still bond perfectly with their babies, for us to believe that this is not possible without labor-inducing hormones. However, with strong evidence lacking either way, you will need to make up your own mind about this.

Asthma and Allergies

Risk: Cesarean delivery increases the risk for asthma and allergies in later childhood and beyond.

We discuss this issue in more detail in chapter 10, "Before They Say It," but in short, this association has been suggested but remains unconfirmed by medical studies. Even research that does make the case for an association between cesarean birth and an increased risk of asthma and allergies is problematic because it almost always includes mixed cesarean data (i.e., both planned and emergency surgeries, as well as planned cesareans at various gestational ages and for various reasons). We know that emergency cesareans and late preterm planned cesareans (those occurring before thirty-nine weeks) introduce increased risks for a baby—specifically respiratory risks—at the time of birth, so it is not beyond the realm of possibility that this increased risk spills over into later life. But the fact remains that we don't know for sure, and we certainly don't know what the likelihood of risk is for babies born at thirty-nine-plus weeks' gestation. This is just another example of a "possible" risk that women must process alongside other "possible," "probable," and "definite" risks associated with other birth types and decide for themselves which risks they are willing to take.

SUMMARY

After everything we've said here, there are a few things we'd like you to take away with you with regard to the safety of your baby, and we'll start with this: we do *not* advocate that all women should or would choose a planned cesarean birth but rather that many will (or would, if they had knowledge of the true risks and benefits of different birth plans and were able to factor that information into their own preferences and tolerances), and that those who do are completely justified in their decision. We want to assure you that the examples of documented injuries to babies that we describe are not for the purpose of scaring women or suggesting that vaginal birth be avoided. They are simply to demonstrate that, overall, serious consequences for your baby are less likely with planned surgery. In fact, whichever birth method you choose, the chances of any of these problems occurring in your pregnancy or birth are very, very low indeed.

It's also important to understand that no matter which birth plan you eventually choose, or how mentally and physically prepared you are for the birth, in the end, there are no guarantees that your baby will be born completely healthy. We argue that statistically, the data show planned cesarean to be safer, but there are still limitations on identifying, preventing, or fixing the problems that naturally occur in pregnancy and birth. And as we've said elsewhere, birth plans can change and health situations can change, so whatever you desire or plan, this can sometimes be derailed.

We'd like to put the whole idea of birth risks for your baby into perspective too, since sometimes the focus of attention on the day of birth itself can become so all-consuming that parents forget about risks or safety in the context of the days, weeks, months, and years that come afterward. This is a particular pet peeve of Pauline's: women who espouse the natural benefits of vaginal birth, labeling cesarean birth "abnormal" or "unnatural," and then make equally controversial life choices for their child after the birth is over. The fact is that having a baby means a lifetime of making difficult decisions and taking risks; getting pregnant and planning your birth are simply the first in a very long line of them. But for you to make these first decisions about which risks you want to take, you need information, and you need data. This book provides you with information about the risks and benefits of a planned cesarean birth so that in the end, your birth plan can be truly *your* informed decision.

Chapter 4

Birth Satisfaction: Cesarean Ranks Highest

Maternal satisfaction has now become one of the most significant outcome factors after childbirth and must be taken into consideration.

—M. S. Robson,
"Can We Reduce the Caesarean Section Rate?"
Clinical Obstetrics and Gynaecology, 2001

"For many women the experience of vaginal birth is among the most fulfilling of their entire life—comparable only to sexuality-related moments of ecstasy—other women come to regard birth as the worst thing that ever happened to them—an experience attended by pain, fear, loneliness, perhaps even long lasting negative consequences."[1]

It would be easy to read the above statement by Dr. Peter Husslein from the University of Vienna, published in the *Archives of Gynecology and Obstetrics* in 2001, and imagine that the second description of women's experiences accounts only for a tiny proportion of vaginal births. But unfortunately, this is not the case. In fact, a very significant number of women experience negative feelings following vaginal birth, and this number is even greater when you include women whose planned vaginal birth results in an emergency cesarean. It is estimated that in Britain alone, ten thousand women per year may develop post-traumatic stress disorder (PTSD) as a direct result of a traumatic birth experience, and as many as two hundred thousand more may feel traumatized by childbirth and develop some of the symptoms of PTSD.[2] And in Australia, researchers interviewing 499 women from four different public hospitals reported that as many as one-third of them identified a traumatic birthing event.[3]

Anecdotally, we would expect that almost every reader of this book is likely to know at least one person in their circle of family and friends who did not have a happy birth experience, and indeed the existence of (and high demand for) national birth trauma groups provides further proof of this reality. In Britain, for example, the charity Birth Trauma Association (BTA) offers help and support to thousands of women, as does a similar organization in Canada, Birth Trauma Canada (BTC). But—and this is very telling—ask each organization how many of the thousands of women who contact them say they were traumatized following a planned cesarean birth on maternal request (i.e., by choice), and the answer is none. Not one single woman, out of thousands, has so far contacted any of these groups to say that she deeply regrets her decision to plan a cesarean birth or that she or her baby have suffered severe birth trauma as a result. In fact, Penny Christensen, executive director of Birth Trauma Canada, says that women who have planned cesareans at their own request get in touch only to say they are happy with the choice they made and want to share their story with women to help them avoid the horror stories being reported by others.[4]

This phenomenon has also been highlighted in Germany, where it was found that PTSD is almost unheard of after a cesarean birth on maternal request.[5] That's not to say that a planned cesarean can *never* be traumatic, and there may indeed be cases of trauma reported in the future, but it does demonstrate that the greatest chance of a woman experiencing mild or severe birth trauma is fundamentally associated with a planned vaginal birth, not a planned cesarean birth.

PLANNED CESAREAN SCORES

It makes perfect sense that if a woman's actual birth experience mirrors the one she imagined and planned while pregnant, her level of satisfaction afterward will be high. This theory is also confirmed in research. For example, an anonymous survey of seventy-eight first-time Australian mothers who had requested and planned a cesarean birth in private maternity hospitals found that they were highly satisfied with their delivery, and in fact, on a scale from 1 (totally unsatisfied) to 10 (completely satisfied), the mean score was a significantly high 9.25.[6]

Similarly, in Sweden, when responses from 91 women who had planned a cesarean birth with no medical indication were compared with 266 women who had planned a vaginal birth (both groups first-time mothers with no known complications), at two days, and again three months after the birth, the cesarean group reported a better birth experience than the vaginal group.[7] In further studies in Scotland, England, Sweden, Iran, and the United States, higher levels of satisfaction, more favorable psychological well-being and mental health, and better physical and emotional adaptation to motherhood have been demonstrated following planned cesarean birth.[8]

UNNECESSARY TRAUMA

And yet, given the above information, planned cesarean birth (particularly when a woman requests it) remains vilified within many maternity centers and by many healthcare organizations around the world. Even when it is evident that cesarean birth by choice enjoys very high rates of post-birth satisfaction, some midwives, doctors, health organizations, and governments still persist in coercing women into enduring unwanted vaginal births—or rather, unwanted *attempts* at vaginal births. Why is this? We believe the answer largely lies in the current lack of coherency, understanding, and communication of specific health outcomes with maternal request cesareans (as discussed in other chapters, the outcomes of emergency, medical, obstetrical, and "no indication" cesareans are all too often pooled together as a single "cesarean" outcome and erroneously used to discredit the legitimacy of maternal request), but that it also lies in a blank refusal by some to look at the available evidence fairly and appropriately.

In the course of our work, we have each encountered medical professionals, including many with influential positions in maternity care, who have revealed their inattentiveness to (and in some cases, willful disregard for) contemporary studies on the subject of planned cesareans. They are not fully informed about the proven benefits of planned surgery at thirty-nine-plus gestational weeks themselves, nor are they capable of making sure the women in their care are fully informed, and so the comparatively high levels of poor satisfaction following planned vaginal births persist, and when things go wrong, women turn to charitable organizations for support—or worse still, suffer in silence.

But why, you might ask, aren't there more vociferous complaints to be heard? Why are so many women simply putting up with this? Why on earth don't we have some kind of feminist revolution on our hands? Well, on the surface, there *are* complaints, and there *are* attempts to change maternity health outcomes. Indeed, there are scores of maternity support groups throughout the world, many of which have proved successful at ensuring the voices of unsatisfied mothers are heard. The problem is that many of these indignant cries focus on the wrong target: the cesarean.

The anti-cesarean sentiment is very strong, and there is a pervading idea that if we eradicate all unnecessary cesareans, the maternal world would be a great deal happier and healthier. But would it? For sure, all the women who desperately don't want a cesarean might well enjoy greater levels of birth satisfaction. But what about the women who want a pro-phylactic planned cesarean and who value their own and their baby's health above any desire to achieve a vaginal birth outcome? Or the women who have no birth preference at all, whose only goal is to go home with a healthy, live baby without sailing dangerously close to the wind?

All these women deserve the uncompromised prospect of a positive birth experience, and for this to happen, cesarean birth should not be auto-matically regarded as a negative outcome, nor should prenatal care be obsessed with achieving normal births for all. Certainly, we agree that in instances where a woman feels that her cesarean birth was absolutely unnecessary, it should be investigated (we don't propose that unnecessary cesareans do not exist; they do), but the idea that one single birth plan — or one type of birth outcome — can satisfy all new mothers and reduce dis-satisfaction rates is fundamentally flawed.

Women, after all, are not homogenous creatures; far from it. What sat-isfies one woman may not satisfy another. Therefore, policies or plans to arbitrarily reduce cesarean rates across the board are both dangerous and unhelpful. They risk lives, polarize hospital staff, and, fundamentally, obstruct healthy progress.

SHORT- AND LONG-TERM SATISFACTION

The focus of maternity policy should be on facilitating positive physical *and* psychological birth outcomes for all mothers and babies, regardless of delivery method, and a good starting point is listening to what each pregnant woman wants and values in her birth plan. If it's a vaginal birth, then provide her with the best support and health professionals to optimize her chances of achieving this, advise her on how to prepare for labor, and be honest with her about the likelihood of success and any increased likelihood of risk (for example, is she more than thirty-five years old? Is she overweight or obese? Is her baby very large?). Likewise, if it's a cesarean birth, stress to her the importance of accurately calculating the baby's gestational age (for example, arranging an early ultrasound), of waiting until at least thirty-nine weeks for delivery, of planning only a small family, of maintaining a healthy weight for surgery, and of possibly arranging help at home for the immediate postpartum period.

It's important to recognize that one woman's satisfaction might be improved by helping her to avoid an unwanted cesarean, whereas another woman's experience might be improved by planning one from the outset.[9] A supportive decision-making approach, rather than a prescriptive and authoritarian one, is far more beneficial for all pregnant women, and in particular for women who have tokophobia, an acute fear of labor and birth. When these women are refused their choice of a planned cesarean, they can suffer higher rates of psychological morbidity than those who achieve their desired birth method.[10] They may also increase their risk of having a negative experience and have difficulty achieving an immediate postpartum attachment to their children.[11] Given that these women already suffer with the psychological distress of tokophobia, this is a particularly troubling example of the negative outcomes that can accompany a coerced trial of labor, and it demonstrates the need to include, assess, and balance the risk of psychological outcomes in different birth plans.

This approach is not only for the sake of the mother. What many people don't realize is that PTSD, birth trauma, and morbidity can all have a potentially detrimental effect on the child too. Maternal bonding may be adversely affected,[12] and even the less serious condition of postnatal maternal anxiety (PMA) has been highlighted as an important risk factor for a child's psychological development.[13] For example, many of us know of mothers who have talked repeatedly about a "difficult birth" in front of the child concerned, and even years later, when the child is an adult, the now customary story of personal culpability continues to be imparted: "He was stubborn even as a baby. He wouldn't come out for days, and I thought I was going to die with the pain."

Interestingly, though, for many women the mere presence of their baby is enough to alleviate any psychological distress that is a direct result of their birth experience. Essentially, the baby provides such a positive new element in their lives that it helps them cope after the birth. Even if they *have* suffered a very traumatic experience, the happiness they feel with their baby has a somewhat healing effect. And this is especially true where there has been what's known in obstetrics as a "near-miss" event—when the baby or mother almost die during the birth. While women who lose their babies are certain to experience severe distress afterward, near-miss women who have a live baby are more protected,[14] most probably because they must simply carry on with the job at hand—being a mom.

BREASTFEEDING AND BONDING

Breastfeeding

A question mark has traditionally hung over the success of bonding and breastfeeding following a cesarean (for those who want to breastfeed), but we believe that, as in so many aspects of risk-benefit comparisons of birth types, planned cesarean delivery has traditionally been tarred with the same brush as traumatic emergency cesarean outcomes.[15] In fact, the breastfeeding organization La Leche League International assures women that it is certainly possible to breastfeed after a cesarean and, furthermore, planning the birth carefully and trying to avoid problems from birth complications might help them achieve success.[16] We don't suggest that the organization is an advocate of planned cesarean delivery on maternal request, or indeed otherwise, but we can't fail to notice an unmistakable parallel between its strategy for breastfeeding success and the nature of a planned cesarean birth. Therefore, we believe that rather than causing potential problems for breastfeeding mothers, a planned cesarean birth is a perfectly natural precursor to breastfeeding and is no more or less guaranteed to ensure success than a planned vaginal birth experience.

Some babies may develop a yeast infection after drinking breastmilk that contains the mother's prophylactic surgery antibiotics, and some women find this experience worrying. However, babies born vaginally can also develop oral thrush, and further research is needed to discover any long-term effects this may have. There is also documented evidence of a significant delay in initiating breastfeeding after all cesareans and an initially lower volume of milk transferred to infants, which researchers think may be related to the surgery. Certainly, these findings should not be ignored, but it is worth noting that this body of research acknowledges and assures women that these early difficulties are relatively short-lived.[17] Also, it has not been established conclusively whether the absence or cessation of breastfeeding after cesareans tends to be voluntary or involuntary (which would be a more accurate measure of the causality of birth method on the breastfeeding result), and of course, there are always other factors involved in breastfeeding outcomes aside from birth type.[18]

Bonding

The idea that bonding might be adversely affected in women who choose a cesarean birth is quite frankly ludicrous in our opinion, and we would suggest that the positive levels of cesarean birth satisfaction presented in the studies mentioned here support this view. Indeed, there is no convincing evidence that a planned cesarean inhibits bonding; some women naturally bond instantly and some don't, and even mothers who have a vaginal birth may not bond straightaway, especially if it is an assisted birth, as this can have a negative impact on the first contact with their baby.[19] Yet French obstetrician Dr. Michel Odent is adamant that the oxytocin released during vaginal birth is a very important hormone of love, and that therefore women having a planned cesarean birth do so without the necessary cocktail of love hormones to facilitate bonding. The situation is better, he claims, for women who have an emergency cesarean at the end of a trial labor, since their love hormones have already been released.[20] Never mind that their emergency surgical birth is associated with some of the worst physical and psychological risks possible for a mother and baby—at least they have their *love hormones* to keep them healthy and happy. All we can say in response to such a concept is this: even if it turns out that his assertion is correct, would this be enough to satisfy *you*?

"CESAREAN NEXT TIME, PLEASE"

One interesting measure of women's faith that a planned cesarean will provide the most desirable and reliable relationship between birth plan and birth outcome is the proportion of maternal request cesareans that occur right from the outset of second pregnancies. This phenomenon is most commonly associated with women whose first birth is a cesarean (whether planned or emergency) and who decide to elect for repeat surgery, but it is also evident in studies of women whose first birth was vaginal. In China, 23.8 percent of women are reported to have changed from preferring vaginal birth to preferring cesarean birth following their first birth experience, citing fear as the most important reason for this.[21] Similarly, in Britain, 24 percent of women who experienced an instrumental vaginal birth said they'd prefer a cesarean birth the second time around,[22] and in Australia, for women who suffered an unexplained stillbirth, this number was 26 percent.[23]

These are not insignificant numbers, and they should not be ignored in an analysis of cesarean benefits. Although the fears of women who are pregnant for the first time might be vulnerable to accusations of overestimating the potential trauma resulting from an imagined vaginal birth, it is far more difficult to dismiss the views of women with actual prior experience. You can reassure them that things will be different this time, that a second delivery is easier than the first, or that their birth was simply mishandled the first time around, but ultimately (as the woman herself already knows by this point), there is no guaranteed predictor for vaginal birth success or satisfaction, whether it's first time, second time, or any other time around, and to claim otherwise is to misrepresent the truth.

FINAL THOUGHT

While it is entirely natural and understandable that a maternity care professional might experience a strong sense of personal and professional satisfaction when the woman in her care succeeds in giving birth vaginally (particularly if some practiced skill has been involved due to unforeseen complications during labor), this should always be secondary to the focus on the woman's satisfaction with her birth process and outcome.

Based on our analysis, we propose that a planned cesarean birth on maternal request provides the greatest likelihood of a high level of satisfaction for the majority of women who make that choice. Given this fact, our book serves as a meticulous plea, based on careful analysis of the current evidence, that planned cesarean birth is therefore a choice that should be recognized, accepted, respected, and provided.

Chapter 5

Doctors Who Support Cesarean Choice

Knowledge is power.
—Francis Bacon, *Meditationes Sacrae*, 1597

DOCTORS WHO CHOOSE

In a letter published in the *British Medical Journal* in 1999, a female doctor writes, "I am very insulted that I am not allowed to make an educated choice to elect for a C-section. My decision not to undergo spontaneous vaginal delivery is made based on my own personal experiences with traumatic deliveries while in medical school: rectovaginal tears, emergency C-sections with death of newborn, fetal distress during labor, etc."[1] Her letter also refers to an oft-quoted survey of obstetricians in London, England, in which 31 percent of female doctors said they would choose a planned cesarean in an uncomplicated pregnancy, compared with only 8 percent of male doctors.[2] She concludes, "Obviously when it is your own pelvic floor that is at risk it affects one's decision making."

We don't know what the outcome of this particular doctor's birth was, and it would be nice to think that she managed to convince her own doctors of the legitimacy of her cesarean preference, but her letter provides an interesting insight into the decision making of a medical professional. As we will demonstrate in this chapter, a healthcare provider's personal experience determines not only their own choices (or their partners'), but also the choices they're willing to offer their patients.

For instance, in the United States, different surveys have reported 6 percent, 21 percent, and 46.2 percent of doctors choosing a cesarean, with reasons for their choice including avoidance of incontinence and pelvic organ prolapse, concern for fetal death or injury, preservation of sexual function, fear of childbirth, or adverse previous birth experience.[3] However, when the birth weight of their baby is expected to be large (8.8–9.9 pounds or more than 10.1 pounds), the maternal request rate of one group of doctors surveyed jumps to 70 percent and 88 percent respectively.[4] The same is true in a number of other countries. In Denmark, where only 1.1 percent of doctors say they'd prefer a cesarean birth, this number increases to 22.5 percent if a big baby is expected.[5] In Ireland, 7 percent of obstetricians would choose a cesarean, rising to 38 percent with an estimated fetal weight of 9.9 pounds.[6] In Australia and New Zealand, the proportion of doctors choosing a cesarean rises from 11 percent to 26 percent if the baby is believed to weigh 8.8 pounds, and 55 percent if 9.9 pounds or more, mainly due to fear of fecal and urinary incontinence.[7] And in Britain, reported rates of 15 percent and 17 percent again rise to 40 percent and 65 percent with these estimated weights.[8]

This is a significant demonstration of doctors' views of cesarean safety with the introduction of just one risk factor. If you imagine factoring in any other risks or reasons to favor a cesarean delivery besides the baby's predicted weight—for example, breech presentation, advanced maternal age, or family history of birth trauma—you can see that in the community of doctors, at least, it wouldn't take long before cesarean delivery became the majority birth plan.

This phenomenon has not gone unnoticed by those concerned with rising cesarean rates. A British study posing the question "Who is responsible for the rising caesarean section rate?" suggests that because doctors evidently favor cesarean birth, there is a need for a change in their attitude before they educate women about cesareans on request.[9] And in Norway, a survey that asked random members of the general public as well as physicians, surgeons, and specialists in obstetrics and gynecology whether their children had been born via cesarean, respective rates of 12 percent, 19 percent, 26 percent, and 27 percent were found. Again, the researchers conclude that the cesarean rate in the general population is unlikely to fall as long as so many doctors have their own children delivered this way.[10]

What concerns us is that many women who are not privy to the knowledge and experience of their doctors, and who in some countries do not even come into contact with doctors unless they are referred by their midwife as high risk, are unaware of the full spectrum of risks and benefits with different planned birth types. Moreover, the women who educate themselves about the risks of planned vaginal birth and decide they would be more tolerant of the risks of planned surgery are then denied the birth plan of their choice. They are instead often coerced into experiencing an unwanted trial of labor.

Do as I Say, Not as I Do

Pauline recalls being told by a doctor in Britain who works in the National Health Service (where maternal request is "not on its own an indication for cesarean" but is under review) that he has witnessed female doctors in his hospital refusing the legitimate maternal request of pregnant women in their care, despite having had their own births via cesarean with no indication. Dr. Murphy has overheard obstetricians saying to each other, "If I were a woman having a baby, I would not allow anyone to even come *near* me with forceps or vacuum," and, "If someone were to try and bring forceps into clinical practice today as a brand-new idea, it would *never* be allowed," only for those doctors to continue delivering babies using those very instruments. This seemingly unprincipled behavior is borne out in research studies as well. For example, in England, "doctors regard management options not normally available to pregnant women as valid choices for themselves or their partners."[11] And in Canada, which also has a public health service, it appears that when forceps delivery is the alternative, doctors would opt for cesarean birth for themselves more often than they would offer this option to the women in their care.[12]

This is interesting because women who know they want a vaginal birth are often advised (in the United States in particular, but also in other countries or private hospital settings where women might be able to choose their provider) to check out the current cesarean rate of their hospital, or more pertinently, that of its individual obstetricians. The idea is that a high vaginal birth rate is a good indication of mothers' likelihood of being supported throughout their chosen birth plan. Of course, this theory ignores the caseload of each obstetrician and hospital, how many high-risk pregnancies they're dealing with, the maternal demographics in that geographic area, and even whether they've had a litigation scare recently, all of which can have a much greater influence on overall cesarean rates than any personal predilection for one type of delivery.

Even so, personal predilection can play a part in maternity care, and in many cases, given the evidence, it makes sense to find out how your provider (or their partner, sister, or daughter) gave (or would give) birth themselves; this suggests which way they're more likely to lean in your risk-benefit analysis.[13]

Influence of Experience

This is especially important if you do have a personal birth preference (obviously, if you are ambivalent about the birth type, then it may be less so). There has been a considerable amount of research into how many doctors are willing to perform a cesarean delivery on maternal request, and it's been shown that personal birth experience can heavily influence their professional position. For example, in a survey where 37.6 percent of Danish doctors said they support maternal request, those who had experienced a noninstrumental vaginal delivery were less likely to agree with maternal request than their peers were.[14] Similarly in Flanders, Belgium, where only 2 percent of obstetricians preferred a cesarean birth, 70 percent said they would never perform a cesarean on demand.[15] And in Scotland, while 15.5 percent of female obstetricians said they would choose to have a cesarean, none of the doctors who had had a vaginal birth said they would choose surgery.[16]

In the United States, the picture of support is varied, but it would be correct to say that compared with many countries, the chances of finding maternal request support are probably higher here than anywhere else in the developed world (although there is the added complication of whether an insurance company will pay for the surgery, even if a doctor agrees to it, which is an issue we cover in our chapter on cesarean cost). Rates of support in surveys, for example, range from as high as 84.5 percent in Maine[17] to two-thirds[18] and "about half" nationwide.[19] Interestingly, female obstetricians here are sharply divided over the issue of maternal request; 36 percent disagree with it, 32 percent support it, and 28 percent say it "depends upon the woman's circumstances."[20] Elsewhere, evidence of support varies considerably too. For example, in Britain, rates of 69–79 percent have been reported; in France, 19 percent; Spain, 15 percent; Germany, 59–75 percent; the Netherlands 17–81 percent; Canada, 23 percent; Australia and New Zealand, two-thirds; and in Israel, almost half.[21]

With regard to gender, again reports vary. Some surveys find that gender has no influence on maternal request support at all, while others find that male doctors are more likely to support pregnant women than their female counterparts. Notably, the opposite of this—female doctors proving more likely to support than male—has never, to our knowledge, been found, which is curious and potentially concerning, given that more women now work as obstetricians than at any time in history.[22] That said, anecdotally, Pauline's obstetrician in New Jersey was female and fully supportive of her patients' birth plans, whether cesarean or vaginal.

Unsurprisingly, litigation plays a role too: "Perceived risk of complaints and litigation is associated with compliance with the requested cesarean."[23] In the United States, fear of litigation is an oft-cited reason for cesareans, but while such defensive medical practice can be unhelpful for maternal autonomy more broadly, it may actually help women in hospitals or countries where cesarean maternal request is currently refused. This is because the cost of litigation is already enormous in cases where a chosen planned vaginal delivery goes wrong, so if a woman demonstrates that her informed request for a cesarean was denied, and then her coerced trial of labor goes wrong, the liability is arguably even greater.

Nature of Their Work

Just as unsurprising is the fact that professional experience has an important influence on maternal request too.[24] Compared with other medical professionals, and indeed with pregnant women, urogynecologists and colorectal surgeons are the most likely to request a cesarean delivery, with rates of 42 percent and 41 percent, respectively.[25] Equally, urogynecologists are significantly more likely to agree with a woman's maternal request.[26] This is because their daily working life consists of treating the damage caused during vaginal birth. Some may argue that their perspective is skewed by overexposure to the potential risks, but we would counterargue that *under*exposure to these risks has its downside too.

Midwives, for example—and certainly the majority of nonprofessional natural birth advocates—are not generally exposed to the long-term consequences of the vaginal births they attend. In 1999, an Australian parliamentary committee report cited a submission to its committee on the subject of patient demand, suggesting that "the adverse consequences of vaginal delivery, especially operative vaginal delivery, were not appreciated by midwives because they were often not apparent in the immediate post-natal period. This influenced midwives' views of the comparative benefits of vaginal as opposed to Caesarean delivery." The submission was made by Dr. Glen Barker, who reportedly said, "Most midwives are largely ignorant about prolapse and incontinence and their relation to childbirth because they do not deal with these problems in their professional lives. This colors their view of the childbirth process and leads them to see a 'natural delivery' with as little intervention (e.g. caesarean section) as possible as being the ideal."[27] We would agree with this, and it has been both of our personal experience that the majority of midwives do not support maternal request cesareans. Instead, in general, they have a far greater level of confidence in planned vaginal birth and its benefits. Obviously, this is helpful for women who want to choose a vaginal birth but less so for those who want to choose surgery, which is why, again, choice of maternity-care provider can be just as important as the choice of birth type.

In summary, high numbers of doctors are choosing (or would choose) to have a planned cesarean birth instead of a trial of labor, and their reasons have nothing to do with being "too posh to push." They are simply making an informed decision about how they want (or would want) to give birth. And all we ask is this: Don't women have the right to know what their doctors know (and do)? Don't doctors have an obligation to impart their full knowledge? And shouldn't pregnant women be empowered to choose their own birth plans in the light of this information?

DOCTORS WHO SUPPORT

This is a collection of comments by doctors that has been communicated to us personally. We feel they enrich the statistics provided above and help flesh out some of the reasons so many doctors support the informed decision to plan a cesarean birth.

Dr. Philip J. Steer, FRCOG
Editor in Chief of *BJOG: An International Journal of Obstetrics and Gynaecology*

People make many choices about their lives, some of which are safe (e.g., going on holiday by scheduled airline) and some of which are less safe (e.g., going on holiday by microlight), but we recognize their autonomy to make individual choices over a wide range of risks. Elective cesarean section is very safe compared with many other things we do in life, for both mother and baby. Cosmetic surgery carries risks, but no one suggests it should not be allowed. We need to know more about the long-term effects of elective cesarean at maternal request, but it seems to me very unlikely that we will find anything that will make them so risky as to be inadvisable.

Dr. Linda Brubaker, MD, MS
Senior Associate Dean for Clinical and Translational Research; Professor, Department of Obstetrics & Gynecology and Urology, Loyola University Medical Center, Chicago; and Director, Division of Female Pelvic Medicine and Reconstructive Surgery

Patients, midwives, and doctors all agree that the perfect birth outcome includes both a healthy infant and a healthy mother. Yet birth, trends and traditional, are being questioned like never before. Women have become assertive in obtaining their healthcare. Most mothers would willingly transfer risk to themselves if it helped their child in any way. However, if the baby is equally safe, and there are differing risks for the mother, it seems most reasonable that she be given this information.

Dr. W. Benson Harer Jr., FACOG
Retired obstetrician and a former president of the American College of Obstetricians and Gynecologists

A paradox: Why is it that we celebrate every medical advance that enhances or prolongs life except cesarean delivery?

The facts to support elective prophylactic cesarean delivery as a rational choice continue to mount in contradiction to the politically correct "truth" that trial of labor has to be better. Cesarean delivery is major surgery and should not be taken lightly, but we tend to forget that cesarean births are the major factor in preventing vaginal births from being fatal events for 1 percent of women and many more babies. Vaginal birth may be nature's way, but nature's way has always been hazardous and still is in nations where cesarean delivery is not a readily available option.

Some critics of elective prophylactic cesarean delivery claim that it is a waste of resources and is more expensive. Such arguments do not take into account costs of later pelvic reconstructive surgery or the massive expense of providing care for a child with cerebral palsy. Latin American physicians claim that a high volume of elective procedures actually allows more efficient use of surgical suits and reduces need for extra staffing and overtime to meet erratic demand . . .

Because most damage occurs with the first vaginal delivery, I would recommend elective prophylactic cesarean delivery be reserved for nulliparous (borne no children) or multiparous (borne two or more children) women who have had major pelvic surgery. I would further restrict it to women who intend to have no more than two children. This means most women in developed nations are good candidates for elective prophylactic cesarean delivery.

Dr. Ralph W. Hale, FACOG
Executive Vice President of the American College of Obstetricians and Gynecologists

Elective cesarean delivery has become a reality in the practice of obstetrics today as more and more of the women who approach delivery have strong feelings that the option of the mode of delivery should be their decision to make unless there are compelling medical indications for a specific delivery method. Their reasons will vary from woman to woman, but whatever decision she may make, the patient needs to know all of the available risks and benefits.

Historically, for many years, elective cesarean was thought to only be for Hollywood women. It was called the "vaginal preservation operation"; that was the name of it back years ago . . . My own personal opinion—and I stand by what I've done—is if you're my patient and you come in to see me and say, "I want a cesarean delivery," and I am sure of your dates and everything, I would offer it to you. I would discuss with you all the rationale, I would explain the risks to you, including the fact that repeat cesareans can have an increased incidence of previa and abruption, and if you still felt you wanted to have an elective cesarean delivery, we'd have an elective cesarean delivery picked on the date that you wanted. I believe a patient should be informed of all aspects, but then it is her choice.

Dr. Duncan Turner
Medical Director of Santa Barbara Obstetrics and Gynecology Associates, California

If a woman wants a cesarean she should get it, and I feel very strongly about this. Obviously I would talk through the pros and cons of surgery and the risks involved, but there are many more elective surgeries today that are much more dangerous — and far less as important as childbirth — and women are able to elect for these. So in my opinion, any reason should be OK — if the woman doesn't want to go through labor, she doesn't want labor pain, she wants to plan around a certain day or she feels that cesarean delivery is safer for her baby . . .

One reason some doctors have been reluctant to give women a cesarean is because historically, they weren't the gold standard and also, they were criticized for doing too many of them. So some doctors think: "If a woman asks for a cesarean and I end up doing more cesareans as a result, then I will have more criticism." But for me, as long as the patient knows what they are getting into, then they should be allowed to have one. I'm a strong advocate of patients doing things their way with the appropriate knowledge. There isn't one treatment that's right for everyone, so informed choices are what are most important. Doing something that a patient does not want is, in my opinion, malpractice.

Dr. Samantha Collier
Former Executive Vice President and Chief Medical Officer, HealthGrades

Surgery is not without risk, and my own personal decision would not be to go through surgery because I don't like the idea of anesthetic. Anecdotally as a physician and study researcher, I would personally probably prefer a vaginal birth because I think recovering from surgery and looking after a newborn isn't pleasant. But that's a personal decision. I don't see why cesareans should be treated as a negative procedure, when there have been technological advances in every other area of medicine which we accept, and where invasive, laparoscopic, and cosmetic surgery is a multimillion-dollar business. I've seen patients die having a nose job or bleed to death having liposuction. With cesareans, yes, there is an absolute risk because it's surgery but it's about 0.000 percent. If I fly in a plane once a year and my risk is x and then because I fly three times in a year my risk triples, this doesn't stop me flying. If the cesarean debate is all about a death risk then women just shouldn't get pregnant . . .

I think that there is maybe too much emphasis on the negative. It's more important that women become more empowered and that they get exactly what they want in healthcare. Who is it for us to decide what a woman should do when both risks are comparable and the cesarean risk possibly even lower? [Vaginal or cesarean] are just two alternatives, and it's not for us to decide, but rather to support a woman and help inform them to make the best decision for them. A woman should be fully informed, and that is our obligation in the medical community. It's about choice and preserving autonomy. Objectively, we can provide you with data, the risks, long-term implications, and possible outcomes for you and your baby. Even taking an aspirin has risks and benefits which we can tell you about but it's up to you to decide.

Dr. Harry Gee (*retired in 2009*)
Former consultant obstetrician at Birmingham Women's Hospital, England, and former Director of West Midlands Postgraduate School of Obstetrics and Gynaecology

An individual who has had a very successful natural birth does not have the right to assert that everyone else can have the same experience. It's a very unscientific and authoritarian way of thinking because you can't generalize like that. My standpoint is that women should be given as much information as they require. We as professionals should facilitate whatever is their decision. This may include elective cesarean. . . . If I've felt that the patient has understood the important points and she still believes a cesarean is right, then I have gone along with the request, and some of my colleagues do likewise too.

Professor James Drife (*retired in 2009*)
Former obstetrician at Leeds General Infirmary, England

It is ironic that a woman's right to refuse a cesarean should be upheld while her right to refuse vaginal delivery is not. She is allowed to refuse a cesarean even though doing so may kill her or her baby. I think women are perfectly able to make up their own minds provided they are given all the facts, and I think they have the right to do so . . . the problem I have with trying to dissuade them is knowing that they too might end up with a difficult vaginal birth. It's not that obstetricians want to encourage more cesareans at all. They rather like doing clever vaginal births; they get to use their skills if it's an instrumental birth and have a sense of achievement at the end. But that may not necessarily be the best thing for the woman.

Dr. Felicity Plaat
Consultant anesthetist at Queen Charlotte's Hospital, London, England

It seems to me that proponents of choice are not actually advocates of real freedom to choose—they want women to "choose" a mode of delivery that they think is best/cheapest/most natural. Women's choice is fine if they chose normal deliveries or home birth but *not* if they want a cesarean. Whatever one thinks, one should be consistent!

Dr. Peyman Banooni
Obstetrician at Cedar Sinai Hospital, Beverly Hills, California

I'm not a proponent of it, and I'm not against it. I think you should have the option of being able to do this, an elective cesarean section, and if you're aware of the information, the pros and cons of both, and you make your own decision, then we'll do whatever it is that you decide is right for you.

Dr. Elmar Joura
Department of Obstetrics and Gynaecology, Medical University of Vienna, Austria

The main end points are healthy children and mothers; the route of delivery is merely a detail. We give so much medical support in birth today that you can't call it "natural" anymore. A very big system protects women and prevents negative effects where possible throughout her pregnancy, and the delivery is just at the end. I tell my patients very early in their pregnancy that they have free choice of their mode of delivery. I give them all the information and then they take a few weeks to go away and think about it. At the end, most of them know what is best for their personality.

Dr. Bryan Beattie, FRCOG
Consultant obstetrician at a tertiary teaching hospital in the
United Kingdom

From an ethical perspective, women should be provided with accurate
unbiased information about the limitations of assessing risk, and the risks
of various interventions available, to allow them to make informed
choices about their pregnancy and place and type of delivery. However,
whilst they should be supported in their choices by obstetricians and
midwives, they and their partners must also be prepared to accept the
consequences of their decisions, bearing in mind their unborn baby had
no choice in the matter. This applies equally to those who choose to have
a homebirth or delivery in a standalone midwifery-led unit where access
to medical care may be too late if things go wrong, or those who have
complications from a maternal choice cesarean section in hospital. That
said, obstetricians and midwives who are opposed to the concept of
maternal choice cesarean section in uncomplicated pregnancies at term
should ask themselves when the last time a baby had to be admitted to a
special care baby unit (SCBU) and compare it to the last admission for a
"low risk" woman who was planning a vaginal delivery.

Chapter 6

Protecting Your Pelvic Floor

Childbirth is a natural event. So are death and earthquakes.
—Anonymous woman's comment on
Birth Trauma Canada website, 2007

You'd think that by now, with all the millions of cesarean births and the billions of vaginal births that have taken place, there would be sufficient evidence available for all doctors and scientists to agree on whether a cesarean delivery offers protection against pelvic floor injuries such as urinary incontinence, fecal/anal incontinence, and pelvic organ prolapse. But they don't.

On the contrary, the debate rages in medical journals, media news commentary, and blogs. One side of the argument quotes one study while the other side quotes another. So what's the truth?

Certainly, pregnancy itself contributes to and is a risk factor for pelvic floor troubles after the baby is born, whatever the delivery method. Most everyone agrees with that, as they do with the fact that advanced maternal age and obesity are risk factors too. There is also agreement that even women who have never had children, or women who have only ever had cesarean births, can develop pelvic floor problems. However, it is our opinion that although these cases exist, they are regularly misrepresented and used as flawed arguments against the fact that the greatest risk factor for pelvic floor problems is vaginal birth. The incidence and likelihood of injuries are significantly increased during vaginal birth, and this association increases with the number of vaginal births a woman has, even though the first delivery is the one most likely to cause the most damage, especially if the woman is older.

For example, a recent study published in the *American Journal of Obstetrics and Gynecology* (AJOG) looked at the long-term risk of requiring surgery for prolapse or stress urinary incontinence up to thirty years after childbirth.[1] The researchers questioned more than sixty-three thousand women who had *only* ever had vaginal deliveries and compared them with more than thirty-three thousand women who *only* had cesarean deliveries, making it one of the largest studies looking into this problem ever. Interestingly, one thing they did not do was separate emergency cesareans from planned cesareans. As we state repeatedly, the contributing factors around emergency cesareans have the potential to cause significantly more injury than planned cesareans, and so the findings of this study might have been even more significant had the vaginal delivery group been compared to a purely elective cesarean group.

Regardless, the findings were absolutely astounding. For example, contrary to commonly held opinion, each successive vaginal delivery increased the risk for prolapse and incontinence; it was not just the first delivery that had the most impact. Women with three vaginal deliveries had double the risk for incontinence surgery and three times the risk for prolapse surgery, compared to women with only one vaginal delivery. And after three vaginal deliveries, compared to women who had three cesareans, the risk was fivefold higher for incontinence surgery and twenty-fold (almost a 2,000 percent increase) higher for prolapse surgery. For women who *only* had cesarean deliveries, the rate of incontinence and prolapse surgery did not rise with more cesareans but actually decreased with successive births. This would seem to indicate that pregnancy per se, which has always been considered a major independent risk factor, does *not* appear to be a major risk factor for stress urinary incontinence and pelvic organ prolapse—at least, not in this study. Instrumental deliveries, on the other hand, were found to be major risk factors, and as expected, vacuum delivery was found to be safer for the pelvic floor than were forceps. After one forceps delivery, the risk for women having prolapse surgery was double that of women having vacuum or noninstrumental vaginal delivery and twenty times that of the (mixed) cesarean group.

This study is particularly deserving of attention because of its size and longevity, but also because it took place in Sweden, which has an excellent research reputation. This is partly as a result of its homogeneous population and also because its single national healthcare system makes excellent and inclusive registries possible. Also, the study looked at the risk of different birth types for women *having* surgery; it did not include those who developed prolapse or stress urinary incontinence without reporting for treatment. Since it has repeatedly been shown that a minority of women with pelvic floor disorders actually seek medical treatment, it is possible the real burden of birth-related pelvic floor damage is even higher than that reported, and the real significance of the difference in long-term pelvic floor health with different birth plans is even greater.

And yet books and websites insist the very opposite is true. Why? A very interesting article published in *Discover Magazine* early in 2010 answers this question just beautifully. During his discussion of the problems inherent with any research, but with medical research in particular, author David H. Freedman makes the point that it is ridiculous that there are so many ostensibly important research studies being published in distinguished journals, and yet many of these studies have diametrically opposed outcomes and conclusions. He tells the story of a police officer who sees a drunken man crawling around under a streetlight on a dark night. The officer asks the man what he is doing, and he replies that he is looking for his wallet. But when the officer asks whether he is sure that this is where he lost it, the drunk answers that he has no idea, but he can see better under the light.

The drunk's insistence on looking where there is better light illustrates the mistake of researching a health topic for reasons that are superfluous to what should be the overriding goal: to discover the truth. As one of Murphy's laws states, sometimes "research scientists are so wrapped up in their own narrow endeavors that they cannot possibly see the whole picture of anything, including their own research."[2] All too often, medical studies involve underlying beliefs and biases or the desire to confirm or contradict previous studies, all of which cause a clustering effect of research efforts and ideas on any given subject. It can also be easier for researchers to stick with one style of research than to experiment with or articulate an alternative method that might produce more accurate and relevant results. There can also be problems with the way the research is conducted. For example, studies may use surrogate outcomes, such as when breech presentation leading to cesarean birth is used as a surrogate in studies of all "planned cesareans." When different surrogates are used in different studies, inevitably, different conclusions are drawn. Similarly, nonvalidated methods of measuring and inappropriate time spans for studying can muddy the waters as well.

Exacerbating the situation further are peripheral influences in the

research industry, including which articles are accepted by medical journals. Dr. Murphy has acted as a peer reviewer for a number of journals,
and one of the questions he is routinely asked in order to determine
whether a particular study might be accepted is whether it is "interesting"
or "topical." But while something interesting and topical can be a good
thing, there is a danger that with a big enough media impact, a less than
robust finding will make its mark on the public consciousness, and it will
take time before another big story is able to restore the balance (two prime
examples are the World Health Organization's recommendation that a
country's cesarean births not exceed 15 percent and the now completely
discredited finding that the MMR jab may have a causal effect on
increased rates of autism). In Christopher Nolan's 2010 movie, *Inception*,
Leonardo DiCaprio's character, Dom Cobb, states that an idea is like a
virus—it grows and it spreads. And so Freedman's article concludes that
we cannot believe individual studies alone, especially those where surrogate markers have been used, but rather instead, we need to look at results
over a long period and stir in a good dose of logic. This approach in relation to the pelvic floor is long overdue. To date, there has been too much
confusion in the literature, hiding of truths, diluting and crowding of outcomes, and effectively, refusal to search for the wallet (pelvic floor
damage) in the place that it was most likely lost (vaginal birth).

So how might we sensibly and logically approach research into
whether pelvic floor damage is predominantly associated with planned
vaginal birth and whether planned cesarean birth has a protective effect?

It's simple: start out by asking what makes the most logical sense. Does
it make sense that vaginal birth damages the pelvic floor? Yes, it does—
regardless of the latest study that concludes the opposite. Does it make
sense that this damage increases a woman's chance of developing undesirable medical conditions? Yes, it does. And does it make sense that an
abdominal cesarean birth, especially one carried out before labor even
starts, significantly limits the risk of serious pelvic floor damage? Again,
yes, and indeed many studies have reached that very conclusion, but often
without getting the attention they deserved.

Also giving sense a helping hand in the planned vaginal versus
planned cesarean birth debate are personal experience and anecdotes. For
example, doctors and other medical professionals who work in the pelvic
floor field day after day, both at the birth and in the immediate or long-

term postnatal period, can't help but bring actual experience into the equation.[3] Dr. Murphy recollects the many births he has watched or assisted in the past in which, during intense pushing by the woman, there was a sudden "give" in the process as a previously stuck baby descended quite rapidly. He cringed, knowing something very bad had happened to the woman's body, but he recalls the events being couched in positive terms by those around him shouting, "Oh, look, the baby is coming! It's here! Congratulations!" Compare this recollection with that of the numerous young women who have come into his clinic over the years with their "blown-open" vaginas. The power of personal involvement with these women and the impact that vaginal birth has had on their lives is rarely incorporated into a statistical analysis—despite being a reality. Similarly, there are the thousands of stories told by women of lives destroyed or blighted by injuries sustained during labor that appear on birth trauma websites, the authors' own websites, and in online chat rooms around the world. These, too, don't necessarily find their way into the finer detail of many comparative birth studies, and yet they serve as powerful examples of what can happen. Here are just some comments that have appeared on the Birth Trauma Canada website:

> "I change my baby's diapers and then I change my own. I'm 23 years old."
>
> "My vaginal delivery was a surgical birth. . . . My crotch looked like a horrible industrial accident."
>
> "When [my sister] needs to have a bowel movement now she has to insert her finger into her vagina to hold her rectum in place. She had to have another operation when her son was three years old so she can control when she urinates. Her husband left her for another woman when her son was a year and a half."
>
> "I looked at my genitals in a mirror when I got home from the hospital and immediately felt sick and faint. It did explain why ibuprofen and ice packs weren't doing anything for the pain. My prenatal course didn't prepare me for how much destruction happens."
>
> "I rarely leave my home anymore. Incontinence supplies cost about $20 every week. If I live to be ninety, that will cost me $57,200."

"I wanted a vaginal delivery to avoid surgery. That was a load of crap."

"My genitals are grotesque. The labia are huge and floppy and parts of them fused together where they shouldn't. . . . I have little flaps of flesh sticking out where the lacerations that weren't sutured healed asymmetrically. There are scar tissue ridges and the opening to my vagina gapes. I'm so ashamed of how hideous I look. Sex is always with the lights out now. Now I understand why women say, 'Not tonight, dear, I have a headache.' The doctor just shrugged and called it 'normal sequelae' and pointed out that if I was that vain I could get cosmetic surgery. More surgery is the last thing I could deal with."

"This will be the third vaginal/anal surgery I've had since having my baby five years ago."

"I was ripped apart stem to stern, shredded to pulp. Like hamburger. . . . When I went for the six-week postpartum checkup, [my doctor says] he wouldn't recommend doing anything to correct the maiming for six months. 'That is the time it takes to really finish the healing process from a vaginal birth,' he says. [I say,] 'Why wasn't I told that before you scarred me for life?' 'Oh', he says, 'then women wouldn't get pregnant, would they, if they knew?'"

"So many people know the truth but no one told me what to expect."[4]

The last two comments in this list are fundamental in any discussion of the pelvic floor, since one of the biggest problems (as addressed in chapter 7, "Lives Destroyed by Vaginal Birth") is that women simply aren't being told the truth about what can happen during a vaginal birth. Their birth educators don't believe it's appropriate or necessary, given that it will only happen to a minority of women. For example, one of Pauline's colleagues, Leigh East, recalls how, during prenatal classes for her second pregnancy, she was being told about her pelvic floor risks and remarked, "This would have been really useful information the first time around." Her instructor promptly replied, "Oh, we don't cover all this in our classes with first-time moms. It would scare them too much." East's reaction was to write her own prenatal information book for women.[5] And while we know that our book, and in particular this chapter, is going to be accused of exaggerating the risks of a vaginal birth and scaring women unnecessarily, we simply don't believe that the alternative—keeping women in the dark—is right either. In the United States, for example, one survey reported that as few as 15 percent of women are even told about the reality of long-term injuries following vaginal birth.[6] And unfortunately, this unethical reality is borne out by women's anecdotal storytelling throughout the world.

"I had no idea this could happen," women repeat to each other, and their doctors, over and over and over again.

So, if you'd rather not know the truth, look away now. But if you want to be fully informed about the pelvic floor, what it does, and how it can be adversely affected during birth, we suggest you read on.

WHAT IS THE PELVIC FLOOR AND WHY IS IT IMPORTANT?

The pelvic floor is exactly what its name implies. Basically, it is a floor, and specifically, it is the floor of the pelvis and the pelvic organs. These organs are the uterus, bladder, urethra, rectum, and sigmoid colon (part of the large bowel). It is also the floor of the whole intra-abdominal cavity and all its organs (e.g., the rest of the bowel).

Like any floor, the pelvic floor provides support and keeps everything above it in its proper place. Without this foundation, the intra-abdominal organs would have nothing to keep them in place and would simply fall through the pelvis (this is discussed in more detail in chapter 18, "The Evolution of Natural Birth and the Future of Cesarean Birth"). However, the pelvic floor is more important than a mere support organ. It is not naturally a passive support structure, and neither is it an unyielding platform. Rather, this organ is tremendously active and vital, and it plays a direct, integrated, and essential part in urination, defecation, sexual function, and childbirth. Indeed, there was even a recent study on breathing with the pelvic floor,[7] a term more usually associated with the diaphragm, and this is because the two are actually very similar. Each one is composed mostly of large muscle areas and closes off the ends of the body's top and bottom cavities.

Crucially, the pelvic floor is essential to the maintenance of urinary and fecal continence, which means that it helps maintain the ability of the bladder and rectal storage mechanisms and prevent inadvertent wetting or soiling. During urination or defecation, the pelvic floor's role changes from support, and the facilitation of continence, to an active and important contribution to these expelling activities. For urination, relaxation of the pelvic floor allows the descent of the bladder neck, which causes a funneling of the upper urethra and helps to initiate urine flow. For defecation, the muscles of the pelvic floor play a role in the amazingly intricate control people have over their bowel movements. Not only does the pelvic floor allow gas to escape while it maintains continence of solid and fluid fecal material, but the timing of such relief is under its direct voluntary control in the normal situation. It also permits the expansion of the lower rectum to allow first the storage of feces, and, when appropriate, the passing.

This amazing ability of the pelvic complex, consisting of anus, rectum, and pelvic floor muscles, can be illustrated with the following example: Imagine holding a mixture of air, water, and sand in your cupped hands and then separating your hands just enough to *only* let the air escape through the cracks. Impossible, and yet the normal pelvis manages this. The problem is that it is critically dependent on the cooperation and normal function of all involved systems. Dysfunction in just one part of the system will lead to problems—in this case, anal or fecal incontinence. Worse still, incontinence of gas cannot be cured, certainly not with surgery, so if a childbirth injury leaves you with such incontinence, you will have it for life. Improvements are possible with diet and physical therapy, for example, but it cannot be cured.

Most important, the pelvic floor prevents the collapse of the pelvic organs into the vagina and helps to minimize or prevent the vagina from being inverted or pushed down and keeps the organs (or their parts) from protruding, bulging, or sagging into the vagina opening. This sagging of the vaginal walls and pelvic organs is called pelvic organ prolapse, and like many words in medicine, *prolapse* comes from Latin. It means the falling down or downward displacement of a part. Other than incontinence, prolapse might also cause inability to completely empty the bladder or bowels, constipation, the need to use fingers to empty the bowels (very common), back discomfort (usually a dull ache), a feeling of heaviness, vaginal discomfort, discharge, bleeding from the rubbing of exposed parts on clothes, recurrent urinary infections, an inability to sit comfortably (because the prolapse is in the way), and difficulties with sex.

In contrast, an intact pelvic floor prevents prolapse complications and helps prevent the uterus from falling through the vagina. Similarly, after a hysterectomy, it helps to prevent the loss of vaginal support, which causes vault prolapse; in effect an inversion of the vagina (imagine an inflated party balloon: if you push your fist on one end you will eventually come out the other by turning the balloon inside out). Straining to urinate or defecate only increases the tendency for these organs to bulge down into the vagina; also, during certain physical and sporting activities, the forces pushing them south are incredible. An intact pelvic floor is essential to prevent any or all these things from happening.

WHY DON'T I KNOW MORE ABOUT IT?

The pelvic floor is one of the most neglected parts of the human body. Its function is essentially unseen and therefore largely taken for granted. That is, of course, unless problems occur, and even then, the affected person can find it difficult to put these problems into words or comprehend what's happening. This is because disorders caused by pelvic floor damage or dysfunction are regarded as embarrassing and definitely not fit for polite conversation; women do not discuss them easily with their doctors, much less with their family and friends.

Consequently, until relatively recently, these disorders have not gained the publicity or resources they deserve and have certainly not generated enough influence in the medical community. Dr. Murphy's previous book (*Pelvic Health and Childbirth: What Every Woman Needs to Know*, coauthored with Carol Wasson in 2003) aimed to educate women about the facts, as have numerous press releases and articles published by Pauline since 2006. But compounding the problem further is the nature of compartmentalized medical specialties—separating different types of incontinence and prolapse, for example. These specialties investigate and treat the various problems related to the pelvic floor, but their separation has also led to the neglect and fragmentation of related research.

Fortunately, the important role played by the pelvic floor in some of our most intimate daily activities is gaining greater exposure. More doctors are speaking out about it, as are more women, as seen in the recent BBC News Online story "My Natural Birth Wrecked My Body."[8] Even so, there remain many more questions than answers, and most frustrating, it is impossible to predict with any real certainty which women will develop pelvic floor problems after childbirth. It might happen to you, but it might not; no one can tell for sure.

UNDERSTANDING THE PELVIC FLOOR

The pelvic floor can probably be best visualized as a strong muscle that covers the opening at the bottom of the pelvis. Anyone who has ever looked at a skeleton might have noticed that the bony pelvis is actually a funnel shape, with a definite wide area at the top and a narrower enclosed funnel lower down. The pelvic floor covers the narrow opening close to the bottom, and in an upright human, it can be best understood if it is visualized as parallel to the ground (a simplistic view, but sufficient for the purposes of explanation here). The pelvic floor is much more than just a muscle or even collection of muscles. It also contains layers of fascia (description to follow), various collagen and elastic fibers, areolar tissue (spongy material made up of thin capillary blood vessels and soft tissue), larger blood vessels, and nerves.

The most important muscles you need to be aware of are the levator ani muscles, which consist of different muscles making up the whole of the large pelvic muscle—one on each side of the pelvis, meeting in the midline. The levator ani muscles are mostly made up of slow twitch fibers and are designed to provide constant and prolonged contraction without you even being aware of it. They do not tire easily, and, unlike ordinary skeletal muscle, they are able to provide constant support. Yet although we are not usually conscious of them, they are under our voluntary control. This is mainly because they also contain a smaller number of fast twitch fibers. These allow quick responses to messages from the brain during episodes of involuntary and increased intra-abdominal pressure, such as when we cough, sneeze, or laugh, and our natural contraction during these episodes serves to counteract the resulting downward pressure on the pelvic floor.

Another crucial aspect of the pelvic floor to understand is the pelvic fascia. This fascial tissue is soft connective tissue that effectively acts as scaffolding for the pelvic floor. If you picture the white layer in your beef steak that seems to be separating different parts of the meat, this is fascia.

As well as surrounding the pelvic floor muscles and providing a framework for them, the fascia also surrounds the various pelvic organs and keeps them each in their proper position.

If there is any damage to the levator ani muscles or if they can no longer support the pelvic and abdominal organ contents, the full weight of these organs, plus the forces generated by a woman's general physical activities, falls on the fascial layers. But perhaps the most important thing to understand about the pelvic fascia is that it does not heal naturally; once torn or otherwise damaged, it cannot heal back to its original condition and must be surgically repaired.

WHEN THINGS GO WRONG

A number of factors can influence the health and longevity of the pelvic floor, and for women in particular they include age (risks at twenty years old are different from risks at forty), weight, number of children, and birth experience. Not all vaginal births lead to the severity of damage described here, and indeed many women's bodies recover with unnoticeable damage, but the process of a baby's passage through the vagina makes it difficult to conclude that there is not at least *some* impact on the pelvic floor, given the physical metamorphosis that is pregnancy and birth.

Damage to the Levator Ani Muscles

Other than being crushed by the baby, tearing naturally, or being cut during an episiotomy, the levator muscles are also sometimes completely torn off from their implantation sites (avulsed), specifically at the points where they attach to the pubic bones and other attachment sites. As discussed above, a muscle can work only when strongly anchored. Even the strongest hydraulic ram (think of construction equipment) will be useless if the ram is not firmly bolted or otherwise attached at its normal anchor points. Unfortunately, it is not currently possible to surgically repair avulsed levator muscles, and of course muscles cannot be repaired if they are absent.[9] These weak, injured muscles are often painful, and chronic pelvic pain can sometimes continue for years after childbirth. Notably, forceps use is a particular risk factor for levator injury.

Another consequence of injured or weakened levator muscles is an increase in the size of the urogenital hiatus—the vagina and genital aperture.[10] It can also lead to a greater risk of prolapse later because the pelvic organs are lower too.[11] During episodes of increased abdominal pressure (for instance, during straining), the bladder neck is lower in women after vaginal birth compared to women who have not had children or women who have had planned cesareans. In fact, studies have found that this positional change occurs in more than 50 percent of women after vaginal birth and is usually persistent, whereas in contrast, there is almost no difference after a planned cesarean.[12] Similarly, a recent French study, which was the first to do comparative MRI (magnetic resonance imaging) evaluations of the levator muscles of first-time mothers who had planned pre-labor cesareans and cesareans after labor had commenced, showed a significant difference in MRI evaluations that were done a few days later. The women whose cesareans were done after labor had commenced were found to have significantly higher numbers of levator abnormalities, indicating the likelihood of nerve injuries or local ischemia (lack of oxygen).[13]

Nerve Injuries

Muscles can also function only if the nerve supply is intact. Without this essential element, muscles degenerate and atrophy (waste away). Damage to nerves can take many forms and does not necessarily have to be permanent or complete. During vaginal birth, there are multiple possibilities for nerve damage within the pelvic area. For example, nerves can be damaged by overstretching, being crushed against a hard object (e.g., a pelvic bone), tearing, or being cut (e.g., during an episiotomy).

Two very important nerves that supply the pelvic floor—the pudendal nerves—are very vulnerable to a combination of crushing and stretching forces. These nerves, one on each side, together with contributions from the spinal nerve roots, play a significant part in the control of the voluntary muscles of the pelvic floor and perineum and are essential to normal pelvic muscle action. While injuries to these nerves can usually repair themselves in time, deficits often remain. If the nerve is not completely severed, full recovery can take place in time, but more severe injuries can lead to the death of nerve fibers and subsequent dysfunction of the muscle they're connected to. Also, pudendal nerves have significant sensory functions, including being the nerve of the clitoris, so it doesn't take much imagination to realize that their injury might affect sexual function as well as general pelvic sensation.

Fascia Tears

Fascia is often the last defense after damaged or torn levator ani muscles have given up the struggle, whether through weakening, injury, or shrinkage, but it can act as the pelvic organs' sole support for only a limited time before it gives way, sometimes suddenly.[14] Women throughout the years have described to Dr. Murphy the precise moment when they felt something "pop," "snap," "tear," or "rip," and they knew something awful had happened. Sometimes they describe feeling pressure from prolapse shortly after this initial sensation. Of course, many fascia tears that happen during vaginal birth occur immediately, but they might also be temporarily compensated for by strong pelvic muscles or the fill-in effect of scar tissue. Then, months or even years later, when the muscles weaken and the scar tissue stretches, the fascia tears are unmasked again. At this later time, women often don't recognize this complaint as a birth injury and therefore don't talk about it as such (to their daughters, for example). This means that the injury is often not connected to birth in scientific medical literature, since in many cases, the follow-up period of study has long passed.

Conversely, but equally unfortunately, even if there is no damage to the pelvic fascia during delivery, some of the same causes of muscle deterioration can also cause tears or stretching of the fascia; even if initially intact, the absence of the pelvic floor muscle support causes the fascial layer to stretch out over time or eventually tear.

Vaginal and Vulvar Injuries

Significant vaginal and vulvar lacerations are commonplace in the labor ward.[15] These lacerations are sometimes difficult to repair surgically, as it can become an impossible puzzle to determine which shredded piece of tissue should be sutured where. If you've ever tried to repair a net or mesh when it's torn asymmetrically (like the material that surrounds a child's trampoline, for example), you can start to imagine the complexity involved in repairing a woman's flesh that has torn in this way. And where some of these laceration repairs can challenge even the most experienced obstetrician, it can be a disaster if an attempt is made with less surgically experienced hands.

Even a minor tear that is repaired poorly can have detrimental consequences, and as with any tear, the effect of a less than optimal repair might not become apparent for quite a while. But the fact is that the vagina and vulva will often never again appear the same as they did before the birth. The vagina might be stretched; the entrance might be open instead of closed; there might be scar tissue, excess tags, roughness, scars, or separations in the labia minora; and the perineum might be deformed, shortened, or completely absent, with only a thin layer of skin separating the vagina from the anal canal. In short, it is not only the function of the vagina, vulva, and perineum that may be affected, but also the aesthetic appearance. Of course, for many women, this is an accepted consequence of vaginal birth; they are able to adapt easily to any changes and do not suffer any long-lasting distress. But for others, such changes are devastating, traumatic, and often physically uncomfortable.

Perineal Damage

The perineum, or perineal body, is the thickened part of flesh between the vaginal and the anal openings (the part that would be in direct contact with a bicycle seat). Multiple small muscles implant here, and these transform into strong units of dense connective tissues, creating an essential scaffold for normal muscle function and support. Most of the muscles involved surround the lower vagina; if the vagina is contracted with one or two fingers placed in it, these muscles can be clearly felt. The external anal sphincter is also attached to the perineal body. Any disruption or dysfunction resulting from a tear here—extremely common during a vaginal birth—or an episiotomy cut could destroy this critical part of the anatomy, with consequences for vaginal, anal, and sexual function.[16] For example, the tight closure of a woman's vaginal opening can be irreparably altered by stretching, tearing, or otherwise damaging these sensitive tissues. And the cavity of the rest of the vagina also changes with damage: with significant stretching and tearing of muscle and fascia, the vagina can be turned into a wide-open, flaccid cavity.

Disruption of the perineum is often associated with tears through the anal sphincters as well. Any partial-thickness sphincter tear is classified as a second-degree tear, whereas a full-thickness sphincter tear is called a third-degree tear. When the tear goes right through the anal sphincter and through the rectal wall, it is called a fourth-degree tear. These terms denoting degrees of tears are often mentioned in the labor ward but have little or no meaning to exhausted and emotionally drained parents. Unfortunately, the long-term results might be devastating.

Urinary Incontinence

An understanding of urinary incontinence is complicated by the fact that there are different types of incontinence, not all related to pelvic floor damage. The most common type is stress urinary incontinence, which is usually a consequence of pelvic floor damage or dysfunction. Typically, stress urinary incontinence involves a squirt of urine while coughing, sneezing, or laughing, and its relationship with vaginal birth has been established for almost one hundred years. In 1919, Howard A. Kelly, the first professor of gynecology at the Johns Hopkins School of Medicine, coauthored a text titled "Disease of the Kidney, Ureters, and Bladder." In it, he noted this association while still acknowledging that it can also occur in women who have never had children:

> The commonest form of incontinence is the result of childbirth, entailing an injury to the neck of the bladder; it is occasionally seen in the elderly nullipara and is most common after the age of 40. It is usually progressive, beginning with an occasional dribble, later becoming more frequent and occurring on slight provocation. In its incipiency, a strain, cough, sneeze or stepping up to get on a tram car starts a little spurt of urine which, in the course of time, initiates the act which empties the bladder.

It is interesting, and not a little disappointing, that despite almost a century of research, our knowledge in this area has not progressed much.

True urinary incontinence is the result of a hole in a urine-carrying organ, most commonly in the bladder with a tract into the vagina but also in the ureter or urethra. With modern obstetric management in developed countries, this is fortunately rare, but in the past, and certainly in the developing world today, obstructive labor and the associated tissue damage and breakdown has commonly led to such fistulas (holes) and, without treatment, to permanent urinary leakage. In developed countries, these problems are usually the result of operative complications (e.g., with pelvic surgery of any kind, including any cesarean or hysterectomy), but crucially, they are at least repaired here, unlike in many situations in the developing world.

More commonly, some women lose bladder sensation immediately after delivery; though the loss of sensation might be temporary, the effect can be long lasting. Likely causes for the initial lack of sensation include the anesthetic (spinal or epidural) and nerve injuries from stretching and crushing during labor and/or delivery, especially instrumental deliveries or prolonged second-stage labor. The reported incidence of this is all over the map, with studies showing an incidence of severe prolonged urinary reten-tion of 0.06 percent and lesser cases of up to 14 percent. In the most severe cases, there is also a danger of bladder rupture.[17] Sometimes the lack of sensation immediately after delivery leads to bladder overdistention (over-filling and stretching) injuries. What happens is that since the woman cannot feel her bladder filling up, she doesn't become aware of the need to urinate and often *cannot* release her urine. If appropriate actions are not taken, such as inserting a catheter, the bladder might stretch farther than it can endure. Subsequently, the nerves in the bladder wall might be irrev-ocably damaged, thus creating permanent long-term problems with uri-nating. In fact, this can also happen following a planned cesarean if the IV and catheter removal are not managed effectively. It is thus very important that the bladder be managed correctly after the delivery, whether it be a normal vaginal birth, an instrumental birth, or a cesarean birth.

Women sometimes take pride in the fact that they can hold their urine for many hours, but eventually the problem might catch up with them. If not managed correctly by learning to void at regular intervals, the bladder may get cumulative injuries over a period of years through repeated over-stretching, and the woman may become dependent on a catheter. This risk is also true in any situation where people might regularly defer voiding longer than physiologically reasonable. Certain professions create situa-tions where people regularly overstretch their bladders, and over time, and with aging, the bladder might decompensate and become unable to func-tion properly. Dr. Murphy often uses the following analogy in clinic to explain the situation in such cases: A normal bladder, at the moment you try to void, is like a party balloon. If you let go of an inflated party balloon's neck, it will rapidly deflate, just as a bladder empties by squeezing the urine out. A hypocontractile bladder, described above, is like a plastic grocery bag. No matter how full of air you inflate such a bag, when you let go of the pinched outlet, not much happens. It stays full. A normal bladder is a plastic grocery bag while filling but changes to a party balloon the moment your brain gives the signal to void. A bladder with severe irreparably damaged nerves is a plastic grocery bag at all times. And there's no party in that.

Fecal and Anal Incontinence

Fecal incontinence is the involuntary loss of liquid or solid stool, whereas anal incontinence includes loss of gas as well. Anal incontinence is therefore the more common of the two and the subject of more research studies in this area. Now, most of us are aware of our rectal sphincter muscle; if we do not actively relax this sphincter we cannot defecate, and the opposite of that is immediately obvious. If the rectal sphincter muscle relaxes when it should not, or if it cannot contract or maintain the necessary contraction when we want it to, involuntary defecation or incontinence is a high probability. Sphincter muscles are, in effect, our safety clamps. They give us control over our bodily functions, and without them we would be at the mercy of every bowel contraction and, indeed, gravity.

In the case of our anal sphincter, there is a compensatory mechanism that can explain why anal and fecal incontinence often only show up years after childbirth, largely in older women. This is something called the puborectalis part of the levator ani muscles, which remains strong enough to stop the descent of a stool mass even if the sphincter itself is damaged. Later in life, however, the inexorable and inevitable loss of skeletal muscle bulk and strength doesn't spare even the puborectalis, and thus the sphincter incontinence is unmasked.

The body's resourcefulness in combating this type of incontinence until older age is a good thing, but it also means there is a dilution of the effect of vaginal birth as an observable risk factor for anal incontinence, especially in young women. Since many women are still able to control their gas and feces following sphincter damage, this particular risk of vaginal birth is easily obscured and therefore still debated. What we'd like to draw attention to here, though, is the flip side of this situation: when a young woman *does* present with fecal or, especially, anal incontinence after her vaginal birth, and when it doesn't improve or go away within a period of months, it needs to be recognized that this woman almost certainly has a far more significant pelvic injury, likely involving her entire pelvic floor (not just her sphincter muscles), which must be investigated and treated.

Impact on Sexual Health

Sexuality is an important life force. Not only are positive sexual experiences some of the most pleasurable of human sensations, but continued enjoyable sexual relations form the bedrock of many long-term relationships, as well as nurturing a healthy and positive self-image. In this context, it's important to understand that a normal and intact pelvic floor is vital for optimal sexual function.[18]

Here's why. During intercourse, the muscles of the pelvic floor play a major role in orgasm; they contract in rhythmic waves and are the main reason for the pulsating nature of any orgasm. The contractions of these muscles in the female are also important for providing a tighter vaginal grip on the penetrating penis, which facilitates both male and female pleasure.

Pelvic floor damage in the sexual context is commonly known as a "stretched" or "lax" vagina. Women seldom present this to doctors as a problem (often due to embarrassment, denial, or focusing on other factors such as lack of sleep or body image), yet questioning of such women and their partners often reveals dissatisfaction with their sexual lives, even though research results are conflicting.[19] Of course, it is not purely the size of the vaginal opening during intercourse that matters (just as the size of the penis is not the most important thing), but a *change* in size can have a negative impact on mutual enjoyment.

For the woman, more often the complaint lies not with her vagina size but with prolapse discomfort or incontinence during intercourse. Women with prolapse are more likely to have levator muscle defects and weaker vaginal closure pressure during contraction of the pelvic muscles, for example,[20] and many women avoid sexual relationships because of these issues. They may also fear further injuring the vagina, or they may feel embarrassed or experience decreased self-esteem and body image. Most men don't complain, partly because they are either so happy to be having *any* sex (even if it's not as great as before), or they are too afraid of insulting and hurting their loved one. And some men don't notice a difference.

But the effects for some relationships are devastating, and in Dr. Murphy's experience, it is the women who suffer most.

THE EVIDENCE THAT VAGINAL BIRTH CAUSES THE MOST DAMAGE

A great deal of confusion and disagreement surrounds whether there is evidence that a vaginal birth is any worse than a cesarean birth or, for that matter, remaining childless. Certainly, there are studies that find little specific association between vaginal birth and urinary incontinence, fecal/anal incontinence, or prolapse. That said, the overwhelming evidence, logic, and experience point definitively to vaginal birth as one of the most significant causes of these problems.

In a 2005 article published in the *Australian and New Zealand Journal of Obstetrics and Gynaecology*, H. P. Dietz and L. Schierlitz, two highly respected researchers in the field of urogynecology, wrote, "On reviewing the available evidence, it appears that there are sufficient grounds to assume that vaginal delivery (or even the attempt at vaginal delivery) can cause damage to the pudendal nerve, the caudal aspects of the levator ani muscle, fascial pelvic organ supports and the external and internal anal sphincter."[21] We also know that biomechanical and imaging studies of the properties of vaginal tissue and the surrounding structures, as well as what happens to these during childbirth, have demonstrated what tremendous loads are placed on them, and how this can lead to permanent and severe damage.[22]

Of course, acute injury doesn't necessarily lead to permanent or later consequences, but research has been unable to accurately predict which injuries are likely to cause future problems, or to whom. And unfortunately, it might be a long time before this is possible—at least not until individual risk predictions based on individual genetic codes are a reality. Even then, issues such as increasing baby birth weight and size and increasing maternal obesity and age will need to be factored in. What we *do* know currently is that the risk for levator and other pelvic floor injuries goes up significantly with increased maternal age,[23] and that this is true for both urinary and anal incontinence.

Urinary Incontinence

Women are anatomically at much higher risk than men for urinary incontinence. Overall, it is estimated that as many as 40 percent of middle-aged women and up to 70 percent of older women will experience symptomatic urinary incontinence,[24] although these figures vary widely from study to study. But this is not related only to childbirth. It is also related to women's short urethra, as well as its anatomical relationship to the vagina. As a result, a significant number of perfectly healthy young women suffer from the occasional urinary leak, just not usually to any serious degree. However, due to this normal incidence of urinary incontinence in young women, women who have not had children, and women who have only had cesarean births (and remember, often the statistics in these studies are not corrected for planned versus emergency cesareans), the effect of vaginal birth on urinary incontinence is often denied, downplayed, or otherwise minimized.

Looked at another way, however, there is very good evidence that a planned cesarean decreases the risk of urinary incontinence more than any other modifiable obstetric factor.[25] Also, it is clearly established in medical literature that assisted vaginal birth (e.g., forceps, vacuum, or both) increases the rates of pelvic floor damage and especially, as shown in a large Canadian study, the likelihood of urinary incontinence, anal incontinence, and prolapse.[26] In fact, its main finding was that cesarean delivery, performed at any stage of labor in the first pregnancy of someone who's never had incontinence, clearly reduces the rate of urinary incontinence. Furthermore, most experts agree that vaginal birth is an established risk factor for stress urinary incontinence with structural and functional damage to the pelvic structures.[27]

It's true that studies have found a high incidence of urinary incontinence during a woman's first pregnancy, with prevalence rates as high as 50 percent reported, and this could be as a result of hormonal changes in the body. But while most of these women recover urine control after the pregnancy, not all do. And unfortunately, a great many of those who *do* recover control have sustained sufficient pelvic floor damage to destine them for future further urinary incontinence anyway, either with or without genital prolapse and anal incontinence. The development of urinary incontinence during pregnancy is a significant predictor for postpartum urinary incontinence, both immediately as well as over the longer term;[28] if the incontinence persists for three to six months after delivery, the risk for persistent incontinence is significantly increased. Similarly, women who recover normal function over the short to medium term might still experience recurrence of incontinence symptoms over the long term.[29]

Another reason the interpretation of urinary incontinence studies is so difficult is the conflicting nature of many findings: for example, while a population-based study of all women in Oregon published in 2009 suggested it is the vaginal delivery itself and not the pushing or engagement of the fetal head that increases the risk of urinary incontinence,[30] an Australian study of two hundred first-time pregnant women in Sydney, who were examined during and after pregnancy, demonstrated it is the deep engagement and pushing that is of importance, and that a cesarean at this late point doesn't allay the risk.[31]

Fecal and Anal Incontinence

Severe anal and fecal incontinence are some of the worst outcomes of pelvic floor damage during childbirth. As mentioned above, the difference between the two is simply a difference in severity; fecal incontinence refers to the leaking of stool, whereas anal incontinence could also include the inability to control gas. In some Third World countries, fecal incontinence is often the result of unrepaired fistulas between the rectum and the vagina, but in developed countries, such severe injuries are mercifully rare. Here the cause is most commonly injuries to the anal sphincter muscle or its nerve, causing weakening of the tight closure mechanism we rely upon to keep gas and stool from coming out. These conditions are common after childbirth, especially with instrumental vaginal births, and it is well proven that anal sphincter injury is the main risk factor for future anal or fecal incontinence.[32] Obviously, planned cesarean completely prevents anal sphincter tears.

One major problem with sphincter injury patients is that if the sphincter is severely injured or is not diagnosed or properly repaired immediately, the later surgical results are dismal. Even in the best hands, the outcome for delayed sphincter repair is usually not very good. As a result, the most common treatment for anal incontinence (even in the presence of partial sphincter injury) involves dietary measures (like increasing fiber), medication to slow the bowels down (like Imodium®), and physiotherapy (to strengthen the levator ani muscles). Usually only if this fails, or if there is a clear defect but the muscle seems to be working, will colorectal surgeons or urogynecologists consider operating.

The risk factors for anal sphincter injury remain in dispute, but they include maternal obesity, vacuum delivery, forceps, macrosomia (large babies), long labor, and abnormal fetal position during delivery.[33] It also remains in dispute whether the risk for incontinence is increased for women *without* anal sphincter injury during delivery. But we do know that unfortunately, anal or fecal incontinence, just like urinary incontinence, can sometimes develop even in young women after a perfectly normal vaginal birth with no obvious risk factors. In these situations, such an unexpected and unpredictable complication is even more devastating for the healthy young woman who least expects it.

Studies estimate the incidence of anal and fecal incontinence after third- and fourth-degree tears to be 40 percent leaking of gas, 20 percent leaking of liquid stool, and 8 percent leaking of solid stool.[34] And a 2010 study published in the journal *Obstetrics and Gynecology* found the cumulative incidence rate during pregnancy and postpartum for anal incontinence to be 10.3 percent. The identified risk factors for postpartum incontinence included vaginal birth, and specifically, this increased the risk for long-term persistent incontinence.[35] The attributable risk—that is, the proportion of the incidence of incontinence among women who delivered vaginally that could have been prevented with a cesarean birth—was found to be 68 percent for urinary incontinence and 58 percent for anal incontinence.

Put another way, this study found that two-thirds of postpartum urinary incontinence and more than half of anal incontinence could be prevented by cesarean births.

Prolapse

Although vaginal birth is not the only cause of prolapse, it is a major contributor and possibly the most significant risk factor. In one study out of Johns Hopkins Hospital in Baltimore, a group of women were followed for up to one year after their first delivery and assessed regarding prolapse. In the vaginal delivery group, the incidence of moderate prolapse was approximately 15 percent, while in the cesarean without labor group, the risk was only 5 percent.[36] Other studies have found much higher relative risk of vaginal birth versus little or no risk attributable to cesarean births.[37] Also, the actual chance of finding severe prolapse in a young woman is significantly higher after a vaginal birth than after a cesarean without preceding labor, and increasing numbers of vaginal births increase the risk.[38]

Bone Fractures

Although much rarer than the other injuries mentioned above, actual bony pelvis injuries such as fractures of the coccyx, sacroiliac joint strain or pain, and symphysis disruption can occur. Symphysis disruption is when the strong connection between the pubic bones (where they come together just above the pubis) is affected by tearing of the ligaments holding them together. Vaginal birth can result in either an acute and sudden rupture of the ligament or a partial separation. The acute complete separation can lead to bladder rupture or severe bleeding, and even a partial separation can lead to severe morbidity, pain, and difficulty with walking. Unfortunately, there is no consensus about treatment. Options include surgery with internal or external fixation (plate and screws), tight corsets for months, or simply waiting it out with prolonged bed rest and immobility. Symphysis disruption is sometimes inflicted by the obstetrical caregiver by cutting the ligaments to cause a separation, but this drastic action is done only in life-or-death situations where the fetus is well and truly stuck and there is no alternative to save it. Possible situations where this might occur include shoulder dystocia and entrapment of the head during breech delivery. In cases like this, it might be impossible to do a cesarean (either at all or in time), and the only option is to get the fetus out vaginally as soon as possible. However, the resultant intervention may leave the mother permanently disabled.

In a way, shocking as this reads, symphysis disruption is just an extreme example of what happens every day in labor wards: various interventions are used to deliver babies who are not coming out easily, thereby inflicting pelvic damage for which there is a price to pay in a woman's later quality of life. Symphysiotomy is extremely uncommon in developed countries, but it is still utilized in some places, especially the developing world, where inadequate access to cesarean is often the unfortunate norm, and it is always mentioned in all standard textbooks as a possible management option for the aforementioned emergencies.

Nerve Damage

Many researchers have proven beyond reasonable doubt that pelvic nerve injuries are common during vaginal birth and also during emergency cesarean births that occur after the second stage of labor (when the cervix has fully opened and the fetal head is ready to come out). During this stage, the mother is usually actively pushing, the fetal head is deep in the pelvis, and the vagina, as well as the pelvic muscles and fascial layers, are maximally stretched. All the factors to cause compression and shearing forces on the pelvic nerves are in play.[39]

We also know that the risk of damage to these nerves is worse during assisted vaginal deliveries.[40] Forceps delivery has a higher risk than vacuum extraction (it is well known to increase the risk for levator injuries, as well as severe perineal tears, with a higher incidence of third- and fourth-degree tears), but the latter is also associated with an elevated risk of third- and fourth-degree tears.

The dilemma is that these operative procedures are, in some cases, essential to save the mother and/or baby's life or to make vaginal delivery possible at all. So in those cases where labor has already reached the second stage (often after prolonged pushing), and vaginal operative procedures are considered, it is to a large degree probably already too late to do a cesarean with the aim of making a meaningful difference to the protection of the pelvic floor (although in practice, this protection is often not considered anyway).

Conversely, researchers have found no nerve damage after planned cesarean births. With planned cesarean births in particular, the fetal head is usually still high in the pelvis, or even above the pelvis, and at any rate, the tremendous compression and stretching forces have not been applied.

IS A CESAREAN PROTECTIVE?

Scheduling a cesarean birth, although protective, does not give any woman a guaranteed lifelong exemption from pelvic floor problems. As we've mentioned, there is indeed evidence in medical studies that women with no children or only cesarean births might develop problems in later life, and that issues unrelated to delivery type such as obesity, aging, constipation, and lifestyle also play major roles.[41] However, protection against problems has been demonstrated in the short and medium term following cesarean birth, as cited in studies throughout this chapter, and these outcomes compare favorably with those of the hundreds of women Dr. Murphy has treated who are truly pelvic disabled. Many of their lives have been irrevocably altered by a singular event, and the physical and psychological stress that pelvic floor damage can cause is often very severe. Therefore, it is our belief that yes, a cesarean is protective against pelvic floor damage, and its comparative protection against the premature onset of problems is irrefutable.

HOW OFTEN IS A CESAREAN PROTECTIVE?

This is a more difficult question to answer, but a type of research helps us do just that by estimating something called the "number needed to treat" (NNT). This is a commonly used measure for assessing the effectiveness of a healthcare intervention—for example, medication or vaccination versus no intervention at all. The NNT is the number of patients who would need to be treated to prevent just one bad outcome, even though everyone else in the group would not have experienced harmful symptoms if left untreated. Any intervention with a high NNT is not generally considered effective (from a cost-benefit point of view, but especially if there are any side effects or complications for those patients who prove not to have needed it) unless the condition targeted is very serious. For example, the blanket vaccination of some very serious childhood diseases is deemed worthy of its high NNT. For less serious conditions, the ideal NNT is obviously one, meaning every treated individual gains benefit and no one is treated unnecessarily. But of course this is not always possible, as these examples of NNT show:

- Taking aspirin to prevent pulmonary embolism (blood clots in the lungs) after hip surgery; NNT is 195.
- Taking aspirin to prevent a heart attack; NNT is higher than 90.
- Using cholesterol-lowering drugs to prevent a heart attack; NNT is 50.
- Delivering breech babies via cesarean; NNT is 30 (lower in some countries).
- Using beta blockers to prevent hospitalization for heart failure; NNT is 24.[42]

You can see that according to this, 194 patients need to take aspirin unnecessarily to prevent one person having a pulmonary embolism, and twenty-nine planned cesareans need to be done to save the life of one breech baby. All these interventions are utilized daily and, for the most part, are unquestioned throughout the world.

In contrast to the above NNT figures, it is estimated that just *seven women* would have to be delivered by planned cesarean to prevent one woman from having a pelvic floor disorder; thus, the NNT is seven. This is a *very* low number compared to many other acceptable and widely used interventions, and it strongly supports this intervention, provided other risks are not unacceptably raised. This NNT analysis came out of a study of 4,458 women, of whom 7 percent had prolapsed; 15 percent, stress urinary incontinence; 13 percent, overactive bladder; 25 percent, anal incontinence; and 37 percent, "one or more pelvic floor disorders." It was found that cesarean birth had a protective effect on the development of all these pelvic floor disorders, similar to the woman never having had a baby at all.[43] That said, we are not advocating that all women have a cesarean so that one in seven of them will prevent a pelvic floor injury; we are simply highlighting the fact that the avoidance of pelvic floor disorders associated with vaginal birth is a perfectly reasonable justification for maternal request cesareans.

STUDY LIMITATIONS

Most medical studies have limitations, and this is nowhere more true than with studies related to the impact of birth on the pelvic floor. Most look at go anywhere in public, could not participate in any sport, could not attend any social events, and could hardly go out for anything (she had absolutely no control over her bowels). All as a direct result of what should have simply been one of the happiest moments of her life: the birth of her first child.

As a result of the prolapse, incontinence problems, and widely stretched vagina, sex had become not only unsatisfactory for both Jessica and Brad, but something that was impossible to even contemplate. The couple had difficulty relating to each other on an intimate basis. Not only had Brad witnessed his wife's vagina ripping and tearing right into her anus and rectum, he was constantly aware of her leaking feces and urine. He could smell it on her. On her clothes. On the sheets. For Jessica, in one instant, she had lost so much. Her femininity. Her dignity. Her husband's intimacy. She was embarrassed, afraid of people noticing her plight, and angry about the unfairness of it all. Every day when she looked at her growing child, she was reminded of the cause of her distress, and although she realized it was not the baby's fault, she couldn't help but feel resentment. She also continuously ruminated about what happened in the labor ward. Did she really need the forceps delivery? Would things have been different if she hadn't had one?

On examination, Dr. Murphy discovered Jessica had the classic damage of a vaginal birth gone wrong. The torn paravaginal defects, where the vaginal support from the pelvic sidewalls are torn off, leaving the upper vagina to hang down. The obviously avulsed (torn off) levator muscles, the uterine prolapse, the sphincter damage, and the herniated rectum. In stark contrast, before the birth, mother and baby were both deemed in excellent health, and Jessica and Brad did everything they were expected to do. They both went to delivery classes, doing breathing, meditation, and relaxation training to help prepare for what was expected to be a completely straightforward delivery.

It's true that perhaps the authors of this book have met with or been contacted by a disproportionate number of women like Jessica, but it's also true that stories like this demonstrate beyond all doubt that the unpredictability of a successful, spontaneous vaginal birth is real. No one knows who is most at risk, when it might occur, or how severe it might be, but pelvic floor damage, natural birth's largely unrecognized Achilles' heel, changes women's lives in a way that most could not ever imagine.

Because they are never told.

there is no point in registering because we cannot go at least one week out of four. I did try returning to my old active lifestyle, but even yoga causes me a lot of pain and makes my prolapse worse. I am now forced to lead a much more sedentary life—definitely no impact activities. Even extended walking sessions become painful.

Since the birth of my child, I have had ongoing battles with depression. I am no longer able to do the things I used to enjoy, and I am not able to take on new things due to the limitations placed on me by my prolapse. Living in constant pain is also wearing on me and affecting my emotional health. In the near future, I will be returning to the urogynecology clinic to start looking into surgery options, likely a hysterectomy. I am in my early thirties and may be losing my uterus. None of the surgeries can fix my issues. They can relieve some symptoms, but possibly they could make things worse. I have a great deal of fear about what my future holds.

One of my biggest struggles is that my life could have been completely normal, if only someone had spent more time with me, helping me work through my options. A C-section would have prevented what will be a lifetime of complications and suffering. This was completely preventable, and that more than anything depresses me so much. I hope my story helps other ladies be more informed as they build their families and hopefully will get more women talking about these important issues. Knowledge is so important, but if no one is willing to talk, how can we as women become knowledgeable about all the possibilities around childbirth?

ALEXANDRA, AUSTRALIA

I am a thirty-nine-year-old Australian woman who gave birth to a beautiful baby girl in December last year. Amelia is now six months old and is my first (and probably my last) baby. I have always been very fit and healthy, but a difficult labor changed everything. I had never heard of prolapse before giving birth, and I have now been diagnosed with a moderate cystocele [bladder hernia] and rectocele [rectal hernia], which is giving me a great deal of grief, as I can no longer do the activities I used to do. I was a runner and a triathlete, growing and eating organic food—in other words, I have a very healthy lifestyle that does not involve any vices such as smoking or alcohol or being overweight.

I have not been intimate with my partner since the birth because of the disgusting and uncomfortable feeling of the rectocele; I also feel less womanly because of it. My partner assures [me] that he still finds me sexually attractive, but I think he now fears initiating sex because he is worried that he will hurt me.

The first half of my labor was wonderful; I labored for many hours without pain relief in a deep bath at the hospital and was completely in the zone for giving birth. The obstetrician came in every two hours in the evening to check on me, and he said that I was fully dilated and that the baby was soon going to arrive. He said that he would check in on me during the following two hours when he was doing his rounds. Between his visits, the midwives kept an eye on me, and my partner was of course there to reassure me. Another two hours passed, and the baby hadn't progressed any further into the birth canal. When my obstetrician returned, he pulled me out of the bath and checked to see what was happening. He then found that the baby had been occipital posterior with an anterior presentation of the head [the baby was rotated so that it faced its mother's front]. I had been completely relaxed and focused until that moment. . . . He said he was going to apply the Kiwi cap and try to get the baby out that way. So then I was given an episiotomy before the pulling began. He pulled and pulled, and I was in absolute agony at that point because I hadn't been provided with any pain relief. I was lying on my back and felt enormous pressure on my tailbone, but still the baby was not progressing. He said that he could only use the cap for twenty minutes, otherwise there was potential for damage to occur to the baby's head. Throughout this ordeal, the baby's heart rate remained calm and steady, but mine was not, as I was petrified at this point! When the cap didn't work, things started happening very quickly. He called in a specialist from another hospital, and then he asked me to sign some disclaimer forms that cleared doctors of any potential litigation. I was wheeled down into the operating room and was given a spinal block. The specialist arrived, and, after crying that I didn't want a cesarean (I had heard so many bad things about cesareans but never heard about damage that can occur with forceps deliveries), he took one look and said that he was pretty confident that he could do a forceps delivery, so my baby girl was born this way. The specialist widened the episiotomy cut further before she was delivered, and then he stitched me back up.

I spent five days in hospital before going home. During the first three weeks, I was just concentrating on healing and bonding with my baby, and I had no idea of the things to come. I had severe trouble walking without pelvic pain during the first three weeks, and the physiotherapist gave me crutches to use until I felt better. I was also given a sacroiliac belt to try to stabilize the hip. These things did help a little, but then on the fourth week I was still bleeding quite profusely, even though the blood seemed a dark, older color. One morning, I felt a strange sensation in my nether regions and went to the toilet. When I went to use toilet paper, the paper suddenly caught onto something hanging out of my vagina. I panicked and rang the hospital, and they sent me to see my obstetrician, who had been present at the birth. I went to his surgery, and he discovered that the entire amniotic sac had been left behind. This was, of course, very distressing, as my uterus had been trying to expel this foreign object for some weeks now. This was also related to the profuse bleeding that I had, and once it was removed, the bleeding almost stopped after another week. Two days after the sac had been removed, I was also able to walk without crutches relatively comfortably. I was never told how or why this could have been related to my troubles, but all I know is that I felt immediately better!

Then about a week later, again I felt something hanging out of my vagina. I panicked and once again went to see my obstetrician. At this point I was feeling very emotionally fragile, and he said that I have prolapse of the uterus and the large intestine. My perineum also seems a lot shorter than it used to be. I didn't understand what all this meant or the implications this would have to my life, as they never talk about this sort of thing at antenatal classes or in books. It is just never talked about. Since that time, I have done a lot of research, [and I have considered having] an operation using [a] sling to suspend everything, but I feel that not enough long-term research has been done to say that this is the ultimate solution. The operation just seems so invasive and the outcome uncertain that I am not sure at this point whether it will be safe for me to have this operation. So for the time being, I am using a pessary, which seems to make things a little better. I still have to use a finger to "prop up" the bowel while I go to the toilet, and I guess it will be a decision for me to make in the future as to whether I can live with this or not. I do miss jogging and being able to jump, and importantly, I miss the intimacy I had with my partner. I guess most of it is a psychological barrier that I (we) need to get past. I don't want to apportion blame to any of the doctors or midwives involved; I just wish that I had been informed of the consequences of what I went through. Education is the key, I think. If I had known that any of this could happen, I would have chosen that cesarean after all. I am, however, aware that you can still get prolapses with a cesarean. Hindsight is a wonderful thing, isn't it?

ANONYMOUS, CANADA

The birth of my first and only child was, what many would say, a textbook delivery. Everything went exactly the way the books say it should. The second stage of labor went perfectly with no need for forceps, vacuum, or episiotomy, and I did not have any tearing. We were discharged twenty-four hours later, and my postpartum period went just as well as my delivery. I never had issues with incontinence, and within five months I was back to the gym, jumping rope and running just as I had been in my prepregnancy days. It wasn't until almost a year later that the problems began. I decided to try a Kegel strengthening device just to keep my pelvic floor strong between children. Soon after I began using it, I started having symptoms of what I now know was prolapse. These symptoms mainly included lower backache whenever standing or sitting for too long, difficulty with bowel movements, and painful intercourse. I was soon diagnosed with prolapse and was told by all of the doctors that the injury was most likely caused during the delivery of my child one year prior. It has been seven months since the initial diagnosis, and I cannot explain in words the profound effect it has had on me and my family. There is not an area of my life that has not been affected. A day does not go by that I do not think about it. I am constantly reminded of it whenever I stand or sit for any length of time or try to jog, exercise, lift my child, go to the bathroom, or have sex with my husband. I spend so much of my time trying to decide what to do in regards to surgery and trying to have another child. The problem is, there are no easy answers or quick fixes. If a cesarean section would have prevented this heartache, I most definitely would have pursued that route.

QUESTION POSTED ON BIRTH TRAUMA CANADA (reproduced here with permission):

[Re: Natural childbirth ten months ago]

Should the appearance of my inner vulva, urethra, vaginal opening be so different compared to before the birth? The urethra is about ½ inch higher up. The vaginal opening, which used to be a small (0–1 cm) opening which I could clench shut at will, now takes up the entire cleft, no matter how many Kegels I do. Basically, it looks like what used to be my inner vulva was completely ripped away by the baby. The inside of my vagina is now the outside: bulges of flesh covered with mucus membranes. What happened to the skin that used to be there? There is a lot more mess in my panties. Water gets in when I bathe (seems unhygienic). I have never seen this discussed in any website. Is this what is meant by the vague items like "you may lose some vaginal muscle tone"??!! More like had my privates replaced by completely different ones. I feel freaked out and alienated from my body now. I did have what the doc described as a 2nd degree tear, which she stitched and okayed at the check-up later.

Sample Answers:

- I felt similar; it's like a "road crash." So perfect before, . . . I know about the bath too; when I stand up I "leak" where water has got in . . . (SORRY TMI). I think it happens to us all, even the celebs that don't have arranged c sections. Just another thing us women have to put up with.
- Yeah, nobody ever tells you about this stuff. I had an episiotomy and then tore all the way through to my rectum. Took them just about as long to sew me up as it took to push out my son. My opening is very large too, sorry. My doctor will actually be repairing it after this one hopefully, and stitching it smaller. I almost need 2 tampons to keep them in, so not cool. I would bring it up with your doctor but some of the changes aren't going to be fixed; that's a lot of trauma for your body to go through. I keep reminding myself of how lucky I am to have my son and another one on the way, but it's still hard. . . .

- OK I have to say I'm SOOO glad I'm not alone in this. Up until I read this thread I thought I was just losing my mind. This is a bit TMI but I'm desperately trying to find answers to this. I have the "bulging" out of my vagina too. It actually sticks out and sometimes rubs on my panties. Hurts and makes the whole thing sore honestly. I've asked my GYN about it and he just blows it off as not knowing what I'm talking about. BUT for some reason when I'm standing up, it sticks out, if I lay down it goes back in? Anyone gone through this? Any tips on what to tell my GYN to get him to understand? It's horrible having sex too; makes it really painful most of the time. When I told him that all he did was give me estrogen cream [but] that doesn't help the big spot that is getting irritated. And no it's not from lack of being "wet" either, it just seems that the actual act makes it hurt. I have one kid who is 18 months so I know I've had plenty of time to recover from childbirth and do Kegels yet it doesn't help.

- I wish someone would have told me the hell my VAG would take, especially because you can schedule C-sections now! I don't care how much longer it would've taken to heal, I hate feeling like a freak in my own skin, and HATE what it has done to my once fulfilling sex life!

- Oh my God I have finally found a bunch of women describing what I thought was a freak show in my pants; I thought something was wrong with my vagina and I had asked the doctor and nurse who all said it looked normal. . . . NO IT DOES NOT. . . . My vagina makes noises when I walk like a sloppy piece of wet meat (sorry this is really gross). I look at it and cannot believe I can see my insides. It has affected my sex life and the way I feel about myself "down there." I'm so glad to find out it's not just in my head as my partner tells me . . . thank you. And I'll definitely look into surgery after number 2.

- I came across this having googled "vagina after childbirth." It has been 2 years since I gave birth for the first time, during which I had an episiotomy and about 10 stitches, and despite no one really explaining it to me, I think it was bad down there as I had a catheter in for 4 days after. I also got shocking hemorrhoids during the birthing process. I've been too frightened to look "down there" for a long time, primarily since an appointment with a GP about 4 weeks after the birth (who held up a hand mirror to show me) pointed out that part of my bowels are coming through my vagina!

She was completely un-fussed and said this was completely common in women who have given birth! I had another look last night due to some slight pain I continue to suffer down there and was quite horrified by what I saw. I too have the bulging out vagina and what looks like lots of excess bits and pieces, together with the remnants of the hemorrhoids. I am only 30, and I was blessed in that I got my slim figure back and do not have any stretch marks—but I feel like I am secretly disfigured. Sex does hurt when pressure is put on the area where the episiotomy was made and makes me not want it. I haven't done any pelvic exercises because the physio told me I was doing them the wrong way and would actually damage my pelvic floor muscles more! So I am at a loss at what to do about any of this. It's comforting to know I am not the only one feeling like a freak!

- So relieved to find this forum. I have been so self-conscious since having my daughter 3 years ago. Nothing looks the same. I can see the inside, which is pretty much outside, definitely looser, and I have the same problem with water getting in, and unfortunately, during sex, a lot more air than before. I had a horrible birth experience, she was stuck for 2 hours, and then this. . . . I know it's horrible, but I honestly wish I had chosen to have a C-section. I've been with my boyfriend now for almost 9 months, and just found out that he noticed a lot more than he said he did. He told me that he had worried that I "had something" that would cause it, and that it was contagious, because he didn't understand how it could look like that after. I am the first woman he's been with to have a child, so in his defense, he would have no way of knowing what to expect . . . but it's still heartbreaking to hear. I wish I had known that I would be THIS different after birth, because I am almost positive that I would've chosen a C-section. I really feel like a monster sometimes. I can't look at myself "down there" without being nauseated, and it is hard to see that while remembering how much nicer I looked before, and nicer I felt. Sex feels different, and while still amazing, I miss that tightness. I love my daughter dearly, and ultimately, she was worth it . . . but I do know that if I ever have another child, I will totally have a C-section.
- I'm getting angry now! I am absolutely devastated this has happened to me also. I'm 21 and have a prolapse after my first baby.

This has ruined my sex life and my confidence. I'm disgusted by what I see in the mirror. Why are we not warned of this? They teach us sex education in schools and how to get pregnant, but they don't teach us the life changing effects we have to live with years after giving birth! This thread should be shown to everyone so that they can make an informed decision about childbirth. I bet it would prevent a lot of teenage pregnancies! Can anyone tell me why nurses and friends/family with experience of childbirth are reluctant to tell us the truth? And if anybody says childbirth is not that bad I know now that they're lying. I have a very small frame and found it VERY painful. I sympathize with everyone who is going through this hell.

CORRESPONDENCE RECEIVED FROM WOMEN

These are a few examples of the correspondence we have received from women via our websites. While we know that this book will anger many, we are comforted by the knowledge that many women appreciate the information, support, and hope we provide, and we are inspired by their courage to speak the truth.

Natalia

I have been married for almost ten years, and fear of vaginal birth had made me reject the idea of having a baby. If I had not had the opportunity to have an elective cesarean birth, I would have missed out on life's most amazing experience: being a mom.

Anonymous

I only wish I'd found you sooner. I suffer from extreme tokophobia [fear of childbirth], and I have had counseling, CBT [cognitive behavioral therapy], and hypnosis, all to not much avail. My partner and I desperately want to start a family, and two years ago to our joy we fell pregnant. My GP had led me to believe that a cesarean would be more than expected for a case such as ours. Unfortunately, the area I moved to refused point blank. At my early scan, I was told in no uncertain terms that I would not be allowed a cesarean and to pull myself together. I sought a second opinion and was told the same thing. After much despair and more counseling, I terminated the much-wanted pregnancy. With no funds for private care, I had resigned myself to never having children, a very distressing thought. You have given me a glimmer of hope and the realization that there are people supportive of elective cesareans.

Nicola

You were so helpful in encouraging my decision to pursue the birth of my choice. I have noticed how many of my friends and colleagues who tried to discourage me from having a cesarean are now saying that I made the right choice, as some are experiencing the common physical problems that develop after a natural birth, and I have absolutely none. One particularly militant friend has admitted being envious of my physical state as she battles with postnatal incontinence.

Natalia

I am thirty-five weeks pregnant, and, although my husband and my doctor support me 100 percent on my decision to have a non-medically necessary elective cesarean, everyone else's negativity toward cesareans keeps making me feel guilty.

Brynne (who had a medication-free vaginal delivery and is a home birth advocate)

I have been under the impression for a very long time that these women who actively sought a cesarean birth were merely figments, much like the bogeyman. What a different perspective, how strange and interesting to see the other side of the coin, and after all, damn it, don't we all want the same thing—to be able to have our birth experience? I am glad these women have you.

Ana

I am Brazilian, but I've been living in Australia for the last seven and a half years (I am also an Australian citizen). I am pregnant with my first baby (thirty-five weeks) and did not realize how controversial this topic was here until I chose to have an elective cesarean. In Brazil, cesareans are very common, and women are not seen as any different for asking to have one. When I made up my mind that this was the way I wanted to have my baby, I was surprised to realize that I am only able to do this because I am going private. It was also surprising to realize how other women can be so judgmental of my choice when all I am asking for is to have the right to choose what I believe is best for me and my baby . . . why should I worry I'll be treated differently when all I am doing is having my baby in a hospital surrounded by a medical team who in my view will be able to provide a safer outcome for my baby? [Your work] makes me feel validated and hopeful that in a near future, women who choose to have cesareans will not have to justify themselves or be afraid to be labeled vain or selfish among other things. Thanks once again. Keep up the great work.

Anonymous

There is so much pressure on women to give in and have a "natural birth" as if it is some badge of honor to go through it with minimum pain relief, and it is only usually women who judge others so horrifically. I want to be armed with the right information and believe that this is a legitimate choice. After reading more vaginal horror stories than C-section ones, the natural perfect birth is quite a myth. Finding positive things about C-sections is difficult, and I wanted to cry when I found [your work].

Chapter 8

Worldwide Cesarean Rates, Attitudes, and Experiences

A lie can travel halfway round the world while the truth is putting on its shoes.
                    —Attributed to Mark Twain (1835–1910)

Birth Category	Birth Type
The good	Vaginal delivery
The bad	Cesarean delivery
The *really* bad	Emergency cesarean
The better (but still bad)	Planned cesarean for a medical or obstetrical indication
And the ugly	Planned cesarean with no indication

Broadly speaking, this is the way choice in childbirth is often portrayed around the world, both in the news media and in the majority of prenatal literature for pregnant women. Indeed, in some countries, unless a woman manages to give birth vaginally—and ideally with no pain relief whatsoever—she can often feel inadequate or that she is a failure as a mother before she's even begun the process of mothering.

Even the most apparently confident and self-assured women can fall prey to the peer pressure that revolves around how their baby enters the world. The Oscar-winning actress Kate Winslet, for example, famously tried to hide the truth about the birth of her first child. As she explained in an interview with *Gotham* magazine, quoted in the *Guardian* newspaper: "I've gone to great pains to cover it up. But Mia was an emergency caesarean. I just said I had a natural birth because I was so completely traumatized by the fact that I hadn't given birth. I felt like a complete failure."[1]

121

The social, cultural, and sometimes moral pressure to give babies the best start in life and get motherhood off on the right track by giving birth naturally (read: "properly") can be overwhelming and even traumatic when it doesn't happen like that. This is not helped by subsequent exposure to disdainful or consolatory looks and comments from peers who have "achieved success" with their births. Even women who choose to have a cesarean (as opposed to wanting a vaginal birth and "failing") can be affected by this attitude. For example, Pauline has witnessed and heard about some new mothers' reluctance to let others join in their baby conversations unless they have a birth horror story to share (anything will do, as long as the experience involved a drama of some kind: being in pain or feeling degraded, embarrassed, shocked, or scared), and she knows of numerous women who have lied about their maternal request cesarean, saying it was for medical reasons or their doctor advised it— just in case they are socially rejected by other mothers. It's almost as if there is an attitude by some women that if they had to go through such a frightful experience, then so should you, and that sharing the worst bits creates a closer bond. More sympathetically, perhaps it's the maternal equivalent of "Show me yours and I'll show you mine," where the problem is that because one of you has nothing to show, the other is left feeling exposed and vulnerable.

But beyond the story comparisons and the often competitive birth spirit between mothers ("Just two pushes and he was out; no pain relief, nothing!"), there is an international birth league at play in which whole countries are held up as virtuous or scandalous examples of birthing styles. Take, for example, the "Netherlands Nirvana," where as many as 30 percent of women give birth at home and hardly anyone has an epidural, let alone a cesarean. Compare this with "China in Crisis," where cesarean rates are rocketing to levels of 46 percent, a quarter of which are for maternal request. Or even worse, "Body-Conscious Brazil," with rates of cesarean birth that can reach more than 90 percent in some private hospitals. And closer to home, with cesareans at a record one-third of all births, growing concerns about the "United States' Soaring Rates" are echoed throughout most of the developed world.

This is because, year after year, as each country's summary of birth methods is entered into a virtual table of results, the media are free to write their annual reports and national comparisons. However, the problem is that the results are almost always measured using the ingrained but fundamentally flawed grading system shown here:

Result	Cesarean Rate by Country	Comments
Summa cum laude	Between 5 and 15 percent	High praise indeed!
Pass	Slightly higher than 15 percent	Good, but could do better.
Fail	Less than 5 percent / Higher than 25 percent	Why? How? Who or what is at fault?

But where does this grading system come from?

Back in 1985, a World Health Organization document titled "Appropriate Technology for Birth" was published in the *Lancet*, stating, "Countries with some of the lowest perinatal mortality rates (PMR) in the world have caesarean section rates of less than 10 percent. There is no justification for any region to have a rate higher than 10–15 percent."[2]

Subsequent handbooks referred to "a minimum (5 percent) and a maximum (15 percent) acceptable level" of cesarean births, and as a result, the World Health Organization's minimum and maximum cesarean recommendations became enshrined in maternity principles and continue to be quoted by natural-birth advocates as the ideal cesarean rate that developed countries should aspire to and not exceed. And by highlighting unfavorable cesarean outcomes (following emergency surgeries or surgeries that have occurred through medical or obstetrical necessity, including premature births), they are able to present an argument for reducing national cesarean rates—but worse, for refusing cesarean births on maternal request where there is no indication.

What we will demonstrate here, however, are the basic flaws in such tunnel-vision strategies to reduce cesarean rates with little or no regard for the much wider picture of maternity health. To begin, here is a prime example of how countries can be simultaneously criticized for their high cesarean rates and praised for their improved birth outcomes.

One of the United Nations Millennium Development Goals has as its target a 75 percent reduction in maternal deaths from 1990 to 2015, and so in 2010, researchers at the University of Washington decided to evaluate

what progress had been made so far. Overall, the news was good. They estimated that in 2008, 342,900 mothers died in childbirth, giving a rate of 251
deaths per 100,000 live births, compared with a rate of 320 per 100,000 in
1990 and 422 per 100,000 in 1980. Unfortunately, they found that not all
countries are on track to achieve the 75 percent reduction by 2015, but of
the twenty-three countries that are successfully reducing the deaths of
mothers, four in particular were mentioned by name as having achieved
"accelerated progress." They were Egypt, China, Ecuador, and Bolivia."[3]

And what do these four countries all have in common? Rapidly
increasing cesarean rates—three of which far exceed the World Health
Organization's 15 percent threshold.

Bolivia's rate has increased from around 4.9 percent nationally to 15.8
percent in hospitals, a huge increase, but having come from such a dangerously low base rate initially, it has not yet crept *too high*.[4] Meanwhile, in
Egypt, the cesarean rate is 27.6 percent (41.7 percent in private hospitals),[5] in China, it's 46 percent, and in Ecuador, it's 40.3 percent in places.[6]
Therefore, ironically, despite their maternal mortality successes, these
countries have been reproached rather than acclaimed for their position in
the cesarean league table.

And the same is true for neonatal mortality (i.e., babies who die before
they are twenty-eight days old). In a recent report, the World Health
Organization stated that to meet the Millennium Development Goal of
"two-thirds reduction in child mortality," some regions need to do more to
reduce newborn deaths. However, the same report described improvements between 1990 and 2009 in some regions, with an overall fall of more
than 25 percent—from 4.6 million neonatal deaths to 3.3 million.[7] No link
is made with rising cesarean rates worldwide, but it is our opinion that
there is likely a significant causal effect.

RATES VERSUS OUTCOMES

The danger, as we see it, is that any country or region that decides to
employ a blanket strategy of reducing cesarean rates might target the statistically safest cesareans first (for example, refusing maternal request or
canceling a planned surgery with an obstetrical indication and deciding to
have a trial of labor first instead), and do little or nothing to reduce the

number of the more dangerous (usually emergency) ones. In fact, the numbers of these may even be increased with such a strategy.

In our view, the emphasis should be on attaining the highest possible percentage of positive birth outcomes, not risking lives or wasting valuable resources trying to arrive at an apparently one-size-fits-all figure. Others agree. There has been very strong criticism of the World Health Organization's 1985 recommendation over the years from medical professionals and institutions alike.[8] For example, in 2006 the United States' National Institutes of Health concluded, "There is no consistency in this ideal rate, and artificial declarations of an ideal rate should be discouraged. . . . Optimal cesarean delivery rates will vary over time and across different populations according to individual and societal circumstances."[9] And in 2008, a newly formed group, the Coalition for Childbirth Autonomy (cofounded by Pauline and renamed Birth Coalition in 2011), publicly called on the World Health Organization to urgently reexamine what it called an "outdated and unsafe" 15 percent threshold. It warned that ongoing attempts to reduce national cesarean rates to these levels were leading to deaths, disability, and trauma for mothers and babies. And it argued that in a developed world where pregnant women are heavier, older, and having fewer and larger babies than at any point in history, an 85 percent safe vaginal delivery success rate is simply unachievable.[10]

NEW GUIDELINES

Then, in 2009, a very interesting thing happened.

Albeit ever so quietly, and without any known announcements to the media (or even to medical journals and periodicals, as far as we know), the World Health Organization finally updated its quarter-century-old cesarean recommendation. In a newly published handbook, it now advises, "Both very low and very high rates of caesarean section can be dangerous, but the optimal rate is unknown. Pending further research, users of this handbook might want to continue to use a range of 5–15 percent or set their own standards."[11]

This very important revision continues:

Earlier editions of this handbook set a minimum (5 percent) and a maximum (15 percent) acceptable level for caesarean section. Although WHO has recommended since 1985 that the rate not exceed 10–15 percent, there is no empirical evidence for an optimum percentage or range of percentages, despite a growing body of research that shows a negative effect of high rates. It should be noted that the proposed upper limit of 15 percent is not a target to be achieved but rather a threshold not to be exceeded. Nevertheless, the rates in most developed countries and in many urban areas of lesser-developed countries are above that threshold. Ultimately, what matters most is that all women who need caesarean sections actually receive them.

In fact, so quiet was the new guidance that it was only through reading an article in the *Irish Times* on October 10, 2009 ("Caesarean Section: A Life-Saving Option"[12]), the first (and only, as far as we are aware) news report on the WHO's lack of empirical evidence for an optional cesarean rate, that Pauline first found out about it. The *Lancet* was duly contacted, and Pauline asked whether it would be updating this information in its next publication, particularly since it was inside the pages of this leading medical journal that the 1985 recommendation had originally appeared. Unfortunately, the answer was no, and an editor there later explained that "at the time of your proposal, as important as it was, it was not considered a priority for publication when compared with other material being considered."

Undeterred, the Coalition for Childbirth Autonomy promptly prepared another press release, "WHO Admits: There Is No Evidence for Recommending a 10–15 percent Caesarean Limit."[13] Disappointingly, this received relatively little media attention (though *Medical News Today* published it online), and it was not until July the following year that the news finally received the media attention it deserved: a front-page mention and three-page spread in the *Times* of London, followed by reports on the BBC News website and others.

CHANGE IS SLOW

Yet even as this book goes to press, you will read media reports that continue to quote the original 15 percent figure as a gold standard—and often without being contradicted when they do so. Evidently, establishing new knowledge and ultimately effecting change can be painfully slow, particularly in areas of healthcare with a long-established authority that is also steeped in social and psychological influence.

As a prime example, even after more than fifteen years of Back to Sleep campaigning (which advises parents that the safest position for a baby to sleep to reduce the risk of sudden infant death syndrome is on its back), so entrenched was the previous advice to place a baby on its tummy to reduce the risk of inhaling vomit that despite the campaign's eventual success, there are still people who believe the latter to be true.

That said, we are not in any way suggesting a campaign for all babies to be delivered by cesarean in the same vein as the advice to lay all babies on their backs. The Back to Sleep example merely illustrates just how slow change can be and how much incontrovertible evidence must be accrued first; studies from the 1940s to the 1980s indicated risk for babies sleeping in the prone position, but it took more than fifty years for this to be widely accepted. What we *are* saying is that women around the world should be allowed to choose their baby's birth route, without prejudice, once the full range of risks and benefits has been fully and individually explained to them.

A WORLD VIEW

Evidently, that is easier said than done. Personal and professional birth experiences can often influence how a doctor or midwife describes the risks and benefits of different birth types, and this in turn can influence women's decision making. We explore the challenge involved in providing women with objective information on the undeniably subjective issue of birth planning in chapter 5, "Doctors Who Support Cesarean Choice," and chapter 17, "Informed Choice: Necessary, Complex, and Challenging," but for now, we're going to discuss what's happening in different regions of the world in relation to birth plans and outcomes, and in doing so, we will explore some of the less publicized information about maternity care and cesarean delivery practice in a variety of countries.

In the process, and in an attempt to move beyond typical news headlines, we hope to provide readers with a broader understanding of the international picture.

We don't purport to offer a comprehensive, standardized review of all types of births in all countries in this chapter. Rather, the aim is to highlight the danger of reducing commentary on international cesarean births to a basic measurement of percentages ranging from low (read: good maternity care) to high (read: bad maternity care). We want to make the reader aware of other facts, figures, and studies, and place them in a social context. We want to rotate the kaleidoscope of cesarean data around a few times to give you a different perspective of cesarean birth on maternal request around the world.

CHINA

There is an old Chinese proverb that goes like this: "To know the way ahead, ask those coming back."

Social and cultural factors are hugely influential in a woman's decision-making process about many things, but the phenomenon of a baby's birth brings to the fore some of the most powerful and instinctive social and cultural forces. This is certainly true in China, where a woman's extended family—with its opinions, stories, and views—plays an important role in her preparation for childbirth. And it has become increasingly apparent that in this country, at least, the mothers coming back from maternity wards seem to be telling other pregnant women that in their opinion, "the way ahead" is planned cesarean birth.

Unique One-Child Policy

Early in 2010, it came to light that at 46 percent, China has one of the highest national cesarean rates in the world, one-quarter of which are carried out on maternal request with no medical indication (that's 11.7 percent of all births). Since then, criticism has rained down on the country's women and doctors for their unhealthy and dangerous attitude toward birth. But the level of outrage is incredible, really, especially once you realize that compared with those of any other nation, Chinese women quite possibly have the most to benefit and the least to risk from a planned cesarean birth.

Why? To begin with, we know one of the greatest risks of a cesarean is the potential consequences for future pregnancies and surgeries. More operations mean more risks. This is why the American College of Obstetricians and Gynecologists and the National Institutes of Health warn that maternal request cesareans are only advisable for women planning small families. With China's controversial one-child policy, for the vast majority of women, this particular risk is reduced. Since there will most likely be only one or two births (some women are permitted a second child), they are therefore within the guidelines of advisable family size with surgery.

Next, we know that small stature may put a woman at higher risk for an emergency cesarean, so it is perfectly reasonable that some Chinese women might decide planned surgery is preferable to the potential outcomes of a trial of labor.[14]

Then there is research that suggests Chinese women have a higher incidence of severe perineal laceration compared to other ethnic groups. This has been attributed in part to a disproportionate relationship between mothers and their newborn babies; small versus increasingly large.[15] Similarly, there is a suggestion that the impact of being overweight might be worse for Chinese women than it is for Caucasian women,[16] and we know that being overweight can increase the risk of adverse outcomes in pregnancy and labor.

Cultural Norms

There is less cultural pressure on Chinese women to give birth vaginally, and therefore they might be less likely to experience feelings of inadequacy or failure that are commonplace in many other countries. This is a big plus in terms of postnatal psychological health; as we discuss in chapter 4, studies have shown greater levels of satisfaction in women who plan a cesarean birth compared with those who plan a vaginal birth. But also, it might make a difference to how women feel socially after the birth. For example, while researchers in Taiwan found no significant differences in perceived stress, self-esteem, or depression among 275 women who'd had either a vaginal or cesarean birth, they did discover a difference in one area—the women who'd had a cesarean birth reported a significantly higher level of perceived social support than those who'd given birth vaginally. The researchers suggest that this could be related, in part, to the "normalizing effect" of China's very high cesarean rate.[17]

Furthermore, another study with a similar number of Chinese women (259) whose first birth experience was an actual or attempted vaginal delivery, at six months after the birth, almost one-quarter of the women (23.8 percent) said they'd prefer an elective cesarean if they had another baby, and the most important reason they gave for this change in preference was fear of vaginal birth.[18] Not fear of the unknown, but fear of an actual experienced event. Since other women's birth stories can be very influential on Chinese decision making, and with the advent of the Internet, these stories are no longer confined to family and friends' word of mouth. The online community is unquestionably large and influential.

Achilles' Heel

Yet despite all of the above, there are two crucial spokes in China's cesarean wheel: the country's obsession with lucky numbers and its hospital remuneration policy for different types of birth.

Every year, we read reports about pregnant women choosing a lucky or auspicious date for the birth of their child (for example, August 8, 2008, or just in time for the new school year entry cutoff date). What's wrong with that? If the birth date chosen occurs after the recommended thirty-nine gestational weeks of pregnancy, then there is indeed no problem. But if the luckiest date happens to fall at the start of the thirty-eighth gestational week, for example, and the surgery is therefore premature, this is an indefensible risk to the baby's health. Should evidence come to light that superstition is overriding safety when it comes to cesarean scheduling, this would seriously undermine the validity of choosing a cesarean in these cases.

Secondly, there have long been concerns about the impact of China's emerging health insurance system and fee-for-service payments to doctors and whether these practices might be a factor in rising cesarean rates.[19] In a report for the *Guardian* in 2007, Jonathan Watts reported that according to Li Ling, an economics professor at Beijing University's China Centre for Economic Research, cesareans command a higher fee for hospitals than vaginal births because they're classed as surgery.[20] This raises questions about the incentive for doctors to encourage surgeries and is one of the reasons why research into this area continues. Of equal concern in China is the disparity in access to quality healthcare. Watts reports that the government's share of what used to be a virtually free healthcare system has fallen following health reforms from 54 percent in 1975 to 17 percent, and that according to James Murray, country director for Plan China (a nongovernmental organization), just 20 percent of China's medical expenditure reaches rural areas, where 70 percent of the population lives.

Therefore, to ensure best health outcomes for mothers and babies, financial incentives should be investigated, but moreover, we think the World Health Organization's interest in China's cesarean rates would be better focused on the lowest percentage rates evident in the most deprived rural areas of the country, than on the more wealthy regions where cesarean rates are highest and deaths are fewer.

Fewer Deaths and Injuries

Throughout China, the number of women dying during childbirth has been decreasing significantly in the last two decades, and there are even fewer deaths in urban areas compared with rural areas.[21] Similarly, the number of babies dying has decreased. Improvements in access to health-care (in some areas) and increased safety of surgery in general have played a role in these reductions, but many Chinese women and doctors view the corresponding increase in cesarean births as having also contributed.

This view is also encouraged by Chinese research, which demonstrates positive cesarean outcomes. For example, the analysis of 3,751 births in a Beijing hospital between 2002 and 2007 found that selective cesarean delivery (43.6 percent of the births) was safer than both induction and spontaneous onset of labor. The groups were all relatively low risk (described as uncomplicated first births at term), and although the cesarean births cost the most and meant a longer hospital stay, there were fewer cases of asphyxia (0.1 percent versus 1.2 percent and 1 percent, respectively) and birth trauma in babies. As for the mothers, hemorrhage, urinary retention, blood transfusion, trauma, and delayed healing all occurred least with a cesarean delivery.[22] And even in a remote and indigent population in China, research has shown that compared with vaginal delivery, a dramatic reduction in babies' deaths has been reported with elective and emergency cesarean deliveries.[23]

Two more studies described an unexpected but continued reduction in the number of babies suffering birth trauma and birth asphyxia during instrumental vaginal deliveries in the last decade and determined that the improvement was due to a change in obstetric practice—namely, "a marked increase" in the emergency cesarean rate.[24]

Precious Child

In China, it has been suggested that a woman's eagerness to have a cesarean birth may reflect her perception of surgery as a means to ensure her baby's safe arrival and to avert the risks of birth complications or stillbirth. Since there will possibly be only one child, and there is the sense of that child being particularly precious, a perceived benefit of planning a cesarean is to reduce some of the unpredictability associated with a trial of labor. Interestingly, the term "precious baby" is often used in the context of couples who have conceived through in vitro fertilization (IVF) in the United States. There can be a greater tolerance of cesarean request in these situations because this baby might be the couple's only chance of ever having a family—although we would echo the sentiment of two New York doctors who point out that we should not assume women who conceive naturally might not be equally willing to choose a cesarean to avoid even remote risks too.[25]

Other, very recent research conducted in China is important in the context of a precious child but relates to the longer-term health of the child rather than to the birth itself. When researchers assessed the emotional and behavioral problems of 4,190 preschool children across 18 counties and 3 cities in China, they reported that the likelihood of childhood psychopathological problems was lowest in children born by cesarean delivery on maternal request, followed by those born by spontaneous vaginal delivery.[26] The highest probability of problems was observed in those born by assisted vaginal delivery. And while further studies are needed to test these findings, this news will undoubtedly be of interest to potential parents.

Who and Why

The profile of a typical woman scheduling a cesarean birth in China suggests that she tends to be educated, professional, wealthy, living in an urban area with access to prenatal care (probably in the west of the country), and slightly older.[27]

Her reasons for choosing a cesarean are likely to include fear of labor pain, lack of delivery confidence, avoiding risks for herself and her baby, making an independent choice, a previous cesarean, advice from her doctor, IVF, and Chinese beliefs regarding date and time of birth and protection of the baby's brain.[28] That said, maternal request is not a universal birth choice in China; there are also many women who feel a cesarean will damage their *yuan qi* (vigor) and cause them to lose energy.[29]

Efforts to Reduce Cesarean Rates

In order to stem the rise of cesareans in China, suggestions have been made for promoting midwifery-led maternity-care models that emphasize birth as a normal process, as currently, most women do not have access to standardized midwifery care.[30] The number of professional midwives employed in the country has been declining since 1996, and midwifery as a profession has been marginalized. Some argue that legislation is needed if the situation is to be reversed,[31] and there have also been calls on medical professionals, public health authorities, members of the public, and the media to help find a solution.[32]

But as we have said elsewhere, while we have few reservations about attempts to reduce rates of *unwanted* unnecessary cesareans, we are concerned that aggressive efforts to lower *overall* cesarean rates[33] may ignore the risk of a potential increase in deaths or serious injuries. We also question the ethics of any strategy that might involve an a priori refusal of maternal request (i.e., wanted cesareans) in a country whose own data demonstrate positive outcomes for both mothers and babies in these births.[34]

For now, though, and in the immediate future, while a significant minority of Chinese women seem to hold the view that the delivery of a healthy baby is not best served by vaginal birth, it is unlikely that this country will witness a sizable fall in its cesarean rate anytime soon.

THE NETHERLANDS

In the fifteenth century, the Dutch humanist Desiderius Erasmus Roterodamus wrote, "The grass is greener over the fence," and we would suggest that this popular proverb is perfect in the context of everything you've probably ever heard about giving birth in the Netherlands. This country is often hailed by natural-birth advocates as the pinnacle of exemplary maternity practice, with cesarean rates that other countries can only aspire to, so some of the facts below may come as a surprise.

But first, a little background information. In contrast with the very small minority of practicing midwives in the United States (in some states, midwifery is actually illegal), midwives have a far more elevated position of authority and influence in the Netherlands, and there is a tradition of midwives being respected and revered. Their training process is more extensive than in many other countries, and they are involved in the vast majority of births. Importantly, they view childbirth as a natural process rather than a medical condition, thereby avoiding unnecessary medical intervention. As an example, it was only in 2006 that fetal scans at around the twentieth week of pregnancy were introduced for all women, as well as extensive blood tests during pregnancy,[35] even though a scan at around this time has been standard in other countries for considerably longer.

Dutch maternity care is separated into two groups: midwives and general practitioners in primary care, and midwives and gynecologists in secondary care. Almost one-third of women (31.3 percent) give birth at home, and the majority of pregnant women (58.5 percent) switch from primary to secondary care, or vice versa, at least once during pregnancy, during labor and birth, or both.[36] This management of pregnant women is designed to identify low- and high-risk births, the status of which can obviously change at any point during the pregnancy and labor. The idea is to make sure babies are delivered in the most appropriate setting; that is, to deliver the largest number of babies as naturally as possible and to seek medical intervention only when absolutely necessary. And for many decades, in the eyes of the world and indeed the Netherlands itself, this appeared to be working most effectively.

That is, until the results of a first-of-its-kind Europe-wide comparative report on the perinatal health of mothers and babies (spanning from twenty-two weeks of pregnancy until seven days after the birth) were published in December 2008 and sent shockwaves throughout the Netherlands' maternity world.[37]

More Babies Die

The report ranked the Netherlands, with 9.8 infant deaths in every one thousand live births, as having one of the highest perinatal mortality rates in Europe, and consistently so.[38] And this is even given the fact that unlike most of the other countries, the Netherlands has limits on what is classified as a "live birth." A baby must be of twenty-two weeks' gestation or more, and if the gestational age is unknown, its birth weight must be five hundred grams. Evidently, if *all* live births were included for analysis, the country's perinatal mortality rate would have been even worse. This shocking news led to urgent calls for further investigation and the introduction of accurate perinatal audits across all maternity services.[39]

And yet fourteen years earlier, in a 1989 letter to the *British Medical Journal* heavily criticizing the Dutch model of maternity care, concerns were already being raised that the Netherlands had no system for the routine audit of obstetric care, and indeed that the country had an unacceptably high perinatal mortality rate.[40] A subsequent study in 1993 concluded that in a group of twenty-nine "preventable" infant deaths, the skills of obstetricians, pediatricians, and midwives were all responsible for blame, and as such, continued education for all workers in perinatal care was recommended.[41]

Reason Mothers Die "Unknown"

The December 2008 European Perinatal Health Report also highlighted another important aspect of the Netherlands' maternity care. In the event of mothers' deaths at or around the time of childbirth, many countries selected the category "Unknown" as a reason for death, but the report mentions just three countries by name as having utilized this category most heavily: the Netherlands (18.8 percent), Belgium (40 percent), and Germany (46.5 percent). It's concerning that the Netherlands has no explanation for why one-fifth of mothers' deaths occur.

"No Blame" Litigation

One reported influence on the provision and development of maternity care in the Netherlands is the comparative lack of litigation in obstetrics, and it is likely that this situation has helped to keep the cesarean rate there relatively low. Dutch doctors have simply not been working under the same litigation pressures as doctors in other countries, and while there continue to be calls for the United States' health litigation system to move toward a system with less blame, with civil litigation claims in the Netherlands increasing in recent years, it's perhaps more likely that the Dutch system could be inching closer to a culture of blame instead.

Move toward Medicalized Birth

To date, research in the Netherlands has not specifically blamed home births for its high rate of newborn baby deaths, but there are suggestions that the attitude of Dutch medical professionals, which may be based on too much confidence in a nonintervention policy, could possibly be partially at fault.[42] Notably, it has been documented that one-third of all planned home births end up being transferred to a hospital, and unsurprisingly, these women experience lower levels of satisfaction than women who planned a hospital birth in the first place.[43] Also, in a recent study of almost forty thousand births, not only was the perinatal death rate "significantly higher" for first-time mothers, but mothers deemed "low risk" during their pregnancies, and whose labor started under the supervision of a midwife, had a significantly "higher risk of delivery-related perinatal death" than mothers whose pregnancies were considered "high risk" and whose labor started under the supervision of an obstetrician — leading the researchers to conclude that "the obstetric care system of the Netherlands needs further evaluation."[44] And in light of all this, there is increasing evidence that at least some changes in Dutch attitudes are taking place.

For example, following the publication of the Canadian "Term Breech Trial" in 2000 (a study that reported safer outcomes for breech babies delivered via cesarean in preference to a trial of labor), the Netherlands' breech cesarean rate increased from 50 percent to 80 percent and, despite some criticism of its benefits, has remained stable thereafter.[45] Moreover, this rapid change in medical behavior by Dutch obstetricians led to a significant decrease in babies' deaths during breech deliveries.[46] Dutch research has also confirmed the findings of many other countries, including the United States, that babies born by elective cesarean have the best health outcomes after thirty-nine gestational weeks.[47]

As far as maternal request cesareans with no indication are concerned, a survey sent out to all nine hundred gynecologists and registrars in the Netherlands reported that doctors' overall willingness ranged from 17 percent to 81 percent, with experienced doctors more willing to perform a planned cesarean than less experienced doctors.[48] Furthermore, a Dutch journal commentary titled "A Request for Caesarean Section without a Medical Indication Should Ultimately Be Granted" argued that "respect for the 'intuition'" of women avoids an undesirable trial of labor with the chance of an emergency cesarean, which will be "perceived as an extremely traumatic experience."[49]

The Future

Traditionally in the Netherlands, there has been a culture of women birthing the way their mothers and grandmothers did before them, so it will be interesting to watch (especially with the availability of information and voices on the Internet) whether the next generation of Dutch mothers are more determined to make their *own* birth choices. Certainly, this idea has been borne out in recent research in which Dutch midwives were asked about their perceptions of the pregnant women in their care. The authors report that midwives saw women age twenty-nine and younger as having more influence in the decision-making process than older women. And crucially, they conclude in their analysis that there might be tension in the future between midwives' own professional ideology and noninterventionist focus and women's choice, which can often lead to an increase in the medicalization of childbirth.[50]

THE UNITED STATES OF AMERICA

One of the most fundamental things to understand when talking about the cesarean rate in the United States is that the data on cesarean births are limited in a most elementary way. This is because despite the helpful system of separating cesarean births into primary and repeat, they are not usually separated into emergency and elective surgeries, which is vital for a clearer understanding of the risks and outcomes of each. Furthermore (although to be fair, this is a criticism of most other countries too, Sweden being the exception),[51] even though we know there are increasing numbers of cesareans on maternal request with no medical indication, this subgroup of surgeries is not identified in the country's birth data either. And frustratingly, when Pauline contacted them a few years ago, the US National Center for Health Statistics said there were no plans to change their policy of cesarean data collation.

One in Three Births Is a Cesarean

With more than four million births taking place each year, the United States' national cesarean rate currently stands at an all-time high of 32.3 percent (for births in 2008), of which 23.5 percent were primary cesareans (2006 data).[52]

Ten years ago, the federal project Healthy People 2010 set the target of reducing cesarean births among low-risk women to a rate of 15 percent for first births and 63 percent for births following a previous cesarean. At the time, the (1998) data were 18 percent and 72 percent, respectively, and the national cesarean rate was 21.2 percent,[53] but as you can see, with the 2010 deadline now past, these rates have gone in the exact opposite direction of the proposed target.

Reasons for this failure to reduce rates include evolving female demographics (mothers are older and heavier, for example), physicians' practice patterns, maternal choice, and for older women, patient and doctor concerns or multiple births. Also, reports of the risks associated with attempting a vaginal birth following previous cesarean surgery, as well as more conservative practice guidelines and legal pressures, are believed to be playing a part. Nevertheless, renewed efforts by local state activists to reduce their cesarean rates have been launched. In Sarasota, Florida, for example, the campaign 20 percent by 2020 describes itself as "an initiative to encourage elected officials, hospital staff, maternity care practitioners and consumers to reduce Sarasota's epidemic cesarean section rates to 20 percent by the year 2020."[54] Similarly, in New Jersey (where both of Pauline's children were born), Worst to First 2010 reports that all but two hospitals in the state have agreed to "re-educate staff" in order to achieve cesarean rates of 10–15 percent and episiotomy rates of 5 percent or less.[55] But it is our opinion that despite good intentions, neither of these cesarean goals can be safely achieved, and again, care must be taken not to risk the health of mothers and babies in the process of trying.

In fact, it's worth mentioning here that in the data recently published by the healthcare ratings organization HealthGrades, the news on cesarean births (and in these two states in particular) was not at all bad.[56] It found that while Florida and New Jersey have the highest rates of both cesarean and "patient choice" cesarean births, they also have the lowest complication rates for cesareans. And across the whole country, Health-

Grades reported that the best-performing hospitals also have higher cesarean rates, and on average, the hospitals with the lowest rates of "inhospital maternal complications" had the highest number of cesareans. Obviously, as with any research of this kind, there are limitations that can affect the accuracy of data collection and analysis, and very general observations like this do not provide the whole story in any given hospital or region, but in the context of cesarean criticism, it's notable that this research hints at some positive cesarean news at least.

Maternal Request

There is much debate about how many women in the United States are requesting a cesarean with no medical indication, and the truth is that nobody knows for sure. The oft-quoted Listening to Mothers survey in 2006 reported a mere 0.06 percent rate of maternal request (just 1 of the 1,600 women surveyed), but in 2003 and 2005, HealthGrades reported rates of patient choice *primary* cesareans across 1,500 hospitals as 1.87 percent and 2.55 percent, respectively,[57] with individual hospital rates ranging from 0 percent up to 7.75 percent. This may or may not be indicative of inconsistencies in the identification and gathering of birth data in hospitals, but again, we don't know. What we do know is that in a 2007 nationwide survey of obstetricians and gynecologists, 58 percent said they had noted an increase in patient inquiries regarding cesarean birth in the past year.[58]

It would be so much simpler, and indeed more accurate, if data were collated both during a woman's pregnancy (i.e., prior to the birth—what is the woman's preferred route of delivery or birth plan?) and after the birth (i.e., how did the birth begin, and what was its ultimate outcome?), but unfortunately, it is not. Pauline's first birth, for example, in a New Jersey hospital, was recorded as an elective cesarean for breech presentation—in effect, an obstetrical indication. However, throughout the vast majority of her pregnancy, she was planning a cesarean on maternal request with her doctor's full support, and on the morning of surgery, her doctor joked, "After all that, you'll never be registered or recorded anywhere as a maternal request cesarean—you of all people!"

Needless to say, this dearth of appropriately attributed data in hospitals leads to difficulties when assessing the health risks and benefits of different intended delivery outcomes. When the National Institutes of Health hosted its "State-of-the-Science Conference Statement on Cesarean Delivery on Maternal Request" in 2006, unsurprisingly, the independent panel concluded:

> [t]here is insufficient evidence to evaluate fully the benefits and risks of cesarean delivery on maternal request as compared to planned vaginal delivery, and more research is needed. Until quality evidence becomes available, any decision to perform a cesarean delivery on maternal request should be carefully individualized and consistent with ethical principles. Given that the risks of placenta previa and accreta rise with each cesarean delivery, cesarean delivery on maternal request is not recommended for women desiring several children. Cesarean delivery on maternal request should not be performed prior to 39 weeks of gestation or without verification of lung maturity, because of the significant danger of neonatal respiratory complications.

The panel added that the NIH "or another appropriate Federal agency should establish and maintain a Web site to provide up-to-date information on the benefits and risks of all modes of delivery."[59]

Unfortunately, five years on, neither the implementation of practical measures that would help gather this very evidence nor the initiation of this potentially invaluable online resource have come to fruition.

Deaths of Babies

There is a tendency for some natural-birth advocates to make a direct link between the number of babies that die in the United States and the corresponding rise in the number of cesarean surgeries taking place. Specifically, they will point to the country's unfavorable record in the worldwide infant mortality ranking as evidence, but it is absolutely not the most appropriate indicator of babies' health to consider when evaluating different delivery methods, as we will try to clarify below.

The infant mortality rate, which is currently 6.75 deaths per one thousand live births (2007), refers to the deaths of all babies under the age of one year.[60] Therefore, it includes causes of death such as sudden infant death syndrome (SIDS), accidental deaths, and other deaths that may be affected by extraneous socioeconomic factors such as poverty or access to infant healthcare. These deaths are in addition to those that occur during or immediately after the birth, but they are included in the overall death rate.[61]

What we should be looking at are deaths that occur *only* at or around the time of a baby's birth.

For example, the neonatal mortality rate, which refers to the deaths of all babies less than twenty-eight days old, is currently 4.42 per one thousand live births (2007). And the perinatal mortality rate, which refers to the number of stillbirths and deaths per one thousand live births from twenty-eight weeks' gestation, up to and including the first week of life, is currently 6.64 per one thousand live births (2005).[62]

Both of these measures of infant deaths are lower than they were in 1980 and 1985, when the cesarean rate in the United States was 16.5 percent and 22.7 percent.[63] This is despite the fact that the percentage of preterm births (which we know increases the risk of infant death) has risen 36 percent since 1984.[64] We're not suggesting all this is exclusively the result of increasing cesarean births. Our perinatology and neonatology colleagues deserve a great deal of credit for improvements in neonatology outcomes. But while it's pertinent to evaluate where the United States ranks in worldwide comparison tables and to strive to improve outcomes further, it is equally important to remember that the overall dramatic declines in infant deaths in the last few decades represent a major public health success and should be celebrated—with cesarean surgery included in this celebration.

Poverty, Obesity, and Deaths of Mothers

The number of women in the United States whose deaths are related to pregnancy and childbirth is 12.7 per 100,000 pregnancies (548 women died in 2007), compared with a rate of 607.9 per 100,000 pregnancies in 1915. Non-Hispanic white women are significantly less likely to die than non-Hispanic black women (10 deaths per 100,000 versus 28.4 deaths per 100,000).[65]

However, even though the maternal mortality rate (MMR) has dramatically fallen over the last century, because there has been very little change in the numbers of deaths over the last twenty-five years, natural-birth advocates are often quoted as making a direct link between the numbers of women dying and the increasing rate of cesarean deliveries.[66] Similarly, women choosing a planned cesarean birth are often warned about or chastised for their irresponsible decision to increase their risk of death in childbirth. But these accusations are not entirely accurate.

It's been known for some time that cesarean birth might be a marker for serious preexisting medical conditions that are associated with an increased risk of death, rather than a risk factor for death itself.[67] The medical condition making the cesarean delivery (elective or emergency) more likely in the first place also makes the risk of surgery greater and more prone to complications, further problems, and death. Think of an inebriated pilot dying in a small aircraft crash. The fact that he was flying a plane isn't the main cause of death (although obviously there are risks involved in flying a plane, and if he hadn't been flying, he may not have died), but it is rather the alcohol consumed before taking to the controls that increased his risk of death.

While this comparison is not an all-encompassing analogy for cesarean birth, it does illustrate how, in their efforts to highlight the risks of cesarean and the benefits of vaginal birth, many study authors and maternity commentators do not recognize a very important distinction when talking about maternal request cesareans in a healthy pregnancy. This, coupled with the aforementioned lack of clarity in hospital data, is why misinformation reigns in the public perception about which birth choices put women at the greatest risk of death.

In a 2008 Lamaze International publication, Ina May Gaskin, a midwife and originator of the Safe Motherhood Quilt Project, suggested that the United States needs to look further afield to find answers to such questions: "Only when we are able to equal the United Kingdom's CEMACH [now CMACE (Centre for Maternal and Child Enquiries)] system of ascertaining and analyzing maternal deaths will we be able to find out the causes of preventable maternal deaths and then set about preventing them."[68] This is because the United Kingdom carries out some of the most comprehensive reviews of maternal deaths in the world, and crucially, CMACE's triennial reviews are enhanced by maternity data that separate elective and emergency cesarean birth outcomes.

Lessons for the United States

This is what the latest (2011) UK review, "Saving Mothers' Lives," uncovered: "Compared with the general pregnant population, the women who died tended to be older and more obese, had lifestyles which put them at risk of poorer health and were more socially disadvantaged."[69] It reported that 49 percent of the mothers who died were overweight or obese, which was a slight improvement on the previous report in 2007, in which just over half of mothers who died were overweight or obese and 15 percent were "extremely obese."[70]

That same review also found that women living in the poorest circumstances were up to seven times more likely to die than women from other demographic groups. These mothers were in poorer health overall, less likely to be in contact with maternity services, and included increasing numbers of refugees and asylum seekers.

The United Kingdom tries to reduce maternal mortality by targeting specific areas of risk. For example, in its 2004 review *Why Mothers Die 2000–2002*, when psychiatric illness was the most common cause of indirect deaths through suicide (thromboembolism, or blood clotting, was the most common cause of direct deaths),[71] targeted efforts to identify women with psychiatric illness in subsequent years meant that the number of suicides reported in 2008 fell to thirty-seven, from fifty-eight in 2004. Similarly, efforts have been made to address obesity in the years between 2007 and 2011, albeit with comparatively less success, and going forward, with genital tract sepsis and cardiac disease currently the most common causes of death, best practice in hospitals will be examined. However, the issue of obesity remains an ongoing challenge.

Obesity Epidemic

The United States faces the same—if not *worse*—challenge as the United Kingdom; for example, recent analysis of the childbirth-related deaths of mothers in New York State found half of those who died were obese.[72] Understandably, medical professionals everywhere are concerned. "Obesity is fast emerging as the public health issue of our generation and its impact on maternity must be taken seriously," said Professor Sabaratnam Arulkumaran, president of the Royal College of Obstetricians and Gynaecologists, in 2007.[73] Dr. Gary Hankins, chair of the American College of Obstetricians and Gynecologists' (RCOG) Committee on Obstetric Practice, agrees: "Obesity has become an epidemic. At this point, 49 percent of non-Hispanic black women are obese, 38 percent of Mexican-American women are obese, and 31 percent of non-Hispanic white women are. And, everything we do in obstetrics is made more difficult and more complex by obesity—from using external monitors to performing surgery."[74]

Some Quick Facts

- The leading cause of all deaths in America is heart disease.[75]
- 36.1 percent of women aged twenty-five and older are obese (with a body mass index, or BMI, of more than thirty).
- 62.1 percent of all adult women are overweight or obese (BMI more than twenty-five).
- Women with a four-year degree or more are less likely to be obese than women who have not gained that level of education.[76]
- 38 percent of US female ob-gyns believe obesity is the most serious health problem facing women today. 78 percent believe it is a great concern.[77]

In a 2005 interview with Dr. Felicity Plaat, a consultant anesthetist at Queen Charlotte's Hospital in London, Pauline asked whether obesity is a potential problem for the advocacy of patient choice and maternal request for *all* women, given the increased risks associated with surgery. Dr. Plaat replied:

> That's an interesting question. From our point of view as anesthetists, yes, obesity is a risk factor; both an important and significant one. We'd rather not give an anesthetic to an obese woman if at all possible, but of course the flip side to that is that you particularly don't want to give an obese woman an emergency anesthetic, especially a general anesthetic, which would be an even greater risk than a planned one.
>
> In fact, anything in an emergency situation is made worse, and if you combine the risks of obesity and general anesthesia, you've got a particularly bad situation. So although a planned cesarean is not advisable for an obese woman, they're the very ones that you don't want to see having an emergency cesarean situation either. . . . Unfortunately, in general, where there is an increased risk of a woman not being able to have a normal delivery, there is an increased risk with the anesthesia in a cesarean too.

Yet given the significant risks of obesity to mother and baby, there has traditionally been a cultural reluctance to bring up the subject of obesity or weight gain (and their effects on mothers' and babies' health) while a woman is pregnant. Dr. Murphy personally experienced a situation in which a patient made a formal complaint after she read that he'd twice referred to her as obese (she weighed about three hundred pounds) in a consult letter written to her family doctor. She said he had "insulted her, had no empathy and was unprofessional"—all because the word "obese" appeared in a formal consultation intended for another medical professional.

Other doctors, including a past president of the American College of Obstetricians and Gynecologists, have spoken about this: "A lot of ob-gyns don't bring up weight with patients. In preconception visits, we talk to patients about genetic risks and immunity to rubella, but rarely do we discuss their weight or diet and exercise."[78] As a consequence, the college has published advice on offering obese women appropriate interventions or referrals to promote a healthy weight and lifestyle, as well as specific advice for women who have had weight loss surgery such as gastric banding or gastric bypass.[79]

Testing Solutions

It is highly probable that reducing obesity in pregnant women would have a positive impact on the numbers of women dying in the United States, and what would be useful going forward (and what we, as well as many doctors, would like to see) is the routine recording of every pregnant woman's BMI on maternity data collection sheets.[80] The benefit of this would be twofold. First, it would more accurately identify maternal deaths that occur in obese or overweight women, but more important, it would provide an unavoidable opportunity for doctors and midwives to discuss weight-related health issues during prenatal visits.

As a final point on this issue, it is worth noting that the high levels of female obesity in America are not solely the fault of women and the food choices they make, and it is not our intention here to blame or disparage women who have issues with their weight. It's no secret that the cheapest sustenance in the country is high in fat, sugar, and salt, due in part to government subsidies in the production of goods such as corn. When Pauline lived in the United States for three years, she was shocked at how expensive fruit and vegetables could be in comparison with the consistently lower prices and special offers on unhealthier foods. For cash- and time-poor shoppers, the temptation for cheap, easy, instant gratification can be too much. Indeed the reality for many, as they commute back and forth from jobs with long hours and low pay, in a society that is completely car-oriented and makes walking or cycling to work impossible for most, is that the lure of a enticingly advertised bargain bucket or dollar deal makes perfect financial sense.

There are no easy answers to all of this, and we don't presume to have them, but just as there's been a turning point in the campaign about the dangers of smoking (you risk your children's health as well as your own), perhaps the same shift in focus when it comes to warnings for pregnant women might work here too—not to scare or criticize, but to address, inform, and take preventive steps for both the mother's and the child's sakes.

Poverty and Healthcare

Unlike Canada and the majority of countries in Europe, the United States does not operate a national health service, free at the point of use. Instead, a complicated amalgamation of health insurance plans exists with myriad costs, benefits, and exclusions, all of which has an impact on birth outcomes. In 2009, a report from Amnesty International estimated that fifty-two million people in the country—more than one in six—have no health insurance. The government-funded Medicaid program provides funding for 42 percent of all births, but still, more than 4 percent of women give birth with no coverage at all, and one-quarter of women do not receive adequate prenatal care, rising to one-third for African American and Native American women.[81] Again, this aspect of healthcare also relates to the key findings in the United Kingdom's review of its maternal deaths, which highlighted worse outcomes for women living in the poorest circumstances. Changes due to be implemented by President Barack Obama's government promise statutory benefits for pregnant women and new mothers, so it will be interesting to see whether these have any impact on maternal health in the country, but in the meantime, poverty in this country remains a maternity risk factor.[82]

Insurance

Health insurance, or rather *quality* of health insurance, is directly related to income in the United States, leaving some women in the poorest sectors of society without adequate care, and by default, without adequate birth autonomy. What this means in practical terms is that although the American College of Obstetricians and Gynecologists has given maternal request the green light (as long as the doctor is happy with the decision), some women either won't be able to afford to pay the copay and excess for surgery, or their insurance companies may refuse to pay any of their costs. One company may not allow maternal request as an adequate indication, another may consider previous cesarean surgery a preexisting condition and refuse to pay for a second, while another may require no justification at all and simply pay out. The problem is that there are so many insurance companies, plans, and options that the process of insurance claims becomes very complicated and potentially obstructive.

Litigation

More than ninety years ago, in 1920, Dr. Paul Humpstone commented, "We have all regretted that we have not done a cesarean in certain cases, but I have yet to regret one that I have done."[83] This sentiment has remained a feature of obstetrics ever since.

In 2006, the American College of Obstetricians and Gynecologists reported that a massive 89 percent of ob-gyns have had at least one liability claim filed against them during their professional careers, with an average of 2.6 claims per doctor. At the time, Dr. Ralph W. Hale, the college's executive vice president, stressed that this is not always a sign of wrongdoing (he said doctors win in court about seven out of ten times), but rather that the high-risk field they work in means that "all too often, doctors are held liable for less than perfect outcomes." The effect of all this is that professional liability insurance premiums have soared in recent years, leaving some areas of the United States without specialist doctors and with anecdotal reports of women with severe complications and even death due to insufficient medical providers.[84]

Numerous studies have reflected the serious impact of this colossal rise in liability premiums, with doctors citing spiraling costs as one of the main reasons they've left or are considering leaving obstetric service. We discuss the impact of this, and indeed the nature of different working practices and models of care in obstetrics, in chapter 10, "Before They Say It," but essentially, as Dr. Thomas F. Heston put it in 2002, "Legalisation Creates Medicalisation."[85] For example, there have been reports of some hospital's cesarean rates rising in the year following a successful lawsuit.

In stark contrast, many European countries practice a rather more no-blame or no-fault system, and although claims for negligence are investigated, the awards patients receive can be relatively modest. One of the reasons they can do this is their national healthcare system, where if a woman or baby is injured during childbirth, their ongoing care will be provided within that system without the need for large monetary payouts. So whereas American doctors and midwives would be hauled into court and sued, this is not always the case for their European counterparts.

Perhaps, if the situation were different, and, as in the United States, each individual medical professional *were* likely to be sued for millions of dollars—especially in the event of delaying or not doing a cesarean—the cesarean rate in countries like Sweden and the Netherlands might climb even faster. We don't know. Either way, that's not to say we condone the overuse of cesarean deliveries due to litigation fears, particularly for women who really want a vaginal delivery. We don't. It's simply that the situation in parts of Europe perfectly illustrates two things:

1. Doctors in the United States, practicing in an omnipresent reality of potential lawsuits, are under immense pressure to get it right *in every single case* or risk financial and professional ruin.
2. When litigation pressure is removed, negligence still occurs, but the women and babies affected must largely rely on state-provided funding for their future care when no (or very low) personal payouts are received.

Doctors' Dilemma

Consider this theoretical case study. An obese woman has been laboring for many hours. Her baby is showing signs of fetal distress, and her labor is being evaluated by one doctor as failure to progress. He advises an emergency cesarean to save the baby's life and reduce its risk of injury or disability. A second doctor maintains that surgery for this woman would be best avoided, given her weight and the ensuing increase in risks with (for example) general anesthesia, blood clots, or wound infection. He advises continuation of labor with assisted vaginal delivery and is confident that the baby can be extracted safely. Unfortunately, neither doctor's decision is fail-safe. The mother or the baby could die or suffer from serious health problems either way. Yet doctors are faced with this type of decision every day, and it often seems as though whichever decision they make, only one thing is certain: they'll come under attack: A cesarean rate too high, and the indication will be branded a lie. A cesarean rate too late or too few, and rest assured that someone will sue.

Finally, on the issue of maternal request cesareans, the American College of Obstetricians and Gynecologists stated in 2003:

> The burden of proof should fall on those who advocate for a change in policy in support of elective cesarean delivery (which replaces a natural process—vaginal delivery—with a major surgical procedure). . . . "Both sides to this debate" must recognize that evidence to support the benefit of elective cesarean is still incomplete and that there are not yet extensive morbidity and mortality data to compare elective cesarean delivery with vaginal birth in healthy women. With better data, there may be a shift in clinical practice.[86]

We believe that our book provides this proof, and that the United States' clinical practice may already be shifting toward recognition that the assessment of risks and benefits in low-risk pregnancies is now so finely balanced as to make it impossible to continue with a presumption of cesarean inferiority.

THE UNITED KINGDOM

There is currently somewhat of a battle going on in the United Kingdom regarding cesarean rates and birth choices, and as 2011 draws to a close, there are likely to be developments in (or indeed changes to) healthcare policy that may well determine (or try to determine) which way cesarean rates will go in the longer term. On the one hand, there is pressure on the government from natural-birth advocate groups to encourage and facilitate more home births for women with low-risk pregnancies (and at a parliamentary group meeting Pauline attended at the end of 2010, home birth was suggested as one strategy for reducing the national cesarean rate), and on the other, a concerted campaign by other birth groups for the current clinical guidelines on maternal request cesareans to be changed (currently, maternal request is "not on its own an indication" for surgery) looks likely to be successful.

The cesarean rate in England (not including its private hospitals, where cesarean rates are much higher) is 24.8 percent (of 650,000 births, of which 14.8 percent are emergency and 10 percent are elective),[87] and maternal request occurs in approximately 5 percent of all births (although with fewer than a third of these requests agreed to, the actual rate reported is 7 percent of all cesarean births).[88] In Wales, Scotland, and Northern Ireland, national cesarean rates stand at 25.5 percent,[89] 24.9 percent,[90] and 29.8 percent,[91] respectively, and similarly, in the neighboring Republic of Ireland, it's 26.7 percent.[92] Each country in the United Kingdom tends to have its own governance and legislation (although there is some overlap when it comes to maternity care policy), but throughout all the regions, there are voices of concern that their rising cesarean rates are creeping far too close to the United States' rate of one in three births. The question is, what should (and what can) be done about it?

Encouragingly, new guidelines have already been drafted to deal with the increased likelihood of pregnancy and birth complications with obesity (including emergency surgery and its associated increased risks for this group of women and their babies), since it's estimated that almost half of all women of childbearing age in England are obese or overweight.[93] The guidelines recommend that women who are pregnant or who are planning a pregnancy understand the health risks of being overweight during pregnancy and the importance of achieving a healthy weight prior to pregnancy. And in a move to address the increased likelihood and risks, particularly of emergency surgery, for older mothers, the president of the Royal College of Obstetricians and Gynaecologists has suggested that alongside education about teenage pregnancies and contraception, schoolchildren should be taught that ages twenty to thirty-five are the best time for a woman to have a baby.[94] But what about the women who choose a cesarean birth?

Maternal Request Debate

In 2004, a guideline on cesarean delivery published by the National Institute for Clinical Excellence (NICE) was criticized for being more political than medical and for presenting an anti–maternal request cesarean position from the outset. The document made it clear that while a woman has the right to refuse cesarean surgery "even when the treatment would clearly benefit her or her baby's health," she does not have the right to choose a cesarean as a potential birth plan.[95]

Around the time of publication, Professor James Drife, then an obstetrician at Leeds Hospital General Infirmary in England (now retired), was particularly vocal about the guideline's flaws in the context of maternal request, likening it to the management of another controversial maternal request:

> The maternal request point is then followed up with rather verbose and threatening language about the woman's concerns being "assessed and recorded" and a recommendation further on that the woman should be offered counseling and cognitive therapy. This attempt to medicalize a perfectly rational point of view is insulting and offensive to women and flies in the face of the evidence that exists.
>
> A woman is allowed to ask for a second opinion about her cesarean choice. This is the same kind of attitude that was taken after the Abortion Act came in. Women requesting abortion could be sent to a psychiatrist, a doctor had the right to refuse her request and she was allowed to ask for a second opinion. The desire to take control of women like this is disgraceful and demeans the whole document.[96]

He was especially concerned that given the nature of the maternity model of care in England, women meet with a midwife when they are pregnant, not an obstetrician (referral to an obstetrician usually occurs only when there is a specific medical or obstetrical indication), and therefore doctors are not able to provide individualized consultation at the planning stage of birth; they tend to get involved only when there are problems.

> Many of the most vociferous anti-cesarean campaigners are basing their beliefs on experiences of birth 20 or 30 years ago and evidence from other countries. They have no idea about modern obstetric practice in hospitals like ours. The propaganda we have to live with is very worry-

ing. You don't get to form a constructive relationship with your patients nowadays because they've been kept away from you during the pregnancy and filled with anti-cesarean points of view.[97]

In May 2009, NICE commissioned an update of its existing cesarean guideline but only a *partial* update that did not include the issue of maternal request in its proposed scope. However, fortunately, it invited interested organizations to register as stakeholders (which Pauline did), and as a result of the feedback and recommendations by these stakeholder representatives, NICE announced in July 2010 that maternal request *would* now be included.

But even better news was to come. In September 2011, following extensive stakeholder consultation,[98] NICE published its final draft guideline, which included the recommendation that *all* maternal request cesareans, including, but not limited to, those due to fear of labor and birth (i.e., tokophobia), should be supported within the NHS. The draft reads, "For all women requesting a CS, if after discussion and offer of support (including perinatal mental health support for women with anxiety about childbirth), a vaginal birth is still not an acceptable option, offer a planned CS. . . . An obstetrician has the right to decline a woman's request for a CS. If this happens, they should refer the woman to an NHS obstetrician in the same unit who will carry out the CS."[99] This wording may change when the actual guideline is published in November 2011, but for now, it signals a welcome move.

Concerns over Cesarean Cost

Because the National Health Service (NHS) in the United Kingdom is paid for by taxpayers, the additional financial cost of surgery versus a spontaneous vaginal birth is frequently raised in discussions about maternal request, and there is nothing wrong with that. But as we explain in chapter 11, the comparison of financial expenditure in maternity care is not as straightforward as some would have us believe. Yes, planned surgery has a price tag, but so does planned vaginal birth, both financially and psychologically. For example, we know that pelvic floor surgeries run into the billions of dollars per year in the United States and that incontinence treatments (including over-the-counter costs for diapers and other incontinence products) are a multibillion-dollar industry, so although the United Kingdom's socialized provision of these remedies may have an arguably lower per-unit cost than in the United States, the overall cost to the system and society is still absolutely massive. Also, while only a certain proportion of these costs will be directly associated with vaginal birth, they are nevertheless undoubtedly more prevalent in women experiencing this birth type than those having a planned cesarean (as we explain in chapter 6) and should therefore be factored into comparative calculations.

Another huge birth cost comes in the form of litigation payments awarded to injured or bereaved families. The NHS Litigation Authority was set up in 1995, and in the fifteen years since, it has handled 11,533 new claims for obstetrics and gynecology with a total value (including costs, payments, and reserves) of £4.4 billion ($7 billion), and, to put this into perspective, in just one year alone (2009–10), a massive £301 million ($482 million) was spent on obstetrics litigation.[100] If you include the actuarial estimate of liabilities in respect of incidents that have incurred but have not yet been reported to the Litigation Authority, billions of pounds more are added to this cost.

Recognition of these figures is hugely important when you consider that as recently as 2009, the NHS Institute for Innovation and Improvement introduced a "programme of reduction of cesarean rates," which promised the outwardly positive benefit of "significant cost savings," even with a "small reduction" in cesarean rates in England.[101] It said that savings of as much as £76.8 million was possible if rates fell from 24 percent to 20 percent, and a reduction in hospital stay from 4 to 2.5 days could be achieved. But clearly, this cost savings is a drop in the ocean when you consider the money that might be saved in litigation costs if *more* cesareans were carried out—namely, the dangerously delayed and/or absent ones.

Currently, there is unfortunately no formal recognition of this cost for predominantly planned vaginal births, and it is kept entirely separate from birth-type comparison tables in the same way the costs associated with long-term health problems are (such as pelvic floor repair and treatments for children's birth injuries, for example). That said, the health economics section of the new NICE (draft) guidance has at least begun to address this issue by citing urinary incontinence as one example of the "downstream" costs associated with vaginal birth. The draft even states, "On balance this model does not provide strong evidence to refuse a woman's request for CS on cost-effectiveness grounds."[102] Evidently, however, there are still more costs that need to be attributed besides urinary incontinence.

And so, efforts continue to be made by individuals and groups to communicate the full breadth of costs involved with a trial of labor to government ministers. Most recently, for example, Pauline contacted the health minister's constituency office following reported discussions in Northern Ireland about whether women who choose to have a cesarean should be made to pay for it themselves.[103] For the most part, this action is to ensure that the politicians who make decisions on healthcare policies are more fully informed than they have been in the past, but there's another reason why it's vital to present them with the actual facts and figures related to birth costs: because if there's one thing both sides of the cesarean debate in the United Kingdom know well, it's that money talks. And never was this truer than in today's economic climate.

What Women Want

Perhaps one of the greatest ironies in the rising rates of cesareans in the United Kingdom is the possibility that the efforts of the country's largest natural-birth advocate group to provide women with greater access to natural-birth choices has actually led to more planned cesareans than home births. Founded in 1956, the Natural Childbirth Association was renamed the National Childbirth Trust (NCT) in 1961, and one of its original aims stated, "As childbirth is not a disease it should take place in the home wherever possible. If impossible the maternity units should be homely and unfrightening and in no way connected with hospital."[104] In the early 1990s, concerned with the state of maternity care and by now having grown into the largest parenting charity in the United Kingdom, the NCT lobbied the government and provided evidence for a Parliamentary Health Select Committee, and its president was invited to join the government's Expert Maternity Group. This group produced a groundbreaking report titled "Changing Childbirth," which outlined choice and involvement in decision making as central principles of maternity care and became embedded in policy for England and Wales thereafter. It stated:

> The woman must be the focus of maternity care. She should be able to
> feel that she is in control of what is happening to her and able to make

decisions about her care, based on her needs, having discussed matters fully with the professionals involved. . . . Women should be involved in the monitoring and planning of maternity services to ensure that they are responsive to the needs of a changing society. In addition care should be effective and resources used efficiently.[105]

However, what no one quite anticipated, but what would nevertheless come to fruition, was that given the choice, many more women decided to choose hospital birth—and indeed surgical birth—than the natural and homely experience the NCT had set out to facilitate and support. Since the "Changing Childbirth" report, the NCT has been heavily involved in the formation and running of the Maternity Care Working Party (MCWP) and the All-Party Parliamentary Group on Maternity Services (APPG) (which were established in 1999 and 2000), and it has continued its focus on promoting normality in childbirth.

A Tool Kit Target

Unfortunately, the drive for more "normal" births (something supported by a number of other maternity groups in the United Kingdom too) is now in danger of becoming less about providing women with the birth they want and more about something altogether different. It assumes what women want, it decides what's best for them, and it ignores birth choices that are outside an ideological normal scope.

In 2007, the Maternity Care Working Party published a consensus statement titled "Making Normal Birth a Reality," which set out the group's "shared views about the need to recognise, facilitate and audit normal birth." But it is Pauline's understanding, having attended two Maternity Care Working Party meetings in 2010, that the definition of normal labor and birth contained within this document was only ever intended by the Information Centre in England to be used as an auditing tool (i.e., a hindsight appraisal of birth processes), and not to be confused with a target or goal for women's birth experiences, as it is here: "Maternity services should aim to increase their normal birth rates toward a realistic objective of 60 percent by 2010."[106]

Aside from the issue of facilitating normal birth as opposed to simply auditing it, what is often not understood about this particular definition of normal birth is that it includes outcomes that may be deemed normal by this group but that are not desirable or even tolerable for a significant number of women. For example, in this particular definition, normal outcomes may include "antenatal, delivery or postnatal complications (including for example postpartum haemorrhage, perineal tear, repair of perineal trauma, admission to SCBU (special care baby unit) or NICU (neonatal intensive care unit))."[107]

Nevertheless, a few years later, at the end of 2009, the NHS Institute for Innovation and Improvement reported on the success of a special "toolkit," designed as an aid for maternity services in England to encourage more normal births and reduce the number of cesareans. The institute stated that there is "a general belief amongst clinicians that maternity units applying best practice to the management of pregnancy, labour and delivery will achieve a Caesarean section rate consistently below 20 percent and will have aspirations to reduce that rate to 15 percent."[108] But the "general belief" and "aspirations" described here have certainly not been Pauline's experience of all doctors' views in the United Kingdom.

For example, Dr. Bryan Beattie, a consultant obstetrician who has worked in British tertiary teaching hospitals for more than twenty years, told us:

> One of the worrying trends in the United Kingdom over the last few years has been the promotion of natural childbirth to the extent that we have also forgotten the risks involved. Even simple things like identification of growth-restricted babies or those presenting as breech are missed as often as they are picked up. Natural childbirth carries a natural risk of death, morbidity, and disability, and obstetricians and midwives deliberately intervene to make it safer. The problem is that they can't always reliably identify which mothers and babies will need that intervention, and even fetal monitoring in labor is still very unreliable. All too often, they have to debrief a mother or a family about an unexpected bad outcome in a so-called low-risk pregnancy.

Choice Is Choice Is Choice

Dr. Beattie makes the point that birth is inherently unpredictable, and that even low-risk pregnancies can become complicated very quickly and without warning. And what's worrying is that even organizations such as the

Royal College of Obstetricians and Gynecologists[109] and the King's Fund[110] continue to suggest that midwife-led care, including maternity care at separate midwife-led birth centers (from which mothers and babies would need to be transferred in emergency situations), is an appropriate strategy for all low-risk women. It isn't. We are not saying that natural birth should not be a choice for women, or that it is never successful or satisfying, but that women should be fully informed of all the risks, no matter how small, and that we shouldn't be fearful of the decisions they may make when this education has taken place. Yes, some will choose to have a cesarean, but just as many, if not more, will still decide to plan a vaginal birth.

Our question is, given the abundant proof that a planned cesarean birth can often have better outcomes for mothers and babies, how can maternity-care professionals in the United Kingdom legitimately talk about offering choice in childbirth and include language in their statements such as "supporting women to have a positive experience of pregnancy and birth," "informed decisions [to] plan for the kind of birth they want," and "evidence-based information,"[111] and yet not include maternal request cesarean in that same discussion? As this book goes to press, we are hopeful, and even tentatively confident, that a change in this situation could introduce the next groundbreaking development in the United Kingdom's maternity-care policy: the confirmed acceptance of maternal request cesarean birth as an indication for surgery.

What will this do to the country's overall cesarean rates? Only time will tell.

CANADA

Canada's national cesarean rate stands at 26.9 percent, although individually, rates vary from one province to another.[112] In general, a strong request for a planned cesarean will be respected, but this is not universally true, and like the situation in the United Kingdom, the outcome of such a request will be dependent on a particular hospital's policy or obstetrician's personal view. Also, contrary to most other developed countries, a parallel system of private healthcare is not available in Canada. Therefore, if a woman's local jurisdiction decides to deny access to planned cesareans, there is no private recourse available to her. Certainly, a prophylactic planned cesarean is almost never discussed without maternal prompt, and this is partly because there is little time or money available for individualized consultation. Many doctors feel that the remuneration for prenatal visits is low, and therefore time spent with women is minimal; nurses do most of the work in many clinics. Also, hospitals are crowded, available operating room time and access is limited, and resources are stretched to chronic or almost crisis levels in some areas. There seems to be little or no appetite for experimenting with any major new ideas, and especially not with those perceived as having unknown implications for staffing and resources.

In fact, "value for money" was one of three buzzwords suggested in the recent Canadian Institute for Health Information report, "Health Care in Canada 2010" ("appropriateness" and "quality of care" were the others),[113] but like many other countries, Canada must be careful not to mistake potentially dangerous short-term cost-cutting plans for properly thought-out approaches providing value for money. For example, in the same report, there is a discussion about how much money could be saved if the primary cesarean rate could be lowered in line with the World Health Organization's recommended range of 5–15 percent, with more women having vaginal births with no interventions instead. The suggested amount that could have been saved in 2008–09 is $97 million, which of course makes a great headline figure, but as a serious target, a reduction from one in five women having a primary cesarean to one in twenty is, in our opinion, unrealistic and would risk poorer health outcomes.

There would appear to be somewhat of a paradox in Canada when it comes to cesareans. The best guess seems to be that only 1–2 percent of women actually request one, but there are concerns that this number is rising, and it's been Dr. Murphy's experience that a majority of individual obstetricians will agree to maternal request cesareans if pushed hard enough and if their local hospitals will allow it. However, this is in contrast to the official line of the Society of Obstetricians and Gynaecologists of Canada (SOGC), which has been steadfast in its commitment to a position of advocating natural birth. Indeed, some Canadian provinces are strongly advocating midwifery practice, with some jurisdictions even paying midwives more than physicians per delivery and prenatal care. And most midwife colleges in Canada have made home birth deliveries obligatory for their members and are vociferously against cesarean birth, both on maternal request but also with obstetrical reasons such as breech presentation or a previous cesarean. It is therefore likely that in some hospital settings, at least, there are, and will continue to be, seriously conflicting views about what constitutes best "quality of care" in Canada's maternity wards.

BRAZIL

It's hard to ascertain exactly what is going on obstetrically in the beautiful country of Brazil, and it would probably be easy for someone to write an entire chapter on the subject of the cesarean culture there, but one thing's for sure: its cesarean rates are unique. Percentages up in the 80s and 90s have been reported in private hospitals, for example, where around one-third of women give birth, and even in public hospitals, where cesarean rates are comparably low, rates of 43–45 percent are commonly quoted.[114] The reasons behind these high rates are multiple and complex, and although women's cultural preferences and obstetricians' self-interest are often blamed, research in the Brazilian city of Salvador da Bahia at least found that a wide variety of political and social factors, and the maternity health system as a whole, may be responsible.[115]

In 1999, research into the rates and implications of cesareans in nineteen Latin American countries was published in the *British Medical Journal*, and it generated considerable response from the journal's readers in the form of letters and comments.[116] One series of correspondence titled "Caesarean Section Controversy" included many insights into what might be happening in Brazil (although of course things may have changed in the last decade). For example, two British doctors point out that while the richest countries in Latin America have the highest rates of cesarean births, they "also have the lowest perinatal, infant, and maternal mortality" —a small but significant detail that is often lost in the hype that surrounds Brazilian surgical births. That said, an obstetrician who worked there for more than ten years says he has "been put under pressure to perform caesarean section many times, from patients, husbands, and relatives." And an independent researcher, having spent two years investigating cesareans in southeast Brazil, describes a number of interesting personal observations, such as the concern that many obstetricians are not trained to facilitate difficult vaginal births with forceps or vacuum assistance because cesarean rates have been so high for so long, and the suggestion that because doctors are paid the same amount for vaginal and cesarean births, there is "no financial incentive" to wait the hours it might take for a vaginal delivery compared with surgery. She also writes about the "status" a cesarean holds in Brazil, where modernity and technology are highly valued, and the notion that in this country, "women's bodies are perceived as sexual rather than maternal, and the genitals as being for sexual intercourse rather than for childbearing."[117]

Research Needed

Research suggests that despite their very high cesarean rates, Brazilian women do not necessarily always *want* a cesarean; they merely perceive it as the lesser of two evils. Reported rates of episiotomy in Brazil, for example, can be as high as 94 percent, and there is the suggestion that many poor women seek a cesarean to avoid poor or abusive standards of care during vaginal birth, including the withholding of pain relief.[118] There has also been research showing an unmistakable disconnect between women's preferred plan and their actual birth outcomes, with many women who said they wanted a vaginal birth but ended up with a cesarean. The authors conclude that "doctors frequently persuaded their patients to accept a scheduled cesarean section for conditions that either did not exist or did not justify this procedure."[119]

Interestingly, the argument has also been made that planned cesarean outcomes in Brazil may only appear better than vaginal birth outcomes because of the "selection bias" that is now commonplace there. Effectively, since there apparently is "an almost universal preference for cesarean sections in low-risk pregnancies" in many parts of the country, it might mean that the remaining women who are planning vaginal births are likely to contain a higher proportion of high-risk cases than would naturally occur.[120] There may be an element of truth in the hypothesis; after all, the irony is that the best candidates for both planned vaginal birth and cesarean surgery are women with low-risk pregnancies. However, it does not change the fact that even when low-risk births alone are compared, there is evidence that a planned cesarean still offers greater predictability of good health outcomes for mothers and babies, and unless this situation changes, it is unlikely that the cesarean status quo in Brazil will change either.

AUSTRALIA

In Australia, the cesarean rate is 31.1 percent, and its neonatal mortality rate is a comparably low 2.8 per one thousand live births.[121] In terms of maternal request, the rules in public hospitals differ from state to state, which means that a cesarean with no medical reason is an accepted birth choice in some but not in others. However, researchers discovered that in 2006, at least 17.3 percent of all planned cesareans and 3.2 percent of all births were on maternal request (which they defined as a primary cesarean birth initiated by the mother with no medical need), making maternal request "an important contributor" to the country's overall cesarean rates.[122]

THE NORDIC COUNTRIES

While there has been a steady rise in the numbers of surgical births taking place in the Nordic countries, they still have relatively low cesarean rates compared with many others in the developed world. For example, out of almost three hundred thousand births in total, Denmark's rate is 21 percent; Finland's, 17 percent; Sweden's, 17 percent; Norway's, 17 percent; and Iceland's, 16 percent (2008 data).[123] And although the way some of the countries define live births is different from that of other countries (which can affect comparative results), the number of babies who are stillborn or die within their first week of life is between three and four per one thousand live births. However, what is also highlighted in these perinatal statistics is that perineal tears during vaginal birth have become more common in the Nordic countries. The reasons given for this are larger babies, fewer episiotomies, and more epidurals, although the National Institute for Health and Welfare report that provides these statistics also mentions that there has actually been a reduction in some of these numbers in recent years. Nonetheless, this situation has interesting parallels with the findings of the United States' HealthGrades study in 2003 (mentioned in chapter 9, "The Politics of Birth"), in which higher-than-expected vaginal complication rates were found in places where cesarean rates were lower than expected.[124]

TURKEY

Turkey's national cesarean rate is a reported 42.7 percent, ranging from 39.3 percent in public hospitals to 61.8 percent in private hospitals.[125] An analysis of births that took place in the 1990s found that cesarean birth was strongly associated with the mother's education and age, place of delivery, access to prenatal care, and household welfare. This implied that women with higher socioeconomic status were more likely to accept a cesarean birth than those with a lower status, which is similar to trends that have been found in other countries. But in terms of maternal request, what's very interesting about Turkey is that although rates among women are high (20.6 percent in a recent survey), the number of medical professionals with this birth preference (with no medical indication) is 45.3 percent. Furthermore, 36.2 percent and 37.8 percent respectively believe that women should have the right to a cesarean delivery on demand.[126]

THE DEVELOPING WORLD

One of Dr. Murphy's nurse colleagues, upon learning that we were writing this book, made a pertinent comment in the context of this particular chapter and maternal request cesareans, and one that we had always planned to address. She complained, "This stand is an arrogant, selfish rich-person stand, while large parts of the world don't even have any maternity care at all. Rather than cater to rich, selfish women, concentrate on improving the lot of those who are completely disenfranchised and are dying in the bush."

This is a very valid point in many respects, and it is absolutely true that vast numbers of the world's maternal population are dying and suffering in childbirth. The International Federation of Gynecology and Obstetrics estimates that worldwide, more than two million women and babies die each year from birth complications.[127] Women who survive with birth injuries often have double incontinence from obstetrical fistulas, leaving them with continuous leakage of urine and feces. This leads to social ostracism, extreme poverty, complete loss of dignity and the ability to care for themselves and their families, and, essentially, a life that is not worth living. But what we're saying in this chapter is that discussions about improving health outcomes with cesarean delivery should not be an either-or dialogue—either we focus on defending the legitimacy of maternal request for women, or we focus on saving lives in the developing world. We need to do both, and indeed we unreservedly support safe efforts to improve the health outcomes of women in underprivileged areas.

But while the irony is not lost on us that as half of the world debates the ethics and merits of the maternal request cesarean with no medical indication, the other half can't access one even when there *is* a medical necessity, it's also true that the disparity between rich and poor countries exists on every other medical, social, and cultural level as well. Most developing-world mothers don't have the privilege of good healthcare, nutritious food, warm houses, or a decent education, let alone further luxuries such as orthodontics, physiotherapy, and psychotherapy. In this light, maternal request cesarean is as legitimate as any other inward-looking discussion on issues that affect our daily lives in the developed world: for example, gas prices, schools, housing markets, diets, or celebrity culture. What's most important to recognize in the context of childbirth is that in addition to all the basic necessities of life such as clean water, medical supplies, essential drugs, and adequate nutrition, it is greater access to emergency obstetric care—namely, cesarean deliveries—that will make any real difference to the world's poorest mothers.[128]

More cesareans will save more lives and result in fewer birth injuries, and so in this respect, our stance on the potential benefits of planned cesarean birth should help highlight the plight of women in the developing world, rather than detract attention from it.

SUMMARY

Cesareans save lives. That's a fact. It's also an undisputed fact that more cesareans are needed in many, many regions of the world and that fewer cesareans are desired in others. But finding solutions for increasing and decreasing cesarean rates is anything but simple, and almost every suggestion is bound up with social, political, and ideological influences that seem to be unique to birth. Who should decide, and indeed, who can say with any accuracy what the correct number of cesareans is? Warren Buffett once wrote about how much clearer things look to investors through the rearview mirror, but that when making investment decisions, they must do so peering through a windshield frequently clouded by fog. The same analogy could be used when it comes to birth plans—and, indeed, for birth policies. It's far easier to look back with hindsight and assess what action was most appropriate (as many law courts do), but much harder to do so during the birth itself.

If we look even farther into the rearview mirror—to 1920, to be exact, the year the prestigious *American Journal of Obstetrics and Gynecology* was first published—we are reminded of the dangers inherent in birth's unpredictability with Dr. Humpstone's words: "No man can hold himself absolutely blameless these days, when after a long trying instrumental birth the baby is born dead. He will always remember that there was a time in that confinement when the baby could have been born alive, and in the retrospect, the mother have been left far less traumatized."[129] Although such outcomes are rare today, the message is still valid. Perhaps in the future, new knowledge will enable doctors to predict even more accurately which women are most at risk for complicated labors, and planned cesareans could then be offered to this group. But until then, doctors are compelled to work on the assumption that all women are at risk and should at least be informed of these risks in order to make an empowered, personal, and considered decision about childbirth. They should not be coerced into decisions inspired by the political, feminist, or economic agendas of the day, or simply because it is the way it has been done in the past.

To be fair, maternity experts at the World Health Organization have a very difficult job trying to police the maternity health of almost two hundred individual countries with a one-size-fits-all approach to cesarean rate advice. In our opinion, it's an impossible task, and one they would do well to relinquish on an international level. The assumption that one cesarean rate range could ever be applicable to an entire worldwide population of women is completely flawed, especially given that even within a single country, rate ranges differ between geographical populations. The maternal environments in individual countries, including mothers' characteristics (young, old, underweight, overweight, short, tall, rich, poor, educated, uneducated), quality of hospital care and medical training, and cultural and social influences, all play their part. And yet it's incredible to think that for almost twenty-five years, so many maternity professionals and groups have been content to accept a "world average" threshold for cesarean delivery, when in almost every other area of health or social development, it's deemed perfectly rational and indeed desirable to strive to reach beyond average outcomes.

As we've explained, the purpose of this chapter is to give a relatively short overview of what is happening in the world and to try to explain some possible reasons for the cesarean trends in each country or region we discuss. We also want to encourage a wider perspective on how cesarean rates in different countries can be presented and compared and why context is so important in the ongoing cesarean debate. We are not arguing the merits of higher overall cesarean rates; we are merely pointing out the reality on the ground. And without doubt, almost all the cesarean trends around the world are pointing toward increasing rates for the future—in spite of concerted and persistent efforts to keep them down. We believe this debate will continue to be waged for years and even decades to come, and what's important to us is that as efforts to reduce overall rates continue, the maternal request cesarean must not be set in the world's sights as the first and easiest target for this reduction.

Chapter 9

The Politics of Birth

If you want to make enemies, try to change something.
　　　　　—Attributed to Woodrow Wilson (1856–1924)

B irth is political. It shouldn't be, but it is. And the sooner you realize this, the better chance you'll have of making sure the birth plan you decide on is *your* choice, not one that's already been decided for you.

But this chapter is not about convincing you that a planned cesarean is superior to planned vaginal birth (yes, it's what we would choose, but that choice won't be the same for everyone); rather, it's about throwing light on maternity policies that are all too often encumbered by a struggle for power and shaped by social, ideological, and political ideals instead of best outcomes for mothers and babies.

PROMOTING NORMALITY

First, it's obvious to us that the words *natural* and *normal* are often ideologically loaded in the context of birth, and in many cases, they are in danger of doing more harm than good. Think about it. If natural (i.e., processed with little or no human intervention) and normal (usually defined as spontaneous vaginal delivery but may include induction, monitoring, anesthesia, and even some medical or obstetrical complications as long as the delivery itself is spontaneous) are birth ideals that every *real* woman should aspire to, that every woman who *trusts her body* can achieve, then how is a woman meant to feel when things don't go according to plan? Is it any wonder we have so many women traumatized by an overriding sense of failure when their hoped-for, idealized, and often promised birth turns out to be *unnatural* or *abnormal*—not to mention the many new mothers so focused on their perceived birth failure that they're left feeling unable to bond with their baby?

It's appalling that so many women end up feeling this way—and absurd, especially when you consider that the overwhelming majority of women choose to give birth in a hospital in the first place, as opposed to at home or in a field somewhere, and so in fairness, barely anyone gives birth naturally anymore. And the idea that certain births, fitting within strict criteria of acceptable measures, are subsequently labeled normal by hospital administrators or birth educators, yet others, deemed to exceed a predetermined standard of medical intervention, are not, is arguably unhelpful. Or at least irrelevant (outside of in-hospital audits, perhaps), since fundamentally, the perception of what's normal in birth will always be individual to each woman. Pauline's births felt completely normal and natural to her, for example.

In fact, we would estimate that in the developed world, the number of pregnant women who *truly* have a natural birth in the biological sense is very low. Most choose to surround themselves with midwives and doctors, and, most important in case of an emergency situation, surgeons. This is because although, yes, birth is a normal physiological process, this does not guarantee success or safety. Death is a normal physiological process too, and if that happens, where is the sense of achievement in realizing normality? Whether or not people are willing to accept it, a natural birth outcome is effectively blind luck, and we think it's irresponsible to suggest otherwise. After all, what most women want is a safe delivery and to bring home a healthy baby; that's what's normal and natural to them.

Nonetheless, the term *natural* is an unquestionably powerful marketing brand, perhaps never more so than it is today. In a world that is increasingly polluted, genetically engineered, chemically modified, and generally fraught with human-made health risks, the presence of the word *natural* goes a long way toward alleviating consumers' concerns and, more important, toward forging their unwavering buy-in to products that have not been unnecessarily tampered with. The same is true when it comes to natural birth. Women are being sold the natural approach as though it is something tangible they can have—just as long as they follow advice, prepare for the big day, and avoid any unnecessary medical interventions that might derail this most desirable outcome. But no matter how good the birth preparation and no matter how ideal the birth setting, doctors and midwives are still only able to optimize women's chances of spontaneous vaginal birth—not to predict or guarantee them.

An injection of realism wouldn't go amiss sometimes. For example, it amazes us that in countries where millions of dollars are spent every year on treating chronic constipation, the same women who are incapable of experiencing the arguably straightforward physiological process of defecating each day are led to believe their bodies will just *know* how to give birth naturally, on their own. This is simply not true. Ethnicity, maternal age, and maternal weight have all been shown to affect the chances of spontaneous birth, for example, and to suggest otherwise or to ignore these facts is completely unhelpful in the management of women's expectations of labor. Equally, the irony in the concept of doing things completely naturally within obstetrics is inescapable. After all, how natural is it to ingest vitamins and extra minerals in doses far higher than the amounts usually acquired through normal diets (which women are advised to do by taking folic acid in early pregnancy) or to undergo various prenatal tests, screenings, and scans? These interventions have indeed been proven to be beneficial, but that does not make them natural. The determination to set the birth aside as something special or sacred that should not be tainted by any unnatural intervention is often difficult to understand.

That is not to say natural-birth advocates have got it all wrong. They haven't. And to be fair, they were right to campaign so vehemently against some of the medical interventions introduced during the twentieth century that were eventually proven not to be beneficial to laboring women (and were indeed identified by many professional medical bodies as detrimental): for example, 100 percent episiotomy rates, "twilight sleep" drugging with the mother strapped to the bed, and numerous unnecessary instrumental deliveries. And where cesareans are concerned, we fully understand the current unease about rising rates of unnecessary cesareans, and we recognize that there are legitimate cases where women feel coerced into having surgery and unsupported in their preferred birth choice, a trial of labor.

The term "trial of labor" is sometimes used in cases where there is reason to believe the woman might end up with a cesarean anyway—for instance, in cases of a previous cesarean (also called VBAC, vaginal birth after cesarean), but all attempts to deliver vaginally are essentially a trial of labor.

What we're saying is that just because cesarean rates are rising, this is not an indicator of a problem with *all* cesareans. Sure, some will be deemed unnecessary after the fact, and many more will be classified as unwanted by the women who have them, but ultimately, the continued increase in surgery has a great deal to do with "the difficulty of minimizing obstetric intervention rates in the face of high expectations for fetal outcome," a challenge discussed by Australian researchers in 2007.[1] Women are simply not very tolerant of risks to their baby's health.

You see, as much as women might think or say they want a natural or a normal birth, they only really want it if it is accomplished with a live, healthy baby at the end—and, as an added bonus, preferably not too much damage to their own body. Women who are able to accept the full-term stillbirth or death of their baby during delivery as a natural event, to be accepted as readily as the birth process itself, are a rarity in the twenty-first century. If things look like they're spiraling rapidly out of control, and their natural birth plan has unraveled irrevocably, the vast majority of modern women demand action and answers, and then, if it comes to it, compensation. Doctors know this and act accordingly.

CRITICISM OF MATERNAL REQUEST

At the very opposite end of the birth choice spectrum to the desire for no medical intervention at all is the desire for complete medical intervention with a planned cesarean before labor. Throughout this book, we argue the merits of a prophylactic cesarean at thirty-nine-plus weeks' gestation and provide strong evidence to support our view. In many quarters, however, there remains absolute disapproval of this birth choice and a relentless effort to impede women's legitimate efforts to exercise it. But how can this be happening, if the evidence in support of maternal request is so sound?

As we touch on in chapter 8, cesarean birth as a whole has long been viewed as a negative outcome (its lifesaving qualities aside, of course), with minimal regard for the differences between planned and emergency surgery. Moreover, maternal request has frequently been regarded in the medical literature as a mere myth. However, in more recent years, as it's become evident that women really *are* choosing cesareans with full knowledge of the risks involved, the focus of some critical opinion has begun shifting somewhat, from denying the existence of maternal request to condemning it roundly.

Worse still, it appears that in desperation to control the birth choices of women, critics of maternal request cesareans with no indication are even willing to resort to conformational bias in their research studies in an attempt to distort the truth—despite the fact that in some populations studied, planned cesareans have been shown to have the safest birth outcomes for babies *and* mothers.

Here is an example of the blatant bias against maternal request that exists.

RESEARCH BIAS

In February 2010, the *Lancet* published an article written by no fewer than twenty-three World Health Organization (WHO) researchers, of whom twenty are doctors, titled "Method of Delivery and Pregnancy Outcomes in Asia: The WHO Global Survey on Maternal and Perinatal Health 2007–08." Its aim was to look at the health outcomes of mothers and babies in light of delivery type in nine countries: Cambodia, China, India, Japan, Nepal, Philippines, Sri Lanka, Thailand, and Vietnam. Of a total of 1,515 planned cesareans with no medical or obstetrical reason that were studied, 1,352 of these took place in China, where maternal request rates are very high. The researchers concluded, "To improve maternal and perinatal outcomes, caesarean section should be done only when there is a medical indication."[2]

Needless to say, the article went viral. Virtually every media news outlet reported on it, and the blogosphere went into overdrive. The key message was this: further evidence shows that women who are "too posh to push" are not only endangering their own lives but their babies' too. And because the research came from the internationally recognized WHO, and appeared in a world-renowned medical journal, many journalists didn't read the full text of the article to check the facts for themselves. Pauline does know of one journalist who *did* read the study in full, and who *did* notice the same inaccuracies she did, only here the conformational bias plot thickens. When this reporter sought to write the story about how the WHO's figures did not tally with the article's conclusion, the reporter's editor prevented publication of the proposed article, and revisions more in line with the WHO's interpretations had to be hastily typed.

Fortunately, another journalist, Nigel Hawkes, who is director of the United Kingdom–based pressure group Straight Statistics, decided to write about the "Funny Figures from WHO" independently and again a few days later, in an article for the *Independent* newspaper titled "A Bad Case of Bias against Caesareans."[3] Hawkes's frustration at the quality of the WHO authors' interpretation of their data is palpable, and he calls their evidence of increased risks in cesareans with no indication "unconvincing." Here's why. In this particular population:

- *Not one* woman died following a cesarean with no medical indication.
- There were *no cases* of neonatal mortality in cesareans with no medical indication up to hospital discharge.
- Babies delivered by planned cesarean had a significantly *lower risk* of death than those born vaginally.
- Assisted vaginal delivery had a significantly increased risk of the mother dying.
- There were *no cases* of hysterectomy in mothers having a cesarean with no medical indication, although there were such cases in other birth types.
- For perineal tears of third and fourth degree, as expected, cesarean birth had a *protective* effect (frustratingly, the actual data for this are not shown in the survey).

Another fundamental failing of the article's conclusions (which Hawkes also points out) is the authors' decision to compare spontaneous vaginal births with planned cesarean births, thereby ignoring the crucial fact that not all planned vaginal births have spontaneous outcomes. Instead, they should have compared all planned vaginal birth outcomes with the outcomes of planned cesareans, since to ignore this fact misses the point of informing women at the planning stage of their birth.

And yet despite all the facts above, the authors decided to single out "the increased risk of maternal mortality and severe morbidity" in cesarean deliveries with no medical indication as the "most important finding of the survey."[4] Hawkes rightly asks, "Did none of the 23 think this an odd conclusion to have reached? Did no one check the arithmetic in the tables, which are full of errors? The *Lancet* is a distinguished journal—were its referees asleep?"[5]

Pauline decided to find out, and in June 2010, she lodged an official complaint with the *Lancet*'s ombudsman, questioning how its peer-review process could have accepted the WHO's article in its current state, containing as it did critical data and interpretation inaccuracies and blatant bias against one birth type. And in September 2010, the ombudsman, Dr. Charles Warlow, upheld Pauline's complaint. He wrote:

I will ask the *Lancet* to:

- Review their process of peer review
- Consider whether all reasonable (ie not libellous etc) comments on an article could be put up on their website and linked to the article in question
- Have another statistician look at this particular paper and proceed accordingly.

It is our understanding that this is the first time in its history the *Lancet* has had its peer review process formally criticized in this way. In December 2010, errors in tables 1 and 3 were corrected and a small change made to table 4; these were noted on its website.[6] The *Lancet* also commissioned a statistician to look at the paper and its peer reviews again and stated that it has been working on creating a website comment feature for some time. However, as of October 2011, and despite further communication throughout 2011, Pauline has received no further statement on the outcome of the statistician's investigations.

THE "BODY OF RESEARCH" AGAINST HIGH CESAREAN RATES

This is not the first time the WHO has been criticized, In 1985, its recommendation for a 15 percent cesarean rate threshold appeared in a consensus document (following a conference) titled "Appropriate Technology for Birth" alongside ideological statements that we contend have no place in evidence-based maternity practice. Here is some example text:

Obstetric care that criticises technological birth care and respects the emotional, psychological, and social aspects of birth should be encouraged. . . . Government agencies, universities, scientific societies, and other interested groups should be able to influence the excessive and unjustified use of caesarean section by exploring and publicising its negative effects on mother and infant.[7]

This is a real pity, or at least it's a real pity that this is what the document is best remembered for, because so much of the document contains advice and recommendations that are to be applauded—and that, unlike the 15 percent cesarean figure, are as relevant today as they were twenty-five years ago. For example:

Every woman has the right to proper prenatal care, and she has a central role in all aspects of this care, including participation in the planning, carrying out, and evaluation of the care. Social, emotional, and psychological factors are fundamental in understanding how to provide proper prenatal care. Although birth is a natural and normal process, even "no risk pregnancies" can result in complications. Sometimes intervention is necessary to obtain the best result.

It's interesting that although we've been able to move beyond other 1985 WHO recommendations that would be impossible to get women's approval of today (such as no maternal request epidurals: "During delivery, the routine administration of analgesic or anaesthetic drugs (not specifically required to correct or prevent any complication) should be avoided."[8]), we've managed to cling so steadfastly to the cesarean one.

And even when, in 2009, the WHO finally admitted it has no empirical evidence for recommending an optimum cesarean rate, disappointingly, its updated handbook left a contradiction in its wake, referring to a "body of research" in support of its unsubstantiated advice:

Although WHO has recommended since 1985 that the rate not exceed 10–15 percent, there is no empirical evidence for an optimum percentage or range of percentages, despite a growing body of research that shows a negative effect of high rates. It should be noted that the proposed upper limit of 15 percent is not a target to be achieved but rather a threshold not to be exceeded. Nevertheless, the rates in most developed countries and in many urban areas of lesser-developed countries are above that

threshold. Ultimately, what matters most is that all women who need caesarean sections actually receive them.[9]

Of course, the last line is most crucial here, but in terms of maternal
request, it is important to us that readers of this book understand what
comprises the WHO's "growing body of research" above, particularly
given that just six months later, WHO researchers were bending over
backward to discredit cesarean birth with no indication—in the face of
their *own data* showing the opposite to be true.

The WHO's handbook cites three medical studies next to the words
"body of research" in the quote above (Deneux-Tharaux et al.,[10] Villar
et al.,[11] and MacDorman et al.[12]), but although each of these selected
studies undoubtedly *does* demonstrate higher risks with cesarean births
(and remember, there are also other good studies that show no difference in risks but were not selected), the absolute risk for individual
women and babies is still very low and could be even lower if recommendations like those described in our chapter 13 are followed (e.g.,
antibiotics, thromboembolism prophylaxis, delivery at thirty-nine-plus
weeks' gestation, etc.). Without question, this narrow selection of
research is insufficient for informing the world's maternity policies,
although of course it provides natural-birth advocates with a very convincing quote to use.

But what's more interesting politically in all this is *why* the WHO
refers only to these three studies in particular. Why does it choose to
ignore another growing body of research that demonstrates favorable outcomes with planned cesarean births? Why is it so adamant that high
cesarean rates are a bad thing? And why is it willing to put its reputation
on the line by clinging to an increasingly unsupported ideology of what
constitutes appropriate rates of cesarean delivery?

We suspect the answer lies largely in the fact that the WHO is trying
to achieve the impossible. What it really wants, and quite rightly and
admirably, is to increase the rates of lifesaving cesarean deliveries in countries where cesarean rates are as low as 1 or 2 percent, where an increase
of just a few percentage points would translate into considerably fewer
deaths of mothers and babies. But understandably, all governments are
very sensitive to criticism, which means that the WHO must encourage
compliance as tactfully as it can. Otherwise, if a country perceives the

WHO's health targets as unrealistic or unachievable, it may have little incentive to strive toward them.

Politically, it also helps if perhaps more than one country, and more than one identifiable group of countries, is having its fingers rapped at the same time—those at the lower end of national cesarean rates *and* those at the higher end. This gives a collective sense that everyone needs to make improvements in their maternity services provisions (for example, in countries like Brazil, which has very high rates of cesareans, and where more research into women's birth autonomy, birth satisfaction, and attitudes to surgery and the female body would be useful), and the WHO has probably enjoyed this ability to straddle such drastically different worlds for a quarter of a century. Perhaps understandably—with its one-size-fits-all 5–15 percent cesarean range now successfully embedded in the international maternity psyche—it proved impossible in the end for the organization to completely refute its time-honored figure: "Both very low and very high rates of caesarean section can be dangerous, but the optimum rate is unknown. Pending further research, users of this handbook might want to continue to use a range of 5–15 percent or set their own standards."[13]

And so it chose instead to open a new, indeterminate range for countries that had obviously been complaining about the established recommendation, and at the same time, to continue to provide validation for countries (and natural-birth advocate groups) that still want to believe, and indeed pursue, the 1985 figure. As we have said, diplomacy is of great importance to the WHO. And this is OK. We wouldn't want to see the chances of improved maternity care in the developing world jeopardized either.

We just want it made clear to women in the developed world what is at play here, and for readers to understand that nothing about the reporting of cesarean delivery is as straightforward as it seems. Even within the WHO itself, where there are staff members with a natural-birth ideology and anti–maternal request agenda, there are also supporters of cesarean choice. In August 2008, a director of the WHO's Making Pregnancy Safer program told Pauline in an interview that he agrees maternal request cesarean is ethically justified following individualized consultation. He said, "A woman should have the right to decide. Why should she not have the right to decide? It should be an informed decision; the doctor needs to give the woman all the information she needs, and then the woman should decide whether she wants a cesarean section or she doesn't want a cesarean section."

But it seems that unfortunately for the WHO, more women are making this choice than it could ever have anticipated, especially in countries like China, but also in North America, Australia, and the United Kingdom. And not just maternal request with no indication, either. In births where medical or obstetrical indications *are* present, and women have the choice between a trial of labor and a planned cesarean, more women are choosing the cesarean in those circumstances. These women are then reported to have greater birth satisfaction than the trial of labor group, and you just have to ask yourself: if women are more satisfied, then why is so much time, energy, and effort being dedicated to trying to diminish this birth choice?

TOO MANY CESAREANS IN ONE WORLD, TOO MANY DEATHS IN ANOTHER

Instead, we feel it would serve more women and babies better if the world concentrated on the WHO's statement that "ultimately, what matters most is that all women who need caesarean sections actually receive them." The situation in the developing world, especially Africa, is absolutely appalling in places. Even women who are fortunate enough to survive childbirth are sometimes left with such devastating pelvic floor injuries that their lives are essentially ended. Leaking uncontrollable urine and/or feces, they lose all dignity and utility, and in this state, they are frequently disowned by their husbands and expelled from their community. They cannot work, have no sexual or reproductive value, and after being kicked out of their natural familial social net, they cannot even support themselves with prostitution.

Natural birth for these women is a disaster, leaving them to exist as some of the most miserable living things on this planet—and all because of the failure of an evolutionary system for human reproduction that cares nothing for individuals, depending on sheer numbers to ensure sustainability of a species regardless of how many die in the process and with no empathy for wrecked lives. Today's situation in parts of the world is no better than the general state of maternal and child health up to the Middle Ages, when women were dying in droves and often had to produce large numbers of children in early life (with not all of them surviving) in order to sustain populations.

As we argue in chapter 8, it would be more appropriate for the world's privileged societies to address the dangerously low rates of cesareans elsewhere with the same vigor that is being applied to managing our high rates. Rather than headlines that read "Too Many Cesareans!" we might see more that say, "Too Few Cesareans!" Yet instead, we have a situation where the WHO and many other researchers, medical professionals, and birth educators have become so focused on the negative aspects of surgery that sometimes they cannot see the forest for the trees.

UNNECESSARY CESAREANS

And what happens is this: the majority of doctors simply ignore the WHO's cesarean rate recommendation. They set their own standards and indeed did so long before being given permission by the WHO in 2009. But numerous birth advocacy groups take the exact opposite action: they publicize the 15 percent figure with a passion and use it as a stick to beat their respective doctors, hospitals, and governments with. Their efforts are in vain, of course—countries in the developed world will never again see such low national rates of cesarean delivery (unless something drastic happens that affects *all* types of healthcare provision)—but it is nonetheless frustrating and distracting.

You will frequently read about "unnecessary" cesareans, for example, but while we agree that there are cases in the United States and many other countries where cesareans might well be classified as unnecessary after the birth (and should indeed be investigated as such), the word *unnecessary* has now become politically motivated and is not the most constructive focus for ongoing cesarean debate.

Even legitimate investigations are often thwarted by unreliable birth records and subjective perspectives on the risks present before or during the birth, but fundamentally, the biggest problem with the "unnecessary" classification is that there is no effort to distinguish between cesareans that are wanted and those that are unwanted. The word *unnecessary* indicates something that in hindsight was avoidable, unwarranted, or inappropriate, but in fact, none of these adjectives fits the definition of a prophylactic cesarean chosen by an informed mother.

POLITICS OF DIVERSION

For some groups, even an acceptance of the fact that there are wanted cesareans is a step too far. So ingrained is it in their own consciousness that "natural" is birth's holy grail that it is virtually impossible for them to imagine that women without psychological problems could desire anything else. Pauline recalls attending a birth conference some years ago at which she was besieged at lunchtime by natural-birth advocates who were both genuinely perplexed by what she had said during the morning's open discussion and eager to help her realize there was really no need to elect for birth surgery—they could help. Pauline felt as though she was being perceived as some rare specimen of womankind (odd, since the whole conference was on the subject of maternal request) that simply required informing and somehow "fixing."

Of course, as we know, Pauline is not alone in her desire to choose a cesarean birth, and there is evidence in the United States that the number of women doing so is actually increasing all the time.[14] The big question now seems to be whether maternal request is having a discernable impact on overall cesarean rates. Answers from research vary; in Australia, for example, it is a resounding yes,[15] and the same is true in China,[16] while the United Kingdom remains unconvinced.[17]

The issue is that in an environment in which high cesarean rates are inherently viewed as bad, and in which it suits powerful birth ideologies to simply group all cesareans together (since this makes the risks appear worse), strategies to reduce this disturbing trend come way ahead of exploring whether such strategies are necessary in the first place. So deeprooted is the WHO's magic number of 15 percent that it is a brave doctor who dares to stick his or her head above the parapet and suggest that the country already has it just about right.[18] As Professor James Drife, a retired British obstetrician, told Pauline in an interview some years ago while he was still working in Leeds, "Most of us don't particularly like arguments, and the political attitude towards cesareans is driven by singleissue campaigners. Most of us get tired of debating endlessly with a point of view that will never change. In the end, we back away because it's a waste of time arguing. It's easier just to keep your head down."

But we are adamant that a blanket target of reducing a country's cesarean rate is, quite frankly, a ridiculous and risky method to adopt. We already know from litigation outcomes that sailing too close to the wind when deciding whether to transfer a laboring woman into the operating room can have disastrous results. But from the perspective of maternal request cesareans, when a healthy woman chooses planned surgery and has the best chances of a safe and satisfactory birth experience, how can it be ethical to deny her this choice?

The fact is, it's not ethical, but it *is* easy. Easier than figuring out practical ways to reduce the numbers of emergency or medically indicated planned cesareans, that's for sure. And so the public's attention is diverted from these messier matters and onto maternal request.

Consider this: to reduce rates of maternal request or to at least stop them increasing any further, you need to do just two things: inform women that it is such a perilous plan that the majority won't choose it in the first place, and say no to the few who do. But in contrast, to reduce the cesarean rates that have the worst health outcomes, cost the most financially, and are most likely to be unwanted, the process is far more complicated and extremely challenging. This is because encouraging overweight and obese women to lose weight prior to conception, for example, or urging more women to have their babies earlier in life is far easier said than done, as is discouraging risk-averse actions by obstetricians (for instance, instrumental intervention or urgent cesarean delivery when there is any hint of possible fetal compromise on any of the monitors) while also discouraging litigious action by bereaved families and their lawyers following unsuccessful planned vaginal births.

THE BLAME GAME

Another politically self-serving and easy method of diverting attention away from the problems inherent with planned vaginal birth, particularly in the maternal landscape that we have today (older, heavier mothers and bigger babies), is to point the finger of blame in a different direction. It makes great media headlines and has the potential to create heroes and heroines in the promotion of a better birth, but does the blame really help women in the long run?

First in the line of fire are doctors. We discuss this more thoroughly in chapter 10, but essentially, obstetricians are frequently painted as lazy, money-grabbing, self-obsessed, surgery-pushing, unethical monsters of the medical profession. They must be, to be doing all those cesareans! Of course, to suggest an entire group of healthcare professionals is in cahoots to purposefully carry out more cesareans is ludicrous, and indeed, this has been neither of our experience, personal or professional, of doctors. There may well be pockets of professional indiscretions, as in any medical specialty, but it is entirely inappropriate to tar everyone with the same brush.

In fact, we would go so far as to say that some groups, despite claiming to be advocates of women's choices, are actually endangering the choices of women when they indiscriminately attack the obstetric profession. This is because obstetrics is going through a not-insignificant crisis in recruitment and retention right now in many countries throughout the world. Young trainee doctors are choosing not to enter a specialty in which they will need to work unpredictable, unsociable hours; pay substantial, often unaffordable insurance premiums; and accept a 76 percent chance of being faced with litigation during their careers, all with the added bonus of being constantly criticized for making extremely stressful lifesaving decisions. While asking the question "Who Will Deliver Our Grandchildren?" in 2005, Dr. Alastair MacLennan and his coauthors underline this point with the words "It has never been safer to have a baby and never more dangerous to be an obstetrician."[19]

Next up is medical intervention. The overmonitoring of a perfectly natural process, the impatience of not waiting for a baby to come when it's good and ready, the acceptance of epidural pain relief when it's not *absolutely necessary*—these are just some of the interventions often blamed for contributing to rising cesarean rates. Never mind that medical intervention throughout pregnancy and birth—fetal scanning, fetal heart monitoring, pain relief, emergency surgery—has proven benefits for women, or that the risk of stillbirth increases in very late gestational ages. When it comes to trying to reduce cesarean rates, the worry is that often, all bets are off.

Then come celebrities. Or rather, society's slavish following of all things celebrity. Women who are "too posh to push" are corrupting the minds of other impressionable women, or so the accusation goes. If the likes of Kate Hudson, Britney Spears, Christina Aguilera, Ashlee Simpson, Victoria Beckham, and Elizabeth Hurley hadn't gone off and had irresponsible cesareans instead of giving birth *properly*, then other women wouldn't be so keen to do it either.

Aside from the fact that this accusation completely ignores that these celebrities most likely had individualized consultations with their doctors about their personal birth plan risks and benefits (the details of which we are clearly not privy to) and came to a joint decision that a cesarean would be the best option, it insults the intelligence of a whole group of women by suggesting that any part of their decision to choose a cesarean is grounded in some kind of celebrity copycat obsession.

That said, whether we like it or not, celebrities do have some bearing on how society acts, but in many ways, and certainly in the case of cesarean birth, the process can be rather chicken and egg. Yes, more celebrities may be having cesareans, but as we know, more women in general are having cesareans. So did the general population really follow a cesarean trend, or were the celebrity cesareans merely included within the more general trend? We think that initially, the latter was true, but that going forward, it is very possible celebrities' cesarean birth experiences will accelerate the general trend. To put this into perspective, a few years ago, when Pauline was first seeking a publisher for a book like this, she recalls being told by other authors that if she were a celebrity with this "new, controversial" message about birth, she would be signed up immediately. This came as no surprise because when it comes to the media and the public's attention, often it takes a celebrity to get a message across, which is why so many charities and charitable causes have famous ambassadors. Singer and actress Natalie Imbruglia, for example, is a spokesperson for the End Fistula campaign and has been very effective in publicizing this important issue. But as yet, no celebrity has spoken out in support of maternal request cesareans. However, it is likely to be only a matter of time.

Finally, women themselves are sometimes blamed for the rise in cesarean rates. The absence of sufficient motivation for a natural birth, a lack of trust in their own bodies, insufficient preparation for the birth, and an imperfect attitude toward the process of labor have all been cited as factors in unsuccessful outcomes. And when you look at the language of natural-birth educators, it is sometimes steeped in personal responsibility and accountability for what happens. For example, Suzanne Arms, founder-director of Birthing the Future, told us:

The knowledge of how to give birth without outside intervention lies deep within each woman. It's cellular knowledge, regardless of how she herself was conceived, her in-womb life, and her birth. Childbirth is as natural as pregnancy or sexuality. In fact, giving birth is very much a sexual process because it is governed by the hormones of sexuality. Like those natural biologically normal processes, what successful childbirth depends upon is an acceptance of the process, not allowing our thinking—and our fears—to inhibit it.

For many women, words like this are completely inspirational (and can help them during the birth), but again, this idea of "successful" versus "unsuccessful" can be damaging for others, especially when you consider that for the most part, women have very limited control over their birth experience. Yes, they can ensure that they are as fit, healthy, and mentally rehearsed for a trial of labor as possible, but beyond that, the idea of failure can be detrimental to many women who see birth as a first test of their ability as a mother. In fairness, natural-birth support groups and the language they use have evolved during a human history where for all but the smallest percentage of time, women risked pregnancy every time they had sex and risked death or serious injury every time they gave birth. Coping mechanisms, including those that involve having faith in the ability of our own bodies, undoubtedly have their place—they're just no longer applicable or indeed helpful in *all* births or for *all* women.

In an interview for Pauline's website in 2005, Dr. Samantha Collier, former executive vice president and chief medical officer at HealthGrades in the United States, said of this phenomenon:

> Natural birth is very cultural, and it's ingrained in us from when we are little girls about how we will do it. How many women have you heard of who end up in tears when they're told they're going to need a cesarean? Some women have a feeling of failure and think, "There's something wrong with me because I'm not giving birth in the way God intended." Women are a lot harder on other women than a man would be; a man's more likely to say, "Carry on, I don't mind which way you do it." But women have certain expectations of themselves and then have the same expectations of others.

This type of pressure, in our opinion, should be ignored. If *you* want to have a vaginal birth, then by all means educate yourself on how to make your experience a good one, but if you don't want one or are not yet sure, we would suggest that you try to ignore peer pressure and be prepared to challenge professional pressure; such pressures might not be relevant to you and your circumstances. And as we write about in chapter 5, unfortunately with doctors, what's good for the goose is not always good for the gander — meaning they may suggest a course of action for you that they would never choose for themselves. Or on the flip side of this, your doctor or midwife may merely want you to make the same birth choice as theirs. But remember, ultimately, your birth plan should be your choice and not someone else's.

POWER STRUGGLE

The problem is that while in many respects it can feel as though we've come a long way in terms of progress, improvements, and achievements in maternity care, the politics at play and the struggle to implement birth ideologies never truly go away. We discuss how different doctors have different attitudes and approaches to birth in our chapter "Doctors Who Support Cesarean Choice," and although many midwives and doctors with different views work amiably and successfully together, others are fundamentally at odds with each other in terms of birth management and perception of birth risks. For example, in Italy, 65 percent of midwives questioned said they considered the rates of cesarean delivery in their hospitals to be too high, compared with 34 percent of obstetricians, and in general, midwives were less inclined to believe in the existence of cesarean benefits for the mother.[20] In the same country just two years later, it was reported that two doctors came to physical blows while arguing over whether a cesarean was needed, and allegedly, the delay in surgery caused by their fight left the mother and baby in intensive care.[21]

But medical staff can also be far more subtle in their efforts to impose their personal opinion on others. Dr. Murphy recalls a situation in a Canadian hospital he worked at where an anesthetist apparently deliberately delayed attending to a woman who had planned a cesarean all through her pregnancy but went into labor slightly before her scheduled surgery date.

He accomplished this by simply being busy with other nonurgent and elective situations (for instance, inserting epidurals when there was time to wait) until it was too late. He effectively caused the woman's labor to progress so far that she was forced to go through a vaginal delivery against her wishes. The reason for this apparent deception? The anesthetist disagreed with the woman's birth choice and felt it was his right to refuse getting involved, but rather than coming out and saying so right away, thereby allowing another anesthetist to step in and help, he purposely stalled and wasted time in order to impose his own ideals onto this vulnerable patient. It is true that unless there is imminent risk to life or limb, doctors' personal ethics or beliefs allow them to withdraw from a course of action they don't agree with, and we are by no means trying to argue against that. However, in the event that a decision to withdraw is the result of such personal opinion or belief, then the doctor should declare it openly, allowing another doctor to step in.

Situations like this do little to serve as proper care for pregnant women, and indeed, researchers have highlighted the need for efforts to reconcile the differing attitudes of members of maternity staff after finding that obstetricians have completely opposing views to midwives and doulas when it comes to attitudes toward use of technology, concerns about the consequences of vaginal birth, and support for home birth.[22] We think women need to be aware of what's going on behind the scenes too, especially with the wide range of birth choices available today, because no matter which specialty of maternity care you turn to for advice, you need to realize that while they most likely have your best interests at heart, they cannot help but bring personal subjectivity into the mix. This is only natural to a certain extent, but what concerns us is when women are pressured to adopt a birth plan based on an incomplete or biased presentation of the facts.

(PERCEPTION OF) CHOICE

Perhaps understandably, advocates of natural birth do not want the facts about the safety of planned cesarean birth revealed, and in truth, many are simply unable or unwilling to accept the facts themselves. We have both had experience in hitting a brick wall during conversations with our professional peers, and given the research that has been brought to bear on planned cesareans even in the last five to ten years, it never ceases to amaze us when we hear statements like "You wouldn't elect to have a hip replacement if it wasn't medically necessary, so why would you choose to have a cesarean for no reason?" This particular example occurred at a meeting Pauline attended with UK health professionals whose role is to inform and advise the government on current maternity policy. This reaction is illustrative of how political birth ideology can be. It is our firm belief that many governments, policy makers, and health professionals are being given incomplete information about the risks and costs of planned cesareans, and this is why the idea that natural birth is best for all women pervades many societies. After all, if we're told enough times that a cesarean is a potentially dangerous killer, who on earth would ask for one, and just as important, who would respect the woman who did?

Leniency is awarded by some doctors if a woman is believed to have tokophobia (a severe fear of childbirth), but there are far too many cases in which even this maternal request is refused. Pauline is personally aware of two women who terminated their pregnancies when this happened (including one who, despite being made to go through rounds of counseling and cognitive therapy, was still unable to convince the person in control of her access to obstetric care—a person who probably only suggested these courses of action in an attempt to convince her to have a vaginal birth, rather than to establish the presence of genuine tokophobia), as well as scores of other women too frightened to become pregnant before confirming that they can have a cesarean. Interestingly (without our knowing whether the availability of a cesarean would have made any difference in her case), the award-winning actress Dame Helen Mirren has said one of the reasons she never became a mother was the fact that she was psychologically traumatized after watching an educational film on childbirth.[23]

Even when tokophobia is accepted as a legitimate reason for surgery, there can be a level of condescension involved that is unnecessary. For example, in a recent Dutch survey, doctors were said to be more willing to accept a maternal request if the woman had an "unfounded, but understandable" fear of birth.[24] The word *unfounded* is superfluous, in our opinion, since the risks associated with a planned vaginal birth are both real and significant, certainly no less than those associated with a planned cesarean, as we discuss in chapters 3 and 6.

Of course, this is where divisiveness rears its head again; there are groups that do not accept this point of view and may never do so. In 2009, Pauline sat down with the leader of the International Cesarean Awareness Network (ICAN, a high-profile birth group based in the United States) for the better part of an hour to talk to her about trying to work together toward genuine choice in childbirth for all women, including VBAC (vaginal birth after cesarean) *and* maternal request cesarean, but the outcome was disappointing. Although the discussion was very amicable, the ICAN leader said she felt strongly that she could never understand or accept a woman's conscious choice of surgery over a perfectly natural process. Similarly, at a previous conference, an activist for another birth advocacy group questioned Pauline about why on earth she would opt for the risks of surgery when natural birth was surely safer. But what emerged during this particular conversation was that this woman had undergone gastric stapling surgery for obesity, a procedure with a much higher risk of death than a planned cesarean, and yet the irony in her line of questioning was completely lost on her. The cognitive dissonance in the attitudes of some birth educators is astounding. Dr. Murphy, too, recalls a conference he attended in Toronto on maternal request cesarean birth, which was picketed by an angry mob of placard-wielding demonstrators — no doubt encouraged by the presence of the media's rolling cameras — forcing the conference participants to slink in through side doors to avoid unwanted confrontation.

Surely any birth support group that values *all* women would serve them better by being open to all different concerns and preferences? After all, how can someone argue for women being given access to a VBAC, with all its established risks but deny maternal request as a valid choice simply because risks exist? It makes no sense to us at all. You either advocate informed birth decision making, or you don't. There is no middle ground.

Birth autonomy should not be exclusive to those women whose choice fits within a prescribed ideology. It's so easy to say yes to the woman who plans a vaginal birth with her first pregnancy, but in fairness, why should lifesaving and life-protecting cesarean surgery be reserved for women who want a natural birth but are thwarted by the very natural challenges they encounter along the way? Isn't this a classic case of having your cake and eating it too? Laboring women should, of course, have access to emergency surgery; it's just the attitude that a cesarean birth should be made available *only* to those with a pressing pre-birth medical indication that we contest. Given what we now know about post-birth medical complications following planned vaginal births, women who want to avoid these possible adverse effects have no less medical *need* than anyone else. They're simply taking preemptive action in their birth choice.

FEWER CESAREANS, MORE COMPLICATIONS

We're conscious that we may be accused of the exact same thing we are accusing others of—that is, exaggerating the risks of one birth plan and underestimating the risks of another—but we will leave it up to you, the reader, to decide. All we would say is that we're not afraid of women choosing to have a vaginal birth, we have no preconceived ideas of what percentage of women might choose one birth or another, and we have no interest in campaigning against vaginal birth choices. If we sound defensive or angry at times, it's because the opposite is true of some people's views about cesarean choice, and this is blatantly damaging lives (this is no exaggeration, as the women who relay their experiences in chapter 7 will attest).

Too many doctors, midwives, and birth educators are not being honest with women. Their focus is on positive vaginal birth outcomes and coping mechanisms for when intervention is required. Describing truly negative examples or worst-case scenarios of what might happen with a vaginal birth is perceived as needless scaremongering, while warnings about cesarean risks of death, serious hemorrhage, or infection is standard fare. Even the language used to describe what might happen and the extent of risks during different births can sometimes be laden with subliminal messages. For example, we've seen forceps described as "'stainless steel salad servers' or 'large sugar-tongs' [that] . . . have curved ends to **cradle** your baby's head. . . . Once the forceps are in place, the doctor will **gently** pull while you push during a contraction" (our bold).[25] And a description of cesarean recovery states, "You may be **plagued** with gas pains from being opened, incisional pain, uterine contractions. . . . You may be **extremely** tired from medications, labor (if you had one), or just in general."[26] And a press release describing the location of a Humanization of Birth Conference that was held just days before the National Institutes of Health conference on maternal request in 2006 begins, "Monterrey, México is the conference site because Monterrey **suffers** from one of the highest rates of Caesarian birth in the world."[27]

But back in 2003, the company HealthGrades carried out research involving primary cesarean rates in almost two thousand hospitals in eighteen US states and found that in hospitals that did fewer than expected preplanned cesareans, there was an association with higher vaginal complication rates, and where the cesarean rate was higher than expected, there were lower rates of vaginal complications. The study authors concluded, "This finding is suggestive of, but not definitive of, inappropriate under-utilization of preplanned first time C-sections in those hospitals. This initial finding is significant, especially if it is correlated with pressure from national organizations to reduce C-section rates. Under-utilization of medically indicated C-sections may be related to poorer maternal outcome and thus hospital quality, which is counterproductive to the goals of a lowered national primary cesarean rate."[28]

They add that further studies may be needed to confirm these findings, and as we illustrate throughout this book, but particularly in our chapter on protecting the pelvic floor, the protective benefits of a planned cesarean in relation to vaginal complications have been confirmed in numerous other studies since. Yet the misplaced attempts by some groups to push the perceived superiority of vaginal delivery at all costs (instead of accepting that it has different, but no fewer, risks than a planned cesarean) continue. This is further compounded by misconceptions over the cost of each birth plan, and as we talk about in chapter 11, it is mothers and babies who suffer the consequences of all this birth politics, no one else.

THE BUSINESS OF BIRTH

On the subject of money, what would a chapter on politics be if we didn't talk about the green stuff a little? After all, pregnancy and birth is a period in most women's lives during which a lot of people stand to make a lot of money, and this truth is as natural as any other process that happens during this time, we assure you.

And yet the curious thing is that in some countries, the people who accuse doctors of wanting to make extra money from doing cesareans are the very same people who stand to lose money if women decide not to plan a vaginal birth. Speaking anecdotally, neither Pauline nor Dr. Murphy's wife attended birth preparation classes ahead of their planned cesareans; Pauline did actually try to sign up and pay for one on cesarean birth at her hospital but was told it had been canceled due to too few participants. But how many women can you think of who went into labor without first signing up for a series of (very often paid for) prenatal birthing classes where they could be told what to do and how to do it? Very few, we would imagine—despite the irony of us all being told that birth is such a normal physiological process we can trust our bodies to know what they need to do naturally.

But birth educators cost money. Doulas can cost money. Prenatal physiotherapy attempting to reduce pelvic floor injury costs money. Private one-to-one midwifery care costs money. In Alberta, Canada, for example, a midwife is paid more (on average) for the prenatal care and delivery of a woman than a doctor is in some provinces. And it doesn't stop there. In the business of birth, some of the larger, more powerful, or more popular birth support groups around the world request membership fees from women or receive funding from advertisers, and they develop relationships with mothers that extend far beyond that special nine-month window of time. Like it or not, natural birth has become a commercial enterprise. And there's a great deal more at stake in the debate over maternal request cesareans than many people realize. Certainly, there is a potential loss of revenue but also of face and of respect; remember that many medical and birth professionals have based their whole career on the premise that natural birth is superior to surgery and that surgical rates must be reduced. As a consequence, the business of birth has also evolved into a battle of birth.

This is because until relatively recently, safety has been king when it comes to birth. Quite simply, the unchallenged safest method of delivery was vaginal birth, which perfectly suited the ideology and teaching practices of many established groups and charities (and in fairness, cesarean surgery used to have a very high mortality rate). But then as surgical techniques continued to improve (e.g., anesthesia and infection control), and natural-birth challenges continued to increase (e.g., older, heavier mothers), the position of vaginal birth as the absolute safest delivery method began to be called into question. Initially, research challenged whether special birth circumstances (e.g., VBAC versus repeat cesarean and breech cesarean versus attempting to turn the baby) were better being managed naturally, and as medical opinion moved in favor of planned surgery, this forced a gradual move toward the language of choice in birth. Yes, there are increased risks with a breech presentation or VBAC, argued natural-birth advocates, but the risks are nevertheless relatively small, and a woman should be allowed to choose to accept these risks.

But now the circumstances of safer outcomes are moving into new territory, which could cause a political shift so scandalous that, as we have described above, there are those who are determined to do everything in their power to stop it. And that is this: the shocking possibility that even in perfectly healthy pregnancies, the balance of risks and benefits has now shifted so far that a planned cesarean birth at thirty-nine-plus gestational weeks is statistically safer than a planned vaginal birth. As abhorrent an idea as this may be to some readers, we truly envisage a time (indeed, in many respects, we believe we're already there) when the crown of safety will pass from vaginal to cesarean birth. And this is why we cannot understand the vitriol that exists toward maternal request; surely if what we predict turns out to be true, it would be better for birth advocacy groups to have been seen to embrace *all* women's birth choices and not just the ones that concurred with their own. Perhaps it's because in fairness, the battle to legitimize maternal request is still ongoing, and incredibly, almost five years after a National Institutes of Health conference concluded that the subject needs more research, we are yet to witness a study of full-term, cephalic (head-down) births that compares outcomes by intention to treat—in other words, two groups of women with healthy pregnancies, one taking the planned vaginal route and the other taking the planned cesarean group—and then assesses all outcomes (although recruitment by Dr. Stephen Robson for such a trial was reported in Australia this year[29]).

A MEDIA BEAST

And so the debate rages on (largely hampered by the absence of a controlled comparison), both in the consulting rooms and corridors of hospitals and in medical journals, media reports, and online chat rooms.

Because it's online communication that commands the most attention these days, we predict the inevitable sea change in attitude toward maternal request cesareans will have its roots there. In fact, it's already started. In a recent discussion thread in which a woman asked other mothers to relate their planned cesarean "Positives and negatives—your experiences please," she interjected the next day to write, "No one's having any negatives!" Mothers' comments included: "Wonderful. Calm, civilized, easy. Staff brilliant, quick recovery, can't fault it." "I always say it was the best decision I ever made." "It was the happiest day of my life and was very calm and pain free." "I have had 2 (by choice), both lovely. . . . Painless and very quick recoveries from both."[30] Of course, this does not mean no one has a bad outcome after a planned cesarean—it just illustrates that there are many happy women out there who made this choice. And Pauline has noticed an increase in the number of journalists who are beginning to question the anti-cesarean status quo (especially those who have interviewed her after having babies themselves, with positive cesarean and/or negative vaginal outcomes), which is important because only when enough journalists realize the truth will the message and attitudes really start to change.

In some ways, it's remarkable that we're not already there. After all, there have been numerous efforts over the years by activists and doctors, including Dr. Murphy, to redress the balance, not to mention the many medical studies we cite in our book that have demonstrated positive cesarean outcomes.[31] But time and time again, good cesarean news is barely reported. Data showing that mothers were least likely to die following a planned cesarean made it into just one British newspaper,[32] for example, while a study that categorically demonstrated a greater risk for urinary incontinence with spontaneous vaginal birth versus cesarean birth was given the headline "Choosing C-Section May Not Prevent Incontinence."[33] Why? Because only mothers who delivered *exclusively* by cesarean experienced a reduced risk. Yet even the slightest hint of bad cesarean news is picked up by the vast majority of media outlets and circulated widely.

One theory for why this happens came to mind while listening to the National Public Radio (NPR) *Fresh Air* program on August 4, 2008, when Dave Davies could be heard interviewing the author and journalist John Darnton about his new novel *Black and White and Dead All Over*. They began by discussing an incident in the novel based on real events, about which

Davies asks, "We've got somebody who has a wonderful story of a priest doing good works in the slums of Boston and you have the executive editor, Skeeta Diamond, shoot the idea down. Why?" Darnton replies, "Well, because, Skeeta Diamond says, 'You know, this is not the time for that kind of story. That's a positive priest story. We're in the midst of a scandal here, and to keep a scandal going, you have to feed the beast. You can't just let it die out by printing a story that goes against a scandal.'"[34] And perhaps the same is currently true of maternal request cesareans.

You see, mainly because of medical studies that compared *all* cesarean outcomes to successful vaginal births *only*, and despite being a lifesaver for millions of mothers and babies when nature failed, cesarean delivery earned the infamous title of riskiest birth type. It became, if you like, the media world's birth beast. As time went on, and newer studies began to separate planned and emergency outcomes, a new generation of beast evolved to take the title of most dangerous and most hated birth: the emergency cesarean. However, this beast proved a rather weak specimen, and although it still roams the media world, it was soon displaced from its position as number one beast. In its place, an even more bloodcurdling creature reared its ugly head: the maternal request cesarean had arrived.

As study after study highlighting risks for the mother and baby landed on media desks, hot steam soared out of keyboards as many reporters and bloggers typed, "Why would anyone choose surgery over natural means?" The beast roared even louder when it came to light that some of the women choosing surgery didn't even have a medical reason for it—no tokophobia, or presumed large baby, or perceived small pelvis—no, not a single one of the usual excuses. Accusatory adjectives and newly created labels to describe such women leaped from many an editor's indignant copy: "selfish," "dangerous," "uninformed," "celebrity copycats," "too posh to push."

Fortunately, individuals like ourselves set out to investigate the origins of this maternal request beast a little further and soon discovered it might be far tamer than first thought. We discovered that at thirty-nine weeks' gestation, healthy mothers planning a small family (including many mothers who were doctors) didn't find this method of birth any scarier than the others. Many actually found it less scary than the birth beast that had been around forever—vaginal delivery. Sure, the advice seemed to be that while this naturally occurring beast was once inescapable for all humankind, we now had the power to tame it. But these women remained unconvinced. They chose instead to cautiously befriend the new beast, maternal request, with the view that when it comes to pregnancy and birth, in theory at least, a beast is a beast is a beast.

In fairness to journalists, though, they've been on the receiving end of a powerful public relations effort on behalf of natural birth for decades. It is only relatively recently that those of us with a personal or professional reason for questioning how things stand or how they are being manipulated to appear have started pushing for greater transparency and accuracy in the medical reporting of birth data. Having witnessed truths being obscured, we now want to see studies being more carefully examined, more critically reviewed, and more judicially presented. And in order for everyone to do this, here are some questions that should be kept in mind when interpreting any birth study's data:

- Are emergency and planned cesarean outcomes separated or combined?
- Is successful spontaneous vaginal birth alone used as a comparison group?
- Does the planned vaginal birth group contain all eventual birth outcomes (e.g., assisted vaginal birth and emergency surgery)?
- Are the planned cesareans separated into those with and without medical or obstetrical indications?
- Are the planned cesareans separated into primary and repeat?
- If the cesareans are planned and without medical indications, are there specific data for thirty-nine-plus weeks' gestation?

In closing this chapter, we leave you with a final example of just how deep politics runs in the world of maternity healthcare—and the lengths some will go to in an effort to bury positive birth news that does not suit their particular agenda. Appearing in *USA Today* in April 2010, an Associated Press (AP) article reported that an editor at the *Lancet* had been pressured to delay publication of a University of Washington study that showed fewer women worldwide are dying in childbirth because it contradicted the much higher estimates of maternal death being presented at a public health funding meeting. Reportedly, United Nations health officials were seeking to raise money to save women's and children's lives in developing countries based on 500,000 women dying in childbirth every year, not the smaller number of 343,000 women stated in the study.[35]

That said, we suspect that in the case of suppressing positive cesarean birth news, politically motivated efforts to reduce surgery rates and promote normality are more to do with preserving a preferred ideology than raising the funds to get the job done.

A MATTER OF PERSPECTIVE

What we want to demonstrate here is that there are many perspectives involved—the physician, the pregnant woman, the hospital, societal and/or cultural bias—and that this whole area of controversy is hugely complex and relatively unexplored. What we do know for sure is this: the existence of planned, elective cesarean births is not a myth, and it is for the most part not being used to cover up unethical, self-interested obstetric practice. Pregnant women choosing a cesarean birth are not all vulnerable victims of a maternity machine that aims to make as much money in as little time as possible through unnecessary surgeries. That is not to say valid claims by women who say they were coerced into cesarean surgery should not be heard; of course they should. But equally, there is a need for acceptance and understanding of the growing number of women who *want* a cesarean birth, many of whom are educated, articulate, determined, and confident about their obstetrician's ethical and moral compass when it comes to their baby's birth.

The moral high ground is a chimera. The panorama is completely different depending on your perspective.

Chapter 10

Before They Say It:
We Answer Our Critics

*Every man has a right to his opinion, but no man has a right to
be wrong in his facts.*
                                        —Bernard M. Baruch (1870–1965)

Almost all books on birth depict vaginal delivery as the most valid, natural, or correct way to bring a child into this world. At best, any deviation from this birth outcome is described as an unfortunate or regrettable turn of events—one to be coped with or consoled about. At worst, it is decried as an unnatural, abnormal, medicalized birth performed by interventionist and financially motivated physicians. Similarly, the maternal decision in a perfectly healthy pregnancy to have a planned, elective cesarean birth is often condemned as the irrational thinking of a deluded, scared, or selfish woman whose birth choice risks endangering the life of her unborn child. And just in case insulting her motherly instinct fails to make the point strongly enough, the critics then change tack and target the woman's sense of self-preservation by explaining how dangerous the procedure is for her and how she is putting her own life at risk. It is almost as if, having established that such a woman is too selfish to listen to grave predictions regarding her baby, these critics decide she might listen to good sense if her own self-interest is threatened. Derogatory phrases such as "too posh to push," and "yummy mummy" have their origins in this environment of thinking and are emblematic of the myriad misconceptions and half-truths surrounding the perfectly legitimate decision to request a cesarean birth.

The fact of the matter is that many natural-birth advocates are themselves guilty of misinformation, bias, and an ideology and perceived reality that are not borne out by the facts of twenty-first-century medicine. Indeed, some of the more extremist natural-birth ideals in existence are potentially more dangerous to the unborn child than a scheduled cesarean birth at thirty-nine-plus gestational weeks. But the aim of this chapter is not to attack other birth choices; it is to defend the choice of a planned cesarean.

Sometimes we get the impression that the emotional reaction to maternal request cesarean by its critics has more to do with personal bias and fear, rather than with the actual arguments for and against it. It is almost as if some of the vehement opposition comes from not only the reluctance to question their own birth choices but also from the fear of losing control over others' birth choices and the fear of being proved wrong. You see, with no choice between vaginal and cesarean, if things don't work out with a planned vaginal birth, there is an ego-preserving security that "it was meant to be"—it was the natural course of events. An example of this fear of positive cesarean outcomes appeared in an article in the *Times-Picayune* of New Orleans titled "More Women Ask for Caesareans," in which a doctor reportedly asks, "Where is this heading? There's no control. I think it's heading to a day when a woman's going to come in and say, 'I don't want to have a vaginal delivery. I want a cesarean section,' and we won't have strong enough data to say, 'It's not in your best interest.'"[1]

Fortunately, in contrast to the sometimes emotional denial that a planned cesarean might be a good choice for some women, academic discussions, research papers, and conference summaries have lately become decidedly less dogmatic. There are hundreds, if not thousands, of peer-reviewed articles that touch on one or more aspects of a planned cesarean birth, either stating that there is a lack of good data to say which birth method is best or confirming that a maternal request or non-medically indicated cesarean might be a safe, valid, or appropriate alternative to a trial of labor. And meanwhile, in a direct reflection of these contemporary views on surgical birth, and regardless of the debate raging around them, increasing numbers of doctors and expectant mothers are voting with their feet—straight into the operating room. Female readers of this book may be assured, if you are considering choosing a cesarean, that while it is still a minority choice, you are certainly not alone in this request. And if, like many of the women we have heard from, you find your decision coming under attack from family, friends, colleagues, medical staff, and even strangers, we hope you'll be able to draw on some of the counterarguments we present here in defense of the most common criticisms of cesarean birth we've encountered.

A PLANNED CESAREAN . . .

. . . is more dangerous for your baby
. . . increases your risk of stillbirth in a subsequent pregnancy
. . . affects your future fertility
. . . limits your family size
. . . affects your likelihood of successful breastfeeding
. . . puts your baby at greater risk for asthma and allergies
. . . is more dangerous for you, the mother
. . . could increase your chances of developing depression
. . . does not protect against damage to the pelvic floor (e.g., incontinence or prolapse)
. . . does not protect against painful intercourse and sexual dysfunction
. . . is not natural or normal — vaginal birth is
. . . costs society more than vaginal birth
. . . (on maternal request) is a myth created by greedy obstetricians who desire to earn more money and make their lives easier
. . . (on maternal request) is dangerously contributing to rising rates of unnecessary cesareans

1. *A Planned Cesarean Is More Dangerous for Your Baby*

Not true — as long as your baby is not delivered before thirty-nine weeks of gestation.[2] There has been a great deal of research in this area, and the guideline on gestational age is the most consistent finding on planned cesarean safety. If your baby is delivered before this date, it has an increased risk of respiratory distress. Therefore, it is vital to keep a note of the date of your last menstrual period and to have an early ultrasound scan, both of which will improve the accuracy of calculating your baby's gestational age. It is also important that you don't try to stretch the boundaries of safety just a little bit this way or that;[3] perhaps you want to accommodate your visiting grandma, your partner's work, or something similar. You may feel like you've had enough of being pregnant and want it to be over with. But it is *not* a good idea to compromise on this issue. If you and your baby are healthy, you and your doctor should schedule surgery *after* thirty-nine weeks' gestation.

We go into more detail on the subject of comparable safety in chapter 3,

"The Safest Birth Choice for Your Baby," but in brief, excluding cesareans that are undertaken prior to thirty-nine weeks' gestation, there is now good evidence that a planned cesarean at full term is safer for babies than a planned vaginal birth.[4] This is mostly because of the risks involved when a planned vaginal birth does not result in a healthy, spontaneous birth outcome. Assisted vaginal birth (forceps, vacuum, or both) and emergency cesarean both introduce greater risks for babies, such as asphyxia, trauma, intracranial bleeds, and shoulder dystocia.[5] A planned cesarean reduces these risks significantly, and this is why, contrary to the criticism above, planned cesarean birth is safer for your baby at full term (thirty-nine-plus weeks).

2. A Planned Cesarean Increases Your Risk of Stillbirth in a Subsequent Pregnancy

This fear-provoking association has been proven erroneous in relation to a planned cesarean birth. In 2003, a highly publicized study suggesting that cesarean birth in the first pregnancy could increase the risk of unexplained stillbirth in the second was published in Britain,[6] but this was subsequently eclipsed by other, larger studies. For example, Canadian researchers found no difference (in a study population of almost 160,000 women) in the incidence of stillbirth between those who had a prior vaginal or a prior cesarean birth (0.27 percent versus 0.3 percent).[7] And newer British research discovered that the increased risk of stillbirth with prior cesarean delivery was "mainly concentrated in the subgroup of explained stillbirths," not the unexplained ones, which is a very important distinction.[8] Likewise, of eleven million births analyzed in the United States, the stillbirth rate was recorded as 0.13 percent with a prior cesarean and 0.15 percent with no cesarean.[9] So evidently, in both groups, the chance of this tragic outcome was equally small, and importantly, no causal relationship was found in either. From these examples alone, it is clear that subsequent stillbirth is not a specific risk for women choosing a cesarean birth plan.

On the contrary, as discussed in chapter 3, by looking at the data, researchers have concluded that if all babies were born no later than thirty-nine weeks' gestation, this could prevent six thousand babies dying in the United States every year.[10] This is not meant as an argument in favor of a blanket policy of cesarean delivery in all pregnancies (as we keep reminding readers, it is not our intention to advocate that all women should choose a cesarean birth plan, only that the prophylactic nature of this plan is wholly justified), but it does highlight how outrageous claims are that a planned cesarean increases the risk of stillbirth, when in fact it could actually reduce the risk. What might be useful is for pregnant women to be made more aware of other reported risk factors for an increased threat of stillbirth (both in primary and subsequent births), which include obesity,[11] babies who are small for their gestational age,[12] ethnicity,[13] short inter-pregnancy intervals, low socioeconomic status,[14] exposure to tobacco smoke in utero,[15] live preterm birth, fetal growth restriction, preeclampsia (pregnancy-induced high blood pressure), abruptio placenta (separation of the placenta from the uterine wall),[16] advanced maternal age, shorter maternal height,[17] and congenital anomalies.[18] Some of these factors are quite preventable, or are at least modifiable.

3. A Planned Cesarean Affects Your Future Fertility

There has long been a question mark over the likelihood that secondary infertility is directly related to cesarean birth.[19] Researchers have for many years pointed toward other possible issues—such as birth experience (positive versus traumatic),[20] social or psychological (as opposed to pathological) problems,[21] emergency surgery,[22] and voluntary decision making[23]—that might be considered more influential on subsequent fertility than the cesarean surgery. Yet amazingly, the myth continues to persist that planning a cesarean could jeopardize a woman's chance of a successful second pregnancy.

So where does this accusation come from? First, it became noticeable to some people (often anecdotally) that many women who either chose a cesarean birth or planned one for a variety of other reasons did not go on to have another baby. Second, there were women whose first cesarean birth resulted in a hysterectomy, and although the vast majority of these occurred during emergency surgeries (essentially outcomes of planned vaginal births), in studies where all cesarean data are merged, these data have been used to demonstrate infertility in subsequent pregnancies with planned cesarean birth.

However, these are the facts:

- There is no link between a planned cesarean birth and a woman's subsequent ability to conceive, as demonstrated in the conclusions of a substantial body of medical evidence.[24]
- Women who are currently most likely to request a planned cesarean birth are slightly older than average and are planning to have only one or two children anyway. Added to which, as women age, fertility problems are more common, as is the use of reproductive technologies,[25] and therefore, increasing age is more likely to affect an older woman's subsequent fertility than the delivery method of her first birth is.
- Fertility rates, regardless of delivery method, are very low in the developed world. In North America, Australia, and Britain, the fertility rate is two children or fewer, and in Europe, too, rates have diminished and large families are declining.
- Due to the increased risks associated with multiple surgeries, the advice given to all women choosing a cesarean birth is to plan only a small family; hence, some women will choose to have only one child for this reason.

4. A Planned Cesarean Limits Your Family Size

This argument is absolutely true—not necessarily physically, but certainly in the interests of good judgment and safety it is. This is because the risks of cesarean birth (both emergency and planned, in this case) definitely increase with successive surgeries, both for you and for your baby, and these are discussed in more detail in chapter 13, "The Risks of Planning a Cesarean." Briefly, though, it is important to be aware that these surgeries put a limit on how many children you can reasonably expect to have before the risks increase to unacceptable levels.[26] And while a small minority of women do have large families born via cesarean delivery with very healthy outcomes, the vast majority of evidence maintains that family size must be seriously considered by women during their planned cesarean risk-benefit analysis.[27] We support the guidance that maternal request is reasonable or logical only for a woman who has made a commitment to having a small family, and in our view, this means preferably only one or two, and certainly no more than three.

5. *A Planned Cesarean Affects Your Likelihood of Successful Breastfeeding*

This rather sneaky attack on women who want to choose a cesarean birth plays on their feelings of insecurity and guilt. "You are a bad mother!" it implies. "You are *choosing* to reduce your chances of successful breast-feeding." Well, relax. It is simply not true, and in fact, there is evidence that your longer hospital stay (surrounded by experts to help you if you need it) could even help your chances of successful breastfeeding.[28] Also, the breastfeeding specialists, La Leche League International, have stated that breastfeeding and bonding are not adversely affected by a planned cesarean birth.[29] There *are* some documented issues with how quickly and how much milk mothers' bodies produce after cesarean surgery (which we talk about in chapter 4), but fortunately, any such issues appear to be short-lived. More important, though, it's essential to point out here that not everyone wants to breastfeed their baby, and sometimes it is not possible regardless of delivery method. All we want to do is to reassure women that a planned cesarean is neither a contraindication nor a hindrance to breastfeeding.

6. *A Planned Cesarean Puts Your Baby at Greater Risk for Asthma and Allergies*

There is indeed some concern that cesarean-born babies are more prone to asthma and allergies later in life (including during childhood). But although this has admittedly been the finding of some studies,[30] it has not been a consistent finding; other studies and reviews dismiss or question the idea of a causal association with birth method,[31] and there is even the possibility that planned cesarean delivery might actually lower the risk of asthma.[32] Obviously, each study has its merits and limitations, but certainly the inconsistency of the overall findings makes us wonder whether the apparent association is real. We believe the observation is most likely incidental and has no real causality — and not simply because it suits our argument, as some readers might suspect.

First and foremost, the fundamental problem with most of the studies we have on asthma, allergies, and cesarean birth is their inclusion of mixed cesarean data — emergency surgery, planned surgery for medical or obstetrical reasons (often performed earlier than the recommended thirty-nine-plus gestational weeks, so the lungs are not yet fully matured and the risk of newborn breathing difficulties is greater), and planned maternal request surgery with no such reasons. Obviously, the first two of these cesarean types are inherently riskier than the latter, and the second type, which often involves premature delivery, has a well-established connection with respiratory illness.[33] In our opinion, the inclusion of this mixed bag of data leads to some of the biggest misunderstandings about planned cesarean outcomes, of which asthma and allergies may well be one. It is *all* pregnant women who should be warned of the potential risk of asthma and allergies, including those who plan to give birth vaginally, because this risk is actually applicable to all birth methods. That said, if indeed it is ever proven beyond reproach that a planned cesarean increases the future risk of a child developing asthma or allergies, then we would still regard it as a factor to be considered during an individual woman's overall risk-benefit analysis. Given the established risks that already exist for babies born vaginally or via emergency cesarean surgery (which include greater risk of death and serious morbidity, for example), we do not presume that the likely risk of asthma and allergies would present the ultimate motivation for planning a vaginal birth instead—at least not for all women.

7. A Planned Cesarean Is More Dangerous for You, the Mother

This reproach is certainly not the case if you stick to the small-family rule already mentioned, but it is also not necessarily true if you compare women's health outcomes as they relate to their original birth plans, not just to their birth outcomes. This is because an emergency cesarean, for example, is usually an outcome of a planned vaginal birth. Obviously, the greatest danger for women giving birth is death, and when it happens, it is an especially shocking and devastating experience for the individual family concerned. But fortunately, it is a relatively rare occurrence in the developed world, and this is because, despite oft-coined phrases such as "women have been giving birth since the beginning of time" and "it's the most natural thing in the world," it can sometimes be very easy to forget just how inexorably linked birth and death have always been and just how many lives have been saved through cesarean surgery. Instead, we read opinions that draw a connection between rising cesarean rates and high rates of maternal mortality—and worse, suggest that women choosing cesarean births may be putting themselves at risk. In fact, data on maternal deaths have shown that women are *less likely* to die following a planned cesarean birth than any other delivery type,[34] and that being over-weight, obese, or very poor is much more likely to significantly affect your risk of death.[35] Similarly, it's actually been shown that when compared with a planned vaginal birth, a planned cesarean can have less morbidity too; it just sometimes means a longer hospital stay after the birth. For example, women recovering from planned cesareans have considerably fewer cases of chorioamnionitis (an infection inside the uterus), post-partum hemorrhage, uterine atony (relaxed uterus muscle, a risk for postpartum hemorrhage), and prolonged rupture of membranes, with no difference in transfusion rates.[36] So, with life-threatening maternal mor-bidity being *similar* in each birth plan group,[37] the cesarean is not neces-sarily safer, but it's not more dangerous either.

That's not to say there are no dangers for women planning a cesarean birth. There are, absolutely. The risks associated with surgery are unequivocal, and just like those of almost every other surgical procedure, they increase with each repeat procedure. We explore all these in more detail in chapter 13, "The Risks of Planning a Cesarean," but for now, we're simply answering the claim that a planned cesarean is categorically more dangerous for women than a planned vaginal birth, which it is not.

8. A Planned Cesarean Could Increase Your Chances of Developing Depression

You might ask, "Who wouldn't be depressed if for nine whole months (maybe even longer) you'd planned to have that perfect, self-affirming nat-ural birth, only to end up with a rushed, impersonal, frightening, and dis-orienting change in plans, possibly in the middle of the night and after hours and hours of labor?" Without question, an emergency cesarean is no fun; it's worse still if it follows unsuccessful attempts at assisted vaginal birth with forceps, vacuum, or even both. When this happens, you end up with double the wounds (vaginal *and* abdominal—and the latter made worse because it's emergency surgery rather than a pre-labor, planned event), double the pain, and double the recovery process, not to mention the associated psychological trauma that may include feelings of anger, guilt, shame, inadequacy, or blame.[38] Compare this with a woman who's elected long before her due date to have a cesarean. She's had time to prepare and research, and she knows almost to the hour when her baby will arrive. During the birth, she is able to be completely in the moment to welcome her baby into the world, and she feels happy that her birth plan has been successful (especially since this was her choice). So, two cesarean births, but two completely different sets of emotions at the end. Importantly, we're not dealing here with the entity of clinical postpartum depression—a real and serious disease that can affect any new mother, regardless of delivery type—but we are addressing the argument that women are more likely to regret or feel depressed after a planned cesarean. This is simply not true, and the research is on our side. If things work out as planned, most women will be happy.[39] If they don't, the risk of dissatisfaction is greatly increased.[40] This is outlined in greater detail in chapter 4, but basically, given the statistical risk of assisted vaginal birth and/or emergency cesarean for women who plan a spontaneous vaginal birth, the overall highest chance of general satisfaction has to be with planned cesarean birth, and even more so when it's on maternal request.[41]

9. A Planned Cesarean Does Not Protect against Damage to the Pelvic Floor

This is probably our greatest point of defiance when it comes to countering many of the commonly held misconceptions about cesarean birth. Absolutely, we believe that a planned cesarean offers protection for the pelvic floor, and we have devoted an entire chapter to explaining why. Yes, it is always possible for critics of cesareans to present examples of women who have had no children, or have had only cesarean births, and yet *still* developed incontinence, prolapse, or some other pelvic floor disorder. In fact, two of the most famously cited studies used to support this point involve research with 149 nuns (evidently, no children involved, and also no or limited sexual activity) and 101 pairs of sisters (where one sister had given birth and the other had not). Both studies found no increased risk of urinary incontinence following childbirth.[42] However, what you don't necessarily hear about these studies is that they assessed *only* urinary incontinence—there was no mention of other pelvic floor disorders such as fecal incontinence or pelvic organ prolapse, for example—and more important,

vaginal birth causes even more damage, many relationships suffer. And as controversial as this may be, we suspect at least some instances of marital infidelity have a lack of sexual satisfaction following vaginal birth at their root. Unfortunately, this theory has elicited little attention from researchers, and this could partly be because the link between vaginal birth and infidelity is largely unrecognized and probably vociferously denied. After all, it is one thing for a woman to admit that less sex or less enjoyable sex has led to her partner's infidelity—this brings with it an element of shared responsibility between the couple having sex—but if she acknowledges that changes to her vagina were involved, this shifts more of the responsibility onto her (or worse, onto their baby). And even if a link *were* to be sufficiently proven (through anonymous surveys with men), society in the main would likely have little, if any, empathy with these men and nothing but sympathy for their wives and partners.

But before this counterargument to the critics becomes too bleak a portrait of post-birth sex, we would stress that even when vaginal damage does affect couples' sex lives, for most couples it is not a problem and most certainly does not lead to infidelity or any sexual dysfunction. Lest we forget, love is a powerful thing and not to be underestimated. We also acknowledge there is evidence of little or no difference in postpartum sexual function between a cesarean birth and a vaginal birth where there has been no significant damage.[53] The problem lies in the complete inability to predict who will sustain damage and who will not, and this unknown quantity remains an important element of some women's risk-benefit analysis. Once a woman knows instrumental vaginal births are associated with the highest rate of long-term sexual dysfunction for women and their partners, and planned cesarean births are associated with the lowest rate,[54] is she prepared to take that risk? And is her partner? Perhaps the answer depends on each woman's own personal attitude to sex before pregnancy and the priority she places on trying to ensure she has no physical changes afterward—and this answer won't be the same for all women. But whatever a woman's perception, decision, or outcome is, we are, having read the body of research on this subject, unwaveringly convinced of two things: one, since sexual problems are so common after having a baby, they need more research and attention than they currently receive,[55] and two, while there are undoubtedly many reasons for decreased sexual function in a woman's life, a planned vaginal birth introduces greater risk to a woman's future sexual enjoyment than a planned cesarean.

11. A Planned Cesarean Is Not Natural or Normal, Vaginal Birth Is

This accusation is more annoying than it is offensive; aside from being rude to women by implying their cesarean birth choice is unnatural or abnormal, it in no way reflects the reality of vaginal birth as it exists in the developed world today. Moreover, it puts vaginal birth on a pedestal that, quite frankly, is not all it's cracked up to be. The fact is that natural or normal delivery in its truest sense means squatting under a bush and hoping the baby comes out alive to a mother who has survived the experience—not something we imagine the majority of women would want to emulate in a contemporary birth plan. Indeed, planned vaginal birth in modern hospitals (where more than 95 percent of women choose to give birth) is as far removed from natural or normal as modern anesthesia is from being hit over the head with a club. Why? Because women are surrounded by a team of health professionals who are ready to intervene at the first sign of problems with a variety of medical apparatuses and techniques at their disposal (e.g., fetal monitoring, forceps, vacuum, twenty-four-hour emergency operating room). Even home birth advocates have to admit the technological availability of dialing 911 to summon emergency ambulatory transfer to the hospital provides a welcome addition to the often unreliable presence of Mother Nature alone.

The trouble is, in our world of branding and marketing, as we discuss in chapter 9, the word *natural* has developed an association (quite rightly in most contexts) with very positive and healthy lifestyle choices—for example, the food we eat, the exercise we do, and the materials we use. Turning our backs on processed, synthetic, or artificial alternatives to everything from food to body parts has led to an almost aspirational desire for more natural ingredients and methods and to disdain for those who choose the easy, lazy, or unhealthy option. But natural *birth* is different. It is an extremely challenging and potentially dangerous endeavor, and there are millions of women in the developing world who would give anything to have access to our levels of "overmedicalization" and "unnatural" birth methods—since it means they'd have fewer deaths and devastating fistulas.

But that's not to say that women should be advised against natural birth, not at all. They should just be given an honest appraisal of what it might involve and the real likelihood of when and why medical intervention may become necessary, based on an individualized consultation. Phrases such as "Birth is a normal, physiological process" and "Your body will know what to do" are less than helpful in prenatal consultations with a forty-year-old woman, with a woman with a BMI of thirty-two, or with a woman with a familial history of birth trauma that includes severe morbidity and mortality, for example. In fact, it is the irresponsible rhetoric by some natural-birth advocates that fuels the feelings of disappointment, despair, and dissatisfaction in so many women whose planned vaginal births fail to live up to their expectations. Yes, some women will enjoy a spontaneous vaginal birth, but if this is in a hospital, it doesn't mean it is "natural"; it simply means they didn't need access to any of the emergency medical facilities available. And in terms of whether or not it's "normal," we think that depends on your personal perception of what's normal and what's not—something that in all walks of life can differ from person to person, family to family, and country to country. Therefore, since the meanings of the terms *natural* and *normal* remain problematic, illusory, and contentious, we propose that they should not be reserved for the exclusive use of vaginal birth. Rather, it should be acknowledged that while vaginal birth is natural and normal for some women, cesarean birth is natural and normal for others.

12. A Planned Cesarean Costs Society More Than Vaginal Birth

When you compare two births in which one woman has a spontaneous vaginal delivery and another woman has a scheduled cesarean delivery, and in both cases, there are no adverse health complications for the baby or the mother, then the cost of the cesarean birth is greater. Unfortunately, real-life birth plans and outcomes for each of these delivery methods are far more complicated than this, as we explore in far greater detail in chapter 11, but in short, establishing which birth type costs more depends on what information is included in comparative models and how individual countries' maternity systems are set up.

Regarding the cost of planned cesarean birth on maternal request, for example, the vast majority of current estimates are flawed, since they include costs from planned cesareans with medical or obstetrical indications (thus, cesareans that *must* be done for a specific reason, often at a premature gestation) and/or emergency cesareans. But more crucially, these cesarean costs are then compared with vaginal birth estimates that repeatedly fail to include the financial impact of

a) *all* planned vaginal birth outcomes, including spontaneous and assisted vaginal births *and* emergency cesareans,
b) the short- and long-term care of all babies injured during these births,
c) all short- and long-term perineal and pelvic floor repairs, as well as any posttraumatic birth counseling that is needed for the mother, and
d) the colossal litigation bills in cases when things go wrong and the baby or mother (or both) is injured or dies.

It goes without saying that there are potential short- and long-term costs associated with maternal request cesareans too; it is, after all, abdominal surgery for the mother, and for the baby, the possibility of inaccurate gestational age measurement always poses a risk for respiratory problems. However, it seems unlikely that these associated costs are considerably higher than those listed for vaginal birth, similar to what we're increasingly finding in terms of health outcomes. In most cases, it is the complications of emergency cesareans and the medical or obstetrical problems necessitating the cesareans in the first place that add significant expense to the cesarean account, while the vaginal birth account is kept misleadingly clear of costly complications. If the comparison of birth plans is fair and true—taking account of *all* outcomes and costs—then it is no longer correct to assume planned surgery is necessarily the more expensive route.[56]

13. *A Planned Cesarean on Maternal Request Is a Myth Created by Greedy Obstetricians Who Desire to Earn More Money and Make Their Lives Easier*

One of the most common accusations made in trying to explain rising cesarean section rates is that unethical doctors, and specifically obstetricians, are responsible. The premise is that obstetricians are essentially greedy and selfish, performing unnecessary cesareans in pursuit of personal gain. It's a crude attempt to smear one of the noblest of medical professions, which we find very distressing.

First Accusation: Greed

"Obstetricians are motivated by money. They can charge more money for a cesarean, write it up as 'elective,' and thereby unethically carry out more cesareans than are absolutely necessary."

In answer to this charge, to begin with, of course physicians don't want to (and shouldn't) work for free, and yes, of course there are bad apples in every walk of life. But to suggest that an entire obstetrical profession is in cahoots in some conspiracy to rob women of childbirth because of monetary reasons is unfair. Let's look at the facts. Professional incomes vary from country to country, and even within countries, there are many different models of physician remuneration. We will certainly concede that if any jurisdiction puts a financial premium on cesarean birth versus vaginal birth, then that is obviously a concern and should be corrected or at least investigated to ensure it is not being abused.[57] However, this is something practicing doctors almost never have any control over. Also, in many countries, and even in the United States, many obstetricians are paid a fixed salary, which means that regardless of how they deliver babies in their care, their pay remains exactly the same.

One monetary incentive that we *would* agree is occurring—at least in obstetrical practices where the doctor making delivery decisions will personally feel the financial brunt of any subsequent litigation claims—is the influence of lawsuit fears and rising insurance premiums. It is no secret that the cost of liability for obstetricians is the highest of *any* specialty in many countries, and indeed, fear of litigation is frequently cited—and criticized—as an important contributor to rising cesarean rates. As you might expect, ideas for a strategy to remove litigation from the decision-making process are in far fewer supply (but isn't that often the case with criticism?). In countries with universal or socialized medical health systems, public-sector doctors and hospitals are less encumbered by litigation fears, at least in terms of the ensuing financial impact. In Britain, for example, a special public body, the National Health Service Litigation

Authority (NHSLA), was founded in 1995 to deal with the litigation purse strings separately from the rest of NHS funding. And Canada has a universal insurer for doctor indemnity; although doctors are individually invoiced according to specialty, the final amount they have to pay is highly subsidized by the provinces. But in the United States, where such universal systems don't exist, some states cannot even employ enough obstetricians because of the litigation issue, and in many more, obstetricians have to pay hundreds of thousands of dollars in liability insurance every year.[58] Essentially, for many doctors having to pay indemnity expenses out of pocket (and especially for those with their own practices), this means one wrong move could be career ending. In fact, there is a saying in obstetrical circles that goes something like this: "You will quickly be sued for the delayed cesarean, or for not doing one, but never for doing it early." It takes no great intellect to see how this entrenched conclusion affects decisions on the labor ward.

Furthermore, in recent surveys conducted in the United States, the average age of retiring from obstetrics was forty-eight years old, with a frequently cited reason being liability or litigation issues.[59] It was also found that 60 percent of respondents had made changes to their practice because of the high risk or fear of claims, and concluded that "professional liability is a vital and enduring concern."[60] But is it any wonder? The cost of premiums averaged 17.8 percent of gross income, which is the equivalent of approximately one dollar of every six the physician earns, before any other practice expenses have been paid. Unsurprisingly, it has been suggested that to "compensate for this expense, costs to patients and insurers must increase,"[61] but equally unsurprisingly, increased costs are unpalatable for everyone in the current economic climate.

Second Accusation: Selfishness

"It is more convenient to do a cesarean in the daytime than it is to deliver a baby at four o'clock in the morning, so obstetricians encourage women to plan surgical births in favor of a more unpredictable trial of labor."

On the face of it, this makes sense, and indeed, Dr. Murphy has experienced just how the initial excitement, sense of importance, and feeling of being needed on short notice at all times of day and night can quickly wear off for newly qualified doctors. Furthermore, it is true that being solely responsible for your own obstetrical patients can often lead to untenable situations in which overworked, exhausted doctors get called into the hospital night after night to deliver babies. This is where circumstances and lifestyle considerations can quickly lead to impaired decision making and real conflicts of interest. For example, cesarean surgery might allow you to get home again quickly, compared with the possibility of sitting around for hours waiting for a vaginal delivery that might end up as an emergency cesarean anyway. This type of thinking is not necessarily self-deluded or selfish. A doctor might argue that she has legitimate conflicts with working through a particular night; it could affect her performance during the next day's scheduled operations and office clinics or simply get in the way of her need to go to bed and repair the accumulated sleep deprivation that already exists. And who would want to have surgery by a sleep-impaired surgeon? It is well known that sleep deprivation decreases cognitive and psychomotor function, which are both critical functions required for medical practice.[62]

It's also inevitable that daytime labor and delivery that go on for hours will interrupt scheduled surgery and clinic consultations; by definition, if a doctor delivers all his own obstetrical patients, he has to be available at short notice, seven days a week. Therefore, although the system described above (conditions under which obstetricians in some countries have traditionally worked for their entire careers) could raise concerns that some cesareans are done too quickly, we would argue that rather than being proof of widespread unethical behavior, it is a remarkable testament to the moral fiber of so many men and women who have worked through the night, and again the next day and night, for years on end. Indeed, Pauline's experience with her doctor was just that: she knew if she went into labor earlier than her scheduled cesarean date, no matter what time of the day or night, either her own doctor or her doctor's surgical partner would be on hand to scrub in, and from a patient's perspective, she took great comfort in this knowledge and perceived it as another planned cesarean benefit.

But from a doctor's perspective, Dr. Murphy strongly believes that in general, individual obstetrical care systems, in which each obstetrician delivers her own patients, are archaic, stressful, and irresponsible, and lead to temptations for abuse and distortion of the decision-making process. Even with the best intentions, doctors who *do* choose to be there for their patients at any time of the day or night are putting themselves under dangerous levels of pressure, especially if they have a large caseload at any given time. But this old-fashioned, grueling idea of always being available around the clock and having hardly any life outside of work is mercifully disappearing. Partly, the change has come about because younger generations of physicians in all specialties, and obstetrics in particular, are simply not willing to sacrifice their lives to their jobs the way previous generations of doctors did. But the most influential reason behind this change has been the gradual (and likely irreversible) move toward shared on-call systems. And doctors who have practiced in this new working environment almost never want to return to the old system.

This is how it works in many cities around the world: obstetricians and family doctors who do obstetrics work in shared call groups and do fixed on-call sessions, just as emergency room doctors have always done (think about the television series *ER*, and you'll understand what we mean). When on call, the obstetrician stays in-house (in premises at the hospital) and basically works continuously from when he gets there until the shift is over. During the course of the shift, the team might consist of obstetricians, residents, midwives, and nurses, with various degrees of involvement and responsibility in the birth process, all of which depends on the culture of the country. In practice, even though individual obstetricians might sign up personal patients at their offices and follow these women throughout pregnancy, the planned vaginal delivery patients are assisted by the person on call during that particular shift when they arrive at the hospital. When this model is taken to its extreme, even electively booked cesarean deliveries are similarly done by whichever obstetrician is on call and onsite.

Of course, for this to work effectively, institutions need rigorous checks and balances, with careful and ongoing assessments so patients can rightfully expect that the doctor who is working when they come in will offer skilled and compassionate care. It also requires a shared vision of best birth practice; in the case of maternal request, for example, there have been cases of women arriving at the hospital for a planned cesarean, only to find that the doctors on duty are unsupportive of their birth plan, in some cases either forcing the woman to attempt vaginal delivery or making her birth experience uncomfortable and unpleasant (as shown in chapter 16, "Cesarean Birth Stories"). But in terms of remuneration, even in fee-for-service practice arrangements, provided that each doctor in the call group recruits patients into the group, the average income across the

Chapter 11

Cesareans Cost Less than You Think

The cost of a thing is the amount of what I will call life which is required to be exchanged for it, immediately or in the long run.
—Henry David Thoreau, *Walden*, 1854

"A cesarean birth is more expensive than a vaginal birth—financially, psychologically, socially, and ecologically. Therefore, maternal request with no medical indication is not an acceptable reason for surgery and should be afforded only to those who are willing to pay for it themselves."

The above is a view that is held by many. From the man on the street through to the highest echelons of government, the perception is that the financial burden of cesareans gives further cause to efforts to reduce—and not increase—them. However, we are confident that by the end of this chapter, we will expose the flaws in this argument and others like it and demonstrate that the cost of a planned cesarean is not a valid reason for denying maternal request—whoever's paying for it.

Let's start with a quiz.

Which types of birth have the highest and lowest financial cost attached to them (as incurred during the birth period only)?
   a) A spontaneous vaginal birth
   b) An assisted vaginal birth (forceps and/or vacuum)
   c) A spontaneous labor followed by an emergency cesarean
   d) An induced labor with attempted instrumental vaginal delivery followed by an emergency cesarean
   e) A planned cesarean that is medically indicated
   f) A planned cesarean with no medical indication

The answer is (∂) and (a).

What do these two birth types have in common, and how do they differ?

The answer is that they both originate as planned vaginal births, but only one of them results in the vaginal birth outcome as planned — the other ends up as cesarean surgery.

CESAREANS ARE NOT BORN EQUAL

And yet it won't come as a surprise to readers when we tell you that to date, the vast majority of research calculating which birth type is most expensive has looked at just two scenarios: a vaginal birth outcome and a cesarean birth outcome. With no regard for the planned mode of delivery and no accounting for the fact that while barely 2 percent of planned cesareans result in an emergency cesarean, around one-third of planned vaginal births result in assisted delivery; emergency cesarean; or even worse, failed attempts at assisted vaginal delivery, followed by emergency cesarean. The conclusions of these mixed-data studies have formed the basis for the view that the promotion or even discussion of maternal request may not be the best use of increasingly limited resources.[1] The inescapable fact that more planned vaginal births end up as the most costly of all births is all but ignored, and worse still, these planned vaginal birth costs are instead often merged with planned cesarean costs by throwing all cesareans into one basket and coming up with a total cost.[2]

Fortunately, though, fresh thinking is emerging. A National Institutes of Health conference panel in 2006, for example, concluded that maternal request costs "cannot be simply extrapolated from current costs associated with cesarean delivery overall, which includes expensive emergent procedures. Planned [cesareans] will have different cost implications that should be modeled explicitly."[3] And in 2008, the American College of Obstetricians and Gynecologists said, "It is not clear whether widespread implementation of elective cesarean birth would increase or decrease resources required to provide delivery services. Comprehensive analysis of costs and benefits for current and subsequent pregnancies" is needed.[4]

This makes perfect sense. Imagine, if you will, the analogy of a shop selling wine. It has just two immediately apparent types in stock, red and white, but the bottles have come from vineyards around the world and are all of a different vintage. As a buyer, you would not expect the price to be determined by the color of the wine alone—one price for red and another price for white. No, you would expect other factors to be taken into account, such as the wine's origin, the grape variety, and the year it was harvested.

In a similar vein, the cost calculations and comparisons of birth types are not as simple as putting a value on just two modes to compare—vaginal versus cesarean. We only need to look at the positive birth outcomes associated with planned cesareans, and specifically maternal request cesareans, once *health* data have been separated appropriately, and it logically follows that the same effect would almost certainly be transferred into *cost* comparisons too.

And indeed it has.

In 2003, two studies confirmed what many of us had been thinking all along. In the United States, a one-year analysis of birth costs at a not-for-profit hospital concluded that since the average cost for all women who attempted vaginal delivery was only 0.2 percent less than the per-patient cost of elective, planned cesarean delivery, "[t]he adoption of a policy of cesarean delivery on demand should have little impact on the overall cost of obstetric care."[5] And in Britain, researchers determined, "A critical evaluation of the costs indicates that there are probably few grounds for denying women their request for cesarean section for economic reasons."[6]

Furthermore, subsequent research has actually found planned cesarean birth to be *more cost-effective* than planned vaginal birth, especially when a fuller picture of health costs related to different birth types is examined. For example, American researchers who included the cost of newborn babies spending time in a neonatal intensive care unit (NICU) warned, "Recommendations for obstetrical practices as well as health care policy on their charges should not assume that Cesarean section deliveries are always costlier than vaginal deliveries."[7] In fairness, this particular study included an unusually high number of babies born vaginally with low birth weights, which is not typical in other studies, but it is nevertheless useful for demonstrating how additional costs not normally evaluated in birth type comparisons can very quickly begin to tip the scales in a less favorable direction for vaginal birth. For example, you can start to imagine what the effect would be if pelvic floor repair costs were factored in too.

Similarly, when Thai researchers looked at the postpartum costs of different birth types (i.e., costs arising from healthcare needed by mothers after the birth), planned cesareans were very slightly more expensive than vaginal births, but only because emergency cesarean costs were excluded from the study completely—and thereby not attributed to the planned vaginal birth group as applicable.[8] If this had been done, the planned vaginal birth group's costs would have soared. Planned cesareans have also been recorded as "significantly less expensive"[9] and "cost effective"[10] in analysis of breech and macrosomic (large) babies' births, and although this might be expected, given that breech presentation and macrosomia are challenging cases with high rates of complications and emergency cesareans, it's worth noting here because these "soft" obstetrical indications for a cesarean are frequent targets in efforts to reduce cesarean rates on the basis of cost-effectiveness too.

IDENTIFYING AND ACCEPTING BIRTH COSTS

But there is sometimes a reluctance to accept that maternal request cesareans may not cost more than a planned vaginal birth (or even cost less), and very often, there is a tendency for investigations to look for answers in the wrong places (or to *not* to look for them in the *right* places), as we discuss in chapter 6, "Protecting Your Pelvic Floor." It's clear that the truth could be better determined if we look in the right places (in this case, the short- *and* long-term costs associated with different birth *plans*), but researchers very often don't choose to do this. For example, when the United Kingdom's National Institute for Clinical Excellence (NICE) published its cesarean guideline in April 2004, it reported a crude cost saving of around £1,257 ($2,000) for every woman requesting a cesarean who could be encouraged to attempt a trial of labor instead, and it suggested a reduction in maternal request rates, whether small or total (i.e., "if all requests for CS were refused"), would be financially beneficial.[11] Inevitably, this news made headlines around the world, and maternal request was slammed again. However, this was not the whole story.

First, NICE admitted its crude estimate of maternal request costs did not take into account any additional costs associated with planning a vaginal delivery against a woman's judgment or request, such as additional

ences, and in prohibiting just one aspect (in this case, maternal request cesarean) simply because it is perceived as a lifestyle choice.

What's really needed is a better understanding of women's reasons for choosing a cesarean, the acceptance and support of these reasons, and the recognition that birth is just another area of healthcare in which different choices and costs exist. Indeed, in other areas of healthcare development, there are established and ongoing precedents in which additional costs are not prohibitive. For example, in the choices between some commonly performed surgical procedures, such as endoscopic (keyhole) surgery versus open surgery, there are *vast* cost differentials, of which the latest version includes the developing area of robotic-assisted endoscopic surgery. Sometimes the robot is used simply because it's available, not because it's any quicker, better, or cheaper.

Meanwhile, in private hospitals, where maternal request cesareans are openly permitted (albeit only afforded by the very wealthy, hence the term "too posh to push"—its opposite being "too poor to pay"), until very recently, a rather different approach has been taken by some. For example, the Birth Unit (which closed in 2010 but was at the Hospital of St. John and Elizabeth) and the Portland Hospital, both located in London, decided to charge higher prices for planned maternal request cesareans than for planned cesareans with medical or obstetrical reasons. Not because they cost more, but simply to discourage women from choosing one. An emergency cesarean still cost the most, but incredibly, a woman with a healthy, uncomplicated pregnancy was charged up to £2,080 (around $3,300) more for her cesarean than a woman with a planned cesarean with medical complications. And this was the norm for at least six years. Pauline first noticed the price discrepancy in 2004 and shortly afterward began questioning hospitals' administrators, both orally and through e-mail, about their rationale for such a policy. In 2008, the director of operations at St. John and Elizabeth explained to Pauline:

> Our priority is offering the safest care for mothers to be, and in our opinion medically unnecessary cesarean sections do provide additional risks that do not occur in normal deliveries. Our pricing structure is deliberately aimed at reflecting our market, which is primarily the non-elective caesarean sections and therefore we do charge a higher rate for those women who chose to have a procedure we do not consider matches our philosophy.

Meanwhile, in the same year, an account director at the Portland Hospital defended its position like this:

> In line with best practice the number of elective caesareans we carry out for non-medical reasons is low. Our responsible pricing structure reflects the increased costs of providing a caesarean section as well as to encourage best practice. It is important, however, that we never deny a woman's informed choice in the provision of her maternity care, as long as that choice is safe.

However, just as we were preparing to criticize this price differential in our book and went in search of the latest cesarean prices at the Portland, we were delighted to find that the new pricing structure for 2011 has been revised and that there is no longer a supplemental fee for maternal request. In communication with Pauline, the new chief executive officer at the hospital, Janene Madden, described what led to this change:

> When looking towards setting our prices for 2011 our aim was initially to keep our package prices simple for our customers to understand. We therefore began by reviewing our cost base for all types of deliveries provided and as predicted there was little or no difference in cost for the Portland to undertake an elective versus a planned medical [cesarean], and if anything a medical caesarean section can be more expensive as the woman is having a medical caesarean for underlying medical concerns. This was not reflected in the 2010 prices.
>
> I believe the pricing differential was put in place a few years ago to discourage women from seeking elective caesarean sections (as it was deemed socially unacceptable) by maintaining the elective price at a higher rate. However we now take a completely different view on modes of delivery at the Portland Hospital, where we encourage provision of correct information to our women and their partners, which ultimately allows the woman to make an informed choice on the way she would like to deliver her baby.

She added, "I must stress the Portland Hospital will support all modes of delivery as long as it is safe for the mother and child and she is well informed of the decision she is making. The regular modes of delivery at the Portland include fully natural deliveries in our water bath through to mobile epidurals and elective caesarean sections."

So this hospital carried out an evaluation of costs and found no reason to continue charging extra for a planned maternal request cesarean, and evidently, it has found nothing in its hospital records to suggest that there may be safety issues with this birth type. In our view, this hospital's renewed approach and attitude toward birth choice and cost is entirely refreshing, and we can only hope that in this respect, other hospital policies around the world (that aren't already operating in this way) will follow suit.

Chapter 12

Cesarean for Sex:
The Ultimate Birth Taboo?

*If you believe in your own sex, and won't have it done dirt to:
they'll down you.*

It's the one insane taboo left: sex as a natural and vital thing.
—D. H. Lawrence, *Lady Chatterley's Lover*, 1928

In the opinion of some critics, the issue of a woman's postnatal sexual health should neither *need* to be nor *want* to be discussed when deciding her preferred birth plan. This is because the largely unchallenged view exists that sex is not adversely impacted by any particular birth type, and furthermore, that there is something distasteful about a mother-to-be considering her sex life in the risk-benefit analysis of which birth might be best for her baby. Well, we're confident the evidence in chapter 3, "The Safest Birth Choice for Your Baby," will eliminate any argument that a newborn's health is compromised by the mere consideration of planning a cesarean birth, and the information we present in this chapter will help answer the question of whether a planned cesarean can be effective in protecting a woman's post-birth sexual health.

For the longest time, Dr. Murphy has approached the argument of whether vaginal birth might have an impact on a woman's sex life by considering simple physical logic. Instances of vaginas stretched beyond recognition, pelvic floor muscles ripped off the bone (sometimes so damaged that there are large gaps in the muscle, or parts of the muscle are simply absent), damaged nerves, and torn fascia layers all come to mind. It is almost inconceivable that such damage would not have any effect on sexual satisfaction for both parties. In cases where the muscles have been torn off their attachments, this can be clearly seen on special ultrasound and magnetic resonance imaging (MRI) scans, but it can also be felt by a trained practitioner's hands when carrying out an internal examination. Even those who have studied this phenomenon as part of their professional training can be completely unprepared for its physical reality. Dr. Murphy always finds it fascinating to observe the shock of recognition on the faces of residents in the urogynecology clinic when they feel it for the first time, and it is as though they hadn't quite believed or hadn't quite imagined, before seeing and feeling it for themselves, that it could be *this* obvious.

Similarly, for women, the change in sexual experience as a result of pelvic floor damage can be quite significant, and for many, a shock. First, since it is well known now that the pelvic muscles play a major role in orgasm (basically, the stronger the pelvic muscles, the stronger the arousal and eventual orgasm[1]), any damage to these muscles might be noticeable. Second, a wider pelvic cavity caused by damaged and weakened pelvic muscles can change the interaction between a woman's vagina and her partner's penis. This is because a man's erection stays pretty much stable throughout life until partial or complete impotence sets in (and even then, there are pills available to help rectify the situation), so any drastic changes in the dimensions of the vagina might lead to changes in the joint interaction. This can range from an increase in the amount of air getting into and out of the vagina, causing a greater likelihood of vaginal farting, to a level of reduced sensation that is detrimental to either or both partners' pleasure. And the fact is that no vagina is ever *tighter* after vaginal birth; quite the contrary, and in any case, vaginas actually have no inherent tightness, which is a very important concept that even many doctors do not understand.

Indeed, misunderstanding of this fact has caused harm to many women during the post-birth surgical repair of a prolapse or "stretched" vagina. This is because the primary problem is not that the vagina itself is stretched (although that could be a secondary development). Rather, the problem is with the muscles. It is the muscles of the pelvis, specifically the levator muscles, that determine the size of the opening in the pelvis and therefore the size or tightness of a woman's vagina. In contrast, the vagina is simply an elastic epithelial tube (in other words, a skin bag) that fills the space available. Therefore, where some gynecologists go wrong during prolapse surgery is that they focus the repair on "the bag," painstakingly trimming, cutting, and sewing in an effort to tighten it, but not realizing that their effort is doomed not only to failure but also to *short-ening* the vagina, which can severely worsen any preexisting sexual diffi- culties. The real problem is that the muscles themselves *cannot* be repaired, and so efforts at surgical correction have to focus on re-creating support for the vagina's inner attachments and on attempting to prevent sagging. In fact, the only part of the vagina that can be tightened (without changing the force vectors in the pelvis such that new problems will inevitably occur) is the very entrance to it, the so-called introitus. Here, the perineum can be surgically re-created by pulling the small muscles of the perineum back together, thereby narrowing the entrance of the vagina.

Unfortunately, even this method does not guarantee resolution, as it often continues to leave a wide-open cavity behind the entrance. Also, this newly tight vaginal opening can suffer from the same problem experienced with a repaired episiotomy scar: pain during attempts to stretch it and con- sequently, pain during sex (dyspareunia). Of course, satisfying sexual function does not depend on size alone—far from it—and we know that human sexuality cannot be reduced to something as banal as "a tight fit." Interpersonal relationships, love, lust, body image, self-esteem, mood, chemistry, the ability to relax and be in tune with your body and your partner's, and simply being in the moment for giving and receiving pleasure—these all play essential roles. But the question here is whether there is a difference between the sexual outcomes of women who have a planned cesarean birth, compared to those who have a vaginal birth.

We believe there is. And although research has yielded conflicting results, including some studies that show no differences between these dif- ferent birth types,[2] overall, we believe the balance of evidence is in cesarean's favor.

PROTECTION AGAINST PELVIC FLOOR DAMAGE

We introduced this chapter with the concept of the stretching or loosening that the vagina may undergo during vaginal birth and how that may relate to underlying muscle damage, rather than simply hormonal changes that will correct themselves. Unfortunately, there are other pelvic floor prob-

lems that may occur as a direct result of giving birth and that may negatively influence sexual function later on.

We are not saying every woman who has a planned cesarean birth will
have better sexual functioning than women who have vaginal births. Such
a statement would be ridiculous and guilty of gross overgeneralization.
Moreover, it isn't the best way of answering the question posed. What we
are saying is that women who have vaginal births are at greater risk for
worse long-term sexual functioning (physically, as measured against their
own pre-birth sexual function) compared with women who have planned
cesarean births. This is because there is sufficient evidence to illustrate
that some of the greatest risks to a woman's sexual health are inherent to
vaginal births, and it therefore follows that these risks are reduced with a
cesarean. Although the risks are not completely negated by delivering a
smaller baby, there are definitely increased risks with larger babies, and as we
point out numerous times, macrosomia (large babies) is becoming more
and more common.

Pain

Sexual health problems are very common after childbirth,[3] and in the
immediate postpartum period, the most common sexual disorder appears
to be pain that occurs as a consequence of perineal trauma during vaginal
birth (for example, tears in the vagina, perineum, anal sphincter, or
rectum[4]), especially with an instrumental delivery.[5] Pain often leads to
avoidance and, eventually, to a lack of libido. The best outcomes are
reported by women with an intact perineum, which is to be expected,
although even a successful spontaneous vaginal birth can result in mild or
severe tearing and pain. In fact, the highest prevalence of significant pain
with intercourse postpartum, and the *most* pain, occurs in women who
have had episiotomies, perineal lacerations, or instrumental births,[6] a difference that has been shown to persist at six months[7] and even two years
postpartum.[8] And yet frustratingly, studies like these, which actually
demonstrate better sexual health outcomes with a planned cesarean birth,
are all too often dismissed as showing only a short-term benefit of around
three to six months. In fact, less painful intercourse[9] and less reported
vaginal "looseness"[10] have been demonstrated as benefits at twelve months.
Even more telling, a survey of more than four thousand British women *six*

years after their births found those who delivered exclusively by cesarean had a much better perception of their vaginal tone (and said the effect for their own and their partner's sexual satisfaction was better) compared to women who had vaginal births.[11]

Incontinence and Prolapse

The effect of prolapse and incontinence on female sexual function has been the subject of increasing research efforts lately too. Unfortunately, the incidence of urinary incontinence during sex is actually very high, including orgasmic stress incontinence (often erroneously interpreted as female ejaculation[12]), and while sympathetic attempts at humor ("What's the matter with a little more lubrication anyway?") can produce a wry smile from some, many women are severely bothered by leakage during sex[13] — or simply the fear of it happening. And there is no disagreement whatsoever in the research into the effects of urinary and fecal incontinence on sexual function; these are universally and seriously negative factors. But although the results of studies into the effect of prolapse seem to conflict, it would seem that symptomatic prolapse *does* have a negative effect on sexual function.[14] These issues are exhaustively discussed in chapter 6, "Protecting Your Pelvic Floor," where we clearly show to what extent vaginal birth is responsible for the majority of cases of prolapse, as well as incontinence.

Pelvic Nerve Damage

The pudendal nerves are the main nerves of the clitoris, one from each side, and the proven fact that pudendal nerves may be injured during vaginal birth (again, see chapter 6, which has more details) will crystallize the possibility of its negative effect on sexual function.[15]

Subtle Anatomical Changes

Not only might the vagina be wider or looser after delivery, but the clitoris may be in a slightly different orientation to the vagina, meaning a woman may have to adjust her position to get an orgasm. And inside the vagina there may also be new little crevices, crannies, bumps, and skin tags.

Dr. Murphy's own experience has also reflected the outcomes of many studies in the sense that whereas some women with prolapse don't seem to be concerned about it, he regularly sees other patients who say they avoid sex completely or almost completely, denying themselves and their partners this experience, with comments about feeling scared, dirty, ashamed, frightened, or grossed out by their prolapse. Almost everyone he sees with urinary or fecal incontinence is significantly affected, sometimes to the point of avoidance of all sexual contact. Worse, the conditions of prolapse and urinary, fecal, or flatus incontinence often occur together to some degree and are sometimes associated with painful or uncomfortable intercourse and depression. When researchers looked at the prevalence of these conditions and their effect on the sexual satisfaction of 208 women in the United Kingdom two years after their births, there was a significant decrease in sexual satisfaction scores by the women who had a vaginal birth in comparison with those who had a planned cesarean. And there was also a significant increase in the prevalence of urinary incontinence, incontinence of flatus, dyspareunia, and subjective depression in women who had a vaginal birth.[16] Since pelvic floor disorders like the ones screened for in this study are common after vaginal birth, the overall attributable sexual dysfunction load must be huge.

Finally, as per our oft-repeated message, planned cesarean births must be compared to *planned* vaginal births, whatever the final birth outcome. No woman is assured of a successful vaginal birth when one is planned, and yet very often, even studies that find no difference in outcomes between successful spontaneous vaginal births and cesarean births will often show worse outcomes for those planned vaginal births.[17]

SEXUAL HEALTH RESEARCH

Unfortunately, despite the studies we have referred to, research on female sexuality, and especially how female sexuality relates to mode of delivery, is a relatively new field. What we mostly have available are validated questionnaires answered by a specific target group of women with a particular condition and then statistically analyzed. Currently, most commonly used questionnaires in the research of female sexual dysfunction include the PISQ-12 (Pelvic Organ Prolapse/Urinary Incontinence Sexual Questionnaire),[18] the FSFI (Female Sexual Function Index),[19] and the FSDS (Female Sexual Distress Scale).[20] In these questionnaires, women's sexual dysfunction is classified as disorders of sexual desire, arousal, orgasm, and pain that lead to personal distress, not distress to their partner. This is because not every woman who doesn't want lots of sex has a sexual disorder—in spite of attempts to classify and broaden the diagnosis of so-called hypoactive sexual desire disorder (HSDD), which is a deficiency or absence of sexual fantasies and desire. This state is only a disorder if it causes distress for the woman or problems in her relationship as perceived by *her*. Therefore, not every woman with decreased libido has sexual dysfunction.

However, this is precisely what makes studying the effect of childbirth on women's sexual health so challenging. Most women, however they give birth, might feel tired, unattractive, or simply completely distracted by their newborn baby's needs for weeks and even months after the birth. Any or all of these things can have an impact on their levels of sexual health and satisfaction and can mean that some women's answers actually mask real physical changes. For example, some women may not feel the desire for sex at all, and since they don't attempt intercourse, they don't know whether anything's changed. Others who *are* having sex might well experience changes in sensation but don't feel any distress as a result. Furthermore, many women, when asked about their sex lives, can be somewhat reticent, and very few women with a postnatal sexual problem report discussing it with a health professional.[21] After all, in a culture where sex is often portrayed as the lifeblood of any relationship and something that everyone wants—and wants a *lot* of—who's brave enough to admit the very opposite? Because of this, any approach to researching birth type associations with sexual dysfunction must take into account the myriad possible issues that may be affecting mothers' sex lives, but also, as we argue in chapter 6, apply a sense of logic too.

More generally, female sexual function has been an obscure and neglected area in the medical research field until relatively recently. Unlike male sexual function—and particularly, dysfunction—which has been the focus of research for many years, women have traditionally been relegated to second-class status. Whereas male sexual dysfunction is relatively easy to diagnose and confirm—there is either a sufficient erection or not, and there is either a satisfying orgasm or not—female sexual function and dysfunction are much more complicated and eminently more nuanced. Unfortunately, traditional chauvinism, research interest (men have always been more interested in their own appendages), and women's reluctance to come forward and discuss sexual issues have all contributed to the silence in the area of female sexual dysfunction research. And indeed in many cultures, women's sexual enjoyment has been something to fear or dismiss, or at least not publicly celebrate or debate.

A PINK PILL

More recently, the situation has been changing, but not necessarily for the good. The interest in female sexual dysfunction exploded after the male equivalent was to some extent swept away with a tsunami of little blue pills. Suddenly all these researchers, all the industry scientists, and all the representatives, buffed with their recent astronomical sales rates of blue pills, were looking for the next marketing winner. What better than to create a brand-new problem to advertise, exploit, and perhaps solve equally successfully with maybe a *pink* pill? In effect, female sexual dysfunction became a business opportunity. This trivialization and obvious promotion of female sexual dysfunction has angered many respected and legitimate researchers, clinicians, ethicists, and feminists, some of whom have spent careers trying to destigmatize and research female sexual dysfunction in a scientific manner. The idea that a simple pill could be the answer is insulting, degrading, and ultimately, very wrongheaded.

This does not mean that the problem doesn't exist. It surely does, and if the increasing openness of women to talk about this is any indication, it is a big problem. However, the complexity of female sexuality has until recently bedeviled not only classification of the problem but also any attempt to measure it, since it cannot easily be reduced into individual, measurable entities, and particularly because it is so heavily influenced by nebulous metaphysical and psychological states like love, partnership, self-esteem, and body image, as well as hormone cycles. In science there is a truism that what can't be measured can't be described optimally. Conversely, if something cannot be described, it cannot be understood, measured, manipulated, or in this situation, treated.

DOWNPLAYED SEX

Female sexuality has always been mysterious. Some ancient traditions mystified it and created pagan mythologies in which it was bestowed with godlike and reverential qualities. Other traditions, which unfortunately still exist, demonize it and try to cut it out, treating it as a societal cancer. We need only to think of the scourge of female genital mutilation (FGM) that is still practiced in many countries in the name of religion, cultural or traditional values, and so-called decency, for example. The message and belief is that female sexual enjoyment is something that requires permanent destruction or at least mistrust. The implicit fear being that sexuality might lead a woman to act independently of the path chosen for her by her family and ultimately her husband—namely, to be a vessel for producing children. Her own life has so little meaning that personal satisfaction simply doesn't feature.

But although we in the developed world have to a large degree moved away from our own puritan past (for example, chastity belts to prevent infidelity and masturbation), we have no reason to be too smug. Female sexuality, and the need for female sexual fulfillment and expression, is still not always treated with the same respect and acceptance as that of the male. Examples illustrating this abound in our culture. Just think: when a young man sleeps around, he is a "stud" or a "ladies' man," but a young woman who does the same is a "tramp" or a "slut." We won't labor this point, but the fact is that female sexuality has been a suppressed, ignored, and feared entity even in the developed world.

Subtle reminders of this discrepancy in sexual power are evident in prenatal and labor wards too. Postpartum sexual health is definitely *not* on the discussion list of most busy obstetricians or midwives in the days and weeks after a woman gives birth. And the topic simply isn't raised as an issue when an experienced obstetrician demonstrates the use of obstetrical forceps or vacuum to a new resident—despite the fact that most doctors are aware and fearful of the damage these instruments can cause and the significantly negative effects on future sexual function that can potentially follow. It might become an issue, however, when they're considering delivery methods in the context of their own bodies or those of their partners (as demonstrated in chapter 5, "Doctors Who Support Cesarean Choice").

LIVES DESTROYED

Female sexual dysfunction occurs especially around two main life events: pregnancy and childbearing, and menopause. Menopausal changes in libido and function, especially the discomfort related to urogenital atrophy (drying, thinning, and shrinking of the vaginal lining) are strongly related to hormonal changes and can be treated quite successfully. Also playing a role may be body image issues and changes in general health and relationships (especially since this is also often the empty nest time in people's lives). But more vexing is the occurrence of prolonged and distressing sexual problems after childbirth that occur among (by definition) younger women who would be expected to have active, satisfying sex lives if they so desired.

And Mother Nature's timing is nothing if not ironic. Writing in 2007, sex educator, relationship expert, and author Dr. Yvonne Kristin Fulbright described how pregnancy is one of the most sexual times in a woman's life, during which she can feel highly aroused. The changes in her body mean that sensitivity is increased; some women even orgasm for the first time in their lives during this period.[22] And yet between Pauline's website and surveys and Dr. Murphy's medical experience and website, there are many examples of young women who can testify to such life-changing differences in sexual function after vaginal birth as to make any orgasmic pregnancy experiences a distant and painful memory. We include some of these in chapter 7, "Lives Destroyed by Vaginal Birth," in which women describe their experiences—heartbreaking accounts of devastating pelvic injuries that secondarily lead to destroyed sex lives, curtailed social lives, damaged relationships, and even career annihilation. In addition, Dr. Murphy recalls a forty-two-year-old woman he treated recently. She had developed severe urinary incontinence during sex after her first vaginal delivery (she never had any problems before that), but it got much worse after the second delivery. The constant and severe leaking during sex destroyed her and her husband's sex life, and this led to other relationship issues, ending in divorce.

These examples are meant to inform women of what *might* happen following a vaginal birth. The intent is not to scare women or to sensationalize worst-case scenarios, and it is also not to insult or cast aspersions on the sex lives of the majority of women who have had a vaginal birth (many of whom are very satisfied, in fact). Rather, the women themselves have told us that they wish someone had informed them of the truth *before* they had children, rather than after, and now they want to do this for readers of our book. And it's not just women who feel this way about birth. Many men express frustration that no one tells them about the possible repercussions either. We already know there are men who experience symptoms of postnatal depression or post-traumatic stress disorder, including flashbacks to the traumatic events of a negative birth experience, and now, slowly but surely, men are beginning to speak out about the longer-term effects of vaginal birth too.

These following examples of men's views, which were posted on the Birth Trauma Canada website, may be offensive to some readers, since they are not the most comfortable read. However, they do help to explain why issues surrounding postpartum sexual health remain taboo and secretive, and why it is so difficult to obtain a true picture of what's going on. Most men don't want to hurt the feelings of the women they love, and many women don't feel brave enough to talk openly about their problems with a doctor.

- My wife had my child three years ago and I have to say OMG did it change. The area between her vagina opening and her anus is all messed up like it ripped and never got fixed. She has a lot of excess skin hanging out. When she spreads her legs it's as if you can see straight down the vagina opening. It's also got dark skin around it. It's also looser, way looser. It used to be the hottest vagina I ever saw. I loved it so much. I still love my wife more than ever, but how do you tell her this is going on? She is too embarrassed to talk to the gyno about it.

- Three of my male friends and I have all found this board independently looking for answers to what has happened to our wives after birth. We found out that we had all found this board after the newest of us Dads asked if sex was different after birth. So let me tell you this, because I could and never would say anything to my wife: We notice. It's different. It's not nearly as good. We know that, because of our love for you, the cost, and the probability of more children, saying anything about the changes would only make you self-conscious, lead towards less sex and an unhappy wife. So don't expect your husbands or boyfriends to tell you that things aren't as good. From what I've seen (two marriages, first children with each), and talked to male friends, it always changes. The look, feel and tightness will never be the same. And that's not to say that sex afterwards is bad, but you should know what's coming. From reading through the posts on here, no one ever tells women the truth and that's not fair. There is no reason that you should have to find a board like this to get the truth from other women after the fact.

- In response to [man above], unfortunately from a male point of view what he says is spot on. Not only can you visually tell a mile away that a vagina has been used to birth a child but if you ever try to have sex with it, you will be severely disappointed. Sex is nowhere near as good, in fact it makes watching television or sleeping look really attractive. This is a very sad but true fact. Childbirth butchers vaginas, just wish more males knew this before committing to a marriage. In my case the changes were so huge I lost all interest in sex and the relationship and it ended in divorce. These days when I date a lady I chat about how much I love children and does she have any? The answer determines if I stay or run![23]

A WOMAN'S CONCERN TOO

A familiar anecdote claims that had the procreation of humankind relied upon *men* giving birth, our world might be much less populated than it is today, and some of the most cynical views go as far as to envision the human race rendered extinct before an alternative birth method could be discovered—but that certainly once it had, cesarean delivery would rank as the number one choice. Clearly, this hypothetical theory of a man's desire to avoid labor pain is impractical to test, but the closest real-life comparison we have (where genitals and procreation are concerned) is when a man has a vasectomy. On the website Vasectomy.com, one of the questions that appears in the top-ten list of questions is whether a man's sex life could be affected, and a related article on the site discusses the "natural concern" of whether a vasectomy might affect his sex drive and whether things will still be the same for him sexually.[24] While obviously childbirth is unique in that the welfare of another human being is intricately involved, there is nevertheless a comparison to be made here. Why, when it comes to assessing the maternal risks associated with vaginal birth (which is an unquestionably more invasive and traumatic experience than a vasectomy), is it also not accepted that a woman's sex life might be a "natural concern" for her too?

Pauline remembers reading an article a few years ago in which a university professor was quoted expressing concern that almost one in six women mentioned fear of tearing or loosening their vagina as a reason for choosing a cesarean, and furthermore, that this many women would do so just to keep their husbands or partners happy.[25] She found this deduction troubling because it assumes (unless women specifically state, "I'm under pressure from my husband to do this") that the desire voiced by these women to protect their future sexual health is not associated with their own satisfaction and pleasure, only that of their husbands. And it strikes us as disconcerting that even in the twenty-first century, in an age where sexual activity and satisfaction are unquestionably important to many people of both sexes, it can still be so difficult to conceive that women may actually place a high value on the quality of their own sex lives. Because many do, and so it's only right that their sexual health concerns are properly recognized, respected, and researched—and communicated without prejudice or attempts to normalize what for them is a real concern.

Chapter 13

The Risks of Planning a Cesarean

Take calculated risks. That is quite different from being rash.
—George S. Patton (1885–1945)

One of the common themes of this book is that there are no guarantees in labor and delivery. No matter how many prenatal classes a woman attends, and no matter how she prepares, studies, or discusses her birth plan choices with various providers, there is no knowing how things will actually transpire. This is simply the nature of obstetric practice—where Heisenberg's uncertainty principle rules supreme and Schrödinger's cat is both dead and alive until you open the crate.

As we have discussed in other chapters, this inherent unpredictability is predominantly a risk with planned vaginal birth, since the outcome of a trial of labor can range from a healthy spontaneous delivery to complications leading to forceps, vacuum, emergency surgery, or even all three. And avoiding this degree of unpredictability is often cited as a benefit of planned cesarean birth. But the question is, for women who are unsure whether to plan a vaginal or cesarean birth, is there any way to assess what their likelihood of experiencing complications may be so they can be better informed about what decision to make?

The answer to this question is dependent on various factors that are patient specific but primarily include a woman's age, ethnicity, and body weight; the estimated size of her fetus; and any previous deliveries she may have had. In summary, older and more obese women have significantly higher risks of experiencing obstructive labor and emergency cesarean as a final outcome, and furthermore, the risks of an emergency cesarean are higher in this group. A macrosomic (larger than average) fetus increases all risks, both to the baby and the mother (for example, shoulder dystocia, physical injuries, and obstructive labor). And finally, if a woman has had previous vaginal deliveries, her chances of another successful vaginal birth are generally improved, provided the fetus is of similar size and positioned normally inside the uterus, although her chances may also be modified by her age and weight. This would all be discussed with her doctor during an individualized consultation.

But in the event a woman already knows a cesarean birth is her preference (or if she reaches this decision over time), she should have no doubt about this fact: a cesarean is a major abdominal operation. Certainly, it is a remarkable testament to modern science and medicine that it has become as safe as it has, and in such a relatively short time, but there are potential complications—most of which are fortunately minor, but some of which, although rare, could be devastating or even life-threatening. Therefore, the decision to undergo elective surgery should never be taken lightly. It should be based on a thorough understanding of the risks involved, with the potential negatives carefully weighed against the potential benefits. The aim of this chapter is to provide women with an extensive and comprehensible explanation of the risks involved with a planned cesarean on maternal request.

RISKS FOR THE MOTHER

Infection

There are two main types of infection after cesarean: a wound infection (also called a *surgical site infection*) and endometritis (an inflammation of the lining of the uterus). Both of these share the same risk factors, and it is not uncommon for both types to occur in the same patient. This makes sense, given that the nature of the procedure involves an incision through the skin and into the uterus. Wound infections are found in 3–23 percent of women following a cesarean birth, and this wide disparity in rates is due to a variety of factors that can affect study results: for example, whether antibiotics were given, the length of the follow-up period after surgery, whether it was a planned or emergency cesarean, and whether medical and obstetrical conditions that increase the risk of infections were accounted for. It is therefore very difficult to give the reader a percentage risk for planned cesarean, since it will differ from location to location, but a good estimate is a risk of about 8 percent for *any* infection with a planned cesarean (including wound infections, endometritis, and urinary infections combined) and about 15 percent or higher with an emergency cesarean.[1]

Wound infections can involve localized inflammation (cellulitis); abscess (collection of pus) formation; or in very rare cases, a serious, often fatal and rapidly spreading infection called necrotizing fasciitis (flesh-eating disease). These all require antibiotic treatment and sometimes surgery, with quite extensive removal of dead and infected tissue in the case of necrotizing fasciitis. Fortunately, this condition is extremely rare, and it is especially unlikely to occur in an otherwise healthy person having a planned cesarean.

Similarly, the risk for endometritis after *all* cesareans is reported to be on the order of about 8 percent but only about 3 percent for planned cesareans in which antibiotics are given before or during the procedure. Most published research does not differentiate between planned and emergency cesareans, and actual risk is dependent on numerous factors, including the length of time the membranes were ruptured (how long since the mother's water broke), the length of labor, the mother's socioeconomic status, and whether antibiotics were given.[2] Endometritis is defined as a fever beginning more than twenty-four hours after or continuing for at least twenty-four hours after delivery, plus uterine tenderness, in the absence of other causes for fever.[3] The first twenty-four hours are excluded, since a fever during this period is very common and not necessarily related to infection. However, endometritis is considered to be the result of an infection inside the uterus and can occur after both vaginal and cesarean deliveries. Since emergency cesareans often occur after a prolonged labor with multiple vaginal examinations and interventions (for example, the placement of monitoring electrodes on the fetus's head), as well as a variable amount of time that the protective membranes are ruptured (thus exposing the intrauterine environment to the vagina and the bacteria that reside there), this is where the highest incidence of endometritis occurs. An increase in the period of ruptured membranes has been found to increase the risk of endometritis even in normal vaginal births, and in cases of preoperative ruptured membranes, the risk is significantly higher — 15.4 percent in one study.[4]

Who Is Most at Risk?

There is no doubt that infections are more common after a cesarean than after a vaginal delivery, since the major difference is that cesarean includes the necessity for a skin incision. However, they are also much less common after a planned cesarean than after an emergency cesarean. This has to do with the increased risk of chorioamnionitis (an infection inside the amniotic fluid) with labor, and especially the prolonged labor that often leads to an emergency cesarean. One of the most important risk factors is the length of time since the waters broke.[5] In such cases, there is also a degree of dehydration, which influences the immune system, as well as repeated vaginal examinations (the longer the labor, the more vaginal examinations) increasing the risk of chorioamnionitis. All of this increases the risks of wound infections as well as endometritis) afterward. And in addition to emergency surgery, socioeconomic status, age, and underlying health conditions are also associated with greater risk.

Other factors found to be associated with a greater risk of wound infections, seroma (a collection of yellowish fluid), or hematoma formation (a localized collection of blood associated with a swelling that can become infected and form an abscess) include the length of the incision, the mother's BMI, and any use of steroids.[6] And less experienced surgeons (residents and other trainees) taking longer to operate, the need for blood transfusions, and anemia are all associated with higher infection rates too.[7]

How Can the Risk Be Minimized?

A number of interventions can help minimize the risk of infection after any surgery, including a cesarean: for example, giving women preoperative antibiotics. Quite commonly, a single dose of cephalosporin antibiotic was given immediately after delivery of the baby and clamping of the cord, since it was felt the exact timing of the antibiotic made little difference, plus there were benefits in preventing the baby from being exposed to the antibiotic.[8] But more recently, it has been considered better to give the antibiotic even before the incision, since doing so has been shown to decrease the risk of infectious complications dramatically,[9] and medical studies have reduced the concern about the effect of antibiotic exposure on the baby.[10] As such, a single dose of broad-spectrum antibiotics an hour or so prior to surgery is now a standard of care before most gynecological procedures, and the American College of Obstetricians and Gynecologists recently published a recommendation that this be done prior to all cesarean births.[11] Also, in a planned cesarean with an otherwise healthy woman, there is really no benefit in giving her multiple doses of antibiotics, unlike in deliveries where an infection is already present (for example, following a prolonged labor complicated by chorioamnionitis that has ended up with an emergency cesarean), in which case multiple doses may be necessary. Other cases in which multiple doses might be better are prolonged surgery and patients with diabetes.

Another way to minimize risk is by ensuring sterility during surgery. Although this seems obvious and is always strived for, there are instances where an emergency cesarean is done in such a hurry—usually for fear of imminent fetal death—that sterility is not the first consideration, and preparation of the surgical area is done hastily out of sheer necessity. In these situations, a surgeon might not even have the time to scrub to the extent they would normally. Fortunately, only a very, very small number of planned cesareans become emergency cesareans, so while this scenario is possible, it is extremely unlikely in a modern hospital.

Finally, modifying medical risks and issues during pregnancy prior to the actual surgery can be helpful: for example, optimizing diabetes management, combating obesity, and promptly and appropriately treating any other infections or medical issues that may occur.

Thromboembolism (Blood Clots)

Although this complication, involving blood clots, is quite rare compared with other birth risks, it nonetheless remains one of the most common direct causes of death in pregnant women in the developed world,[12] and as such, it should be taken very seriously. That said, blood clots can develop during or after pregnancy, and in fact, two-thirds of clots in veins and half of clots in arteries develop during pregnancy, with the rest after delivery. A pregnant woman is about four times more likely to develop thromboembolism than when she is not pregnant, and overall, about two women in every thousand experience thromboembolism in pregnancy. This is worth knowing because although cesarean delivery is considered a risk factor for thromboembolism, the incidence after all cesareans, including emergencies, is still only quoted as being between two and five women per thousand,[13] which is comparable with the state of simply being pregnant. Overall, thromboembolism causes about 2.8 maternal deaths in every one hundred thousand deliveries of all types.[14]

The most common kind of thromboembolism occurs in veins, and 80 percent of these occur in the legs, where it is called deep vein thrombosis (DVT). The other 20 percent affect the lungs, which happens when a blood clot in the leg dislodges and then travels downstream like a floating piece of cork in a pipe, migrating through the veins, toward and through the right side of the heart, and ending up in the narrower lung vessels, where it cannot go any further—causing a disruption of blood flow back to the heart. The consequences of this can be as mild as an irritation or a cough, but if severe enough, it can also cause death, sometimes instantly. This more dangerous type of thromboembolism is called a pulmonary embolism, since it occurs in the lungs, but although most pulmonary emboli have their origin in the leg veins, where they start off as a DVT, fortunately, they are much rarer than clots in the legs. Pulmonary embolism is estimated to occur in about 0.45 per one thousand births in women with no previous thrombotic events.[15] Also, just like DVT, most pulmonary embolisms can actually be successfully treated with the daily administration of special blood thinners like heparin or Coumadin® (also called warfarin).

In summary, it is estimated that only about 0.5 percent of all cesarean births (not just planned cesareans) result in a woman developing a blood clot, and many of these women have other identifiable risk factors for thromboembolism.[16] Furthermore, the absolute majority of these are treated successfully. It's also important to note that while thromboembolism is indeed a serious potential complication of a planned cesarean section—and this risk should not be understated—the truth is that thromboembolism is a risk with *all* deliveries, regardless of mode, and can actually happen more frequently during pregnancy and before the birth than it does afterward.

Who Is Most at Risk?

Thromboembolism is more common in women who have certain conditions affecting their blood-clotting mechanisms. There are, for example, certain inherited conditions called thrombophilias, which basically just means "having an increased likelihood of blood clotting." Women are also at increased risk who have sickle cell disease, heart disease, lupus, a multiple pregnancy, diabetes, hypertension, bleeding, infection, a history of smoking, or who are overweight/obese or less mobile following surgery. Ultimately, however, clots are not predictable. What we do know is that thromboembolism occurs more frequently after an emergency cesarean than it does after a planned cesarean in a healthy woman, and therefore, just as for almost every other risk, there are many studies in which the risks of a planned cesarean are skewed by the failure to separate these two vastly different procedures. And, of course, when the complication occurs in an emergency cesarean, it is not appended to the list of risks associated with the originating planned vaginal birth.

How Can the Risk Be Minimized?

A number of preventable measures are usually taken in modern hospitals to reduce the risk of blood clots, such as using blood thinner medication or special compression stockings called sequential compressive devices (SCDs). SCDs are basically bandage-like wrappings containing pockets; they are placed around the legs and then inflated with a special pump. This creates a compressive effect on the legs and in so doing pushes the blood up the legs and increases the circulation. Injectable blood thinners, on the other hand, work to interrupt the normal clotting mechanism of blood, and ordinary heparin or a special type of low-molecular-weight heparin (which is considered safer) are most often utilized. The problem is that either form of heparin can also increase the risk of bleeding, meaning there is effectively a trade-off between the two risks. Certainly the balance of benefit is clearly in favor of giving heparin to women with the risk factors mentioned above, but for a healthy, normal-weight woman undergoing a planned cesarean, it is less clear how many women would receive unnecessary heparin to prevent one clot.[17]

Amniotic Fluid, Air, and Fat Embolism

One of the most serious events that can occur during labor and delivery or shortly after delivery is an amniotic fluid embolism. Just as the name implies, this is an event in which amniotic fluid enters a woman's circulation. Not only does it act like a foreign substance (which doesn't mix with blood and interrupts the oxygen-carrying and transferring capacity of blood); it also contains various active substances that start a chain re-action, resulting in often life-threatening effects. Severe consequences such as stroke, heart attack, respiratory failure, disorder of the clotting control mechanisms, or indeed any combination of these are possible, and about 20 percent of all cases end in maternal death. Fortunately, this is a very rare situation, with an estimated and reported incidence of two to three women in every one hundred thousand deliveries, but it is nonethe-less devastating for the families who are affected.[18]

Air embolism is a similarly potentially dangerous event with a very high rate of death (50–80 percent) from serious cases, but fortunately, the risk of a serious air embolism incident is very rare, since it takes a surprisingly large amount of air to actually cause trouble, and most commonly, smaller amounts get filtered out by the lungs before the air can cause trouble. An air embolism occurs when air enters the vascular circulation through open vascular channels and makes its way through the lungs to the right side of the heart. A cesarean is among a large number of surgical procedures or medical interventions in which the risk is increased, and in this case, the air enters the circulation through the open vessels inside the uterus where the placenta was removed. Other, nonsurgical situations in which this might occur include scuba diving and chest trauma, and there have even been case reports of fatal air embolism after oral sex, always during pregnancy.[19]

Another type of embolism is fat embolism. The mechanism is exactly the same as above and the outcome similar, except it is fat that enters the vascular circulation, rather than air. This is very rare in cesarean patients but is potentially deadly. It can also be associated with (but by no means limited to) liposuction, tummy tucks, and other cosmetic procedures, as well as orthopedic procedures and severe trauma (for instance, vehicle accidents, especially with fractures), so this complication is not specific to cesarean by any means.[20]

Who Is Most at Risk?

Women who are pregnant with multiples, who are of non-Caucasian eth-nicity, or who have had an induction of labor or a cesarean birth have been found to be most at risk for amniotic fluid embolism.[21] For air and fat embolism, there are few specific risk factors other than the speculative ones mentioned above.

How Can the Risk Be Minimized?

Minimizing the risk for these complications is very difficult. Serious cases are very rare, and these remain occasionally catastrophic events that, for the most part, cannot be predicted or prevented. For air embolism, the risk with a planned cesarean can be decreased if the surgeon shortens the time it takes to close the uterus, minimizes manual removal of the placenta (instead waiting until it releases spontaneously), and does not deliver the uterus through the incision. The latter is commonly done, especially by inexperienced surgeons, to facilitate suturing. Although the increased risk of air embolism caused by delivering the uterus through the skin incision is very small, it is still a known risk, and in Dr. Murphy's opinion, it is almost never necessary to do this. The incision can easily be sutured with the uterus safely inside the abdomen, where drying of and damage to the ovaries can also be prevented.[22]

Hemorrhage (Excessive Bleeding)

This is a risk with both cesarean and vaginal birth, and aside from uncertainty over whether estimates of measuring obstetric bleeding are particularly accurate in comparative studies,[23] it is increasingly rare to see studies that suggest a greater risk of hemorrhage or bleeding with a planned cesarean birth, and indeed, increasingly common to read that there is little difference or even a lower incidence compared with planned vaginal birth.[24] Again, the reason for this is that many planned vaginal births end up as assisted deliveries or emergency cesareans, both of which have a higher risk. In general, the overall population risk for serious maternal bleeding during birth is about 0.45 percent.[25] The risk for excessive blood loss after a planned cesarean is about 2.1 percent, and after an emergency cesarean, 3.3 percent.[26]

A less serious, but certainly annoying, complication after any surgical skin incision is a hematoma. This basically involves a collection of blood, usually partially clotted, underneath the incision and can cause swelling, pain, or bruising of the overlying skin—or, if it gets infected, an abscess.

Hematomas often drain by themselves, either through the incision or by slowly being reabsorbed by the body. This spontaneous drainage can sometimes be scary for a woman after a cesarean, since the blood might suddenly start coming out through an opening in the incision, causing her to panic and think she is bleeding dangerously. What in fact is happening is that the previously clotted blood has liquefied and is now oozing out. Despite the woman's consternation, this situation provides great relief for her doctor, for whom the possible need to reopen the incision and manually drain the hematoma has just decreased tremendously. If drainage is required, nurses are often asked to irrigate the cavity where the hematoma once was in order to remove all infected material and make sure it empties out completely. Sometimes the cavity is packed with gauze, but sometimes it is left open.

Who Is Most at Risk?

There are a number of known risk factors for excessive bleeding during a planned cesarean birth. Women with clotting disorders, such as Von Willebrand disease and other hemophilias, have a greater risk of bleeding, as do women with an abnormal placentation during their pregnancy, such as a low-lying placenta (placenta previa), and even more so with an ingrown placenta (placenta accreta) or detached or torn placenta (abruptio placentae). More generally, women with a high BMI are at greater risk too. This is best understood by realizing that any surgery is more complicated and difficult in overweight and obese patients. Similarly, multiple surgeries increase the risk of bleeding; it goes up with each successive cesarean birth. Again, this is because more surgeries mean more difficulty, but also because there is more internal scar tissue that now has to be cut, rather than simply separated, to reach the baby. There is also, very importantly, a higher risk of various placental problems. In addition, women with numerous previous cesareans are usually older, with uteruses that are not as capable of contracting strongly, which means more likelihood of bleeding.

Finally, in cases of emergency cesareans, the risk is elevated if hours of labor contractions tired out the uterus or if an infection is already present. For a planned cesarean, these risks are obviously not applicable,[27] which is important to highlight here.

How Can the Risk Be Minimized?

Preoperative testing of a woman's blood-clotting function is useful in cases where there is a history of a previous problem or a family history and during and after the subsequent treatment of any blood-clotting disorders, such as correcting abnormal blood-clotting factors or platelets. In cases where there is any family or personal history of abnormal bleeding, a hematology consultation would be appropriate, and it is also worth having the woman's blood crossmatched and ready in case it is needed. It is also routine to stop bleeding by using drugs that cause strong uterine contractions (e.g., oxytocin or prostaglandins). This is one of the most important ways to stop uterine bleeding, not only after a planned cesarean but after any delivery. And it should go without saying that choosing an experienced surgeon who will perform the cesarean speedily and expertly will also minimize the risk of bleeding.

Abnormal Placentation

Any previous uterine intervention—for example, multiple D&Cs (dilation and curettage), but also a planned cesarean delivery—increases the risk of abnormal placental position and development in a future pregnancy,[28] and this is precisely why women are advised to have only one, two, or a maximum of three cesareans(most doctors advise two).

Normally, after the baby has been delivered, the placenta separates easily and quickly from the inner wall of the uterus, and then the muscular part of the uterus compresses. The contraction of the muscle fibers pinches the blood vessels that fed the placenta, and the bleeding stops. It turns off the tap, so to speak. But if for any reason the placenta doesn't release quickly or completely, the danger exists that the uterus might not be able to contract effectively at all, causing open blood vessels to continue bleeding unimpeded, with the obvious risk that uncontrolled bleeding entails.

Placental problems are not common, per se, but they can be very serious, and there is evidence that the number of women affected by them is increasing. What we don't know, due to a lack of related research, is how many *planned* cesareans are affected. To date, research that has assessed placental risk in repeat cesarean deliveries has included *all* types of primary cesarean births, including those that were emergency surgeries after hours of labor, and we know from other areas of risk that outcomes are usually much worse where an emergency cesarean is involved. That said, as it stands now, it is important that every woman, including those having just one or two *planned* cesarean births, is fully aware of the placental complications that could happen. Namely:

Placenta Accreta, Increta, and Percreta

These are conditions where the placenta has grown into the uterine muscle in a way that prevents complete (or even any) separation or removal. The three conditions differ only in the degree to which the placenta has grown into the uterus muscle, with accreta the least deeply ingrown and percreta where the placenta has grown completely through the uterus wall. There are only three choices when this happens, and they involve carefully removing parts of the placenta that might not be as stuck, initially leaving the entire placenta alone inside the uterus, or doing an immediate hysterectomy after the cesarean with the placenta still inside the uterus. Trying to remove the placenta usually leaves shredded placental residues and open blood vessels, causing a significant risk for bleeding, whereas leaving the placenta might require manual removal later, when the placenta has degraded and liquefied to some degree and the blood circulation through the placenta has ceased. Obviously, a hysterectomy will preclude any further pregnancies.

Although an ingrown placenta can occur after a vaginal birth too, the risk is increased after a cesarean. The main reason for this is that since cesarean delivery causes a scar in the uterus, a placenta that comes to lie on the inside of the scar doesn't have normal uterine tissue to interact with but instead, scar tissue. The end result can be an abnormal implantation. And because the risk increases further with each subsequent cesarean, the risk of an ingrown placenta is one of the main reasons for limiting family size with planned cesarean births. Also, because surgery can interfere with the contraction of the uterus, especially the lower part of the uterus where this problem usually occurs, and because uterine contraction is the main mechanism to stop bleeding after delivery, the risk for bleeding in these situations is further increased.[29]

How Can the Risk Be Minimized?

The most important way to minimize the chances of these complications developing is an almost entirely preventive method—that is, restricting the number of cesarean births and, therefore, pregnancies. We recommend that ideally two planned cesarean births are optimal from a safety point of view. Dr. Murphy was once involved with a patient who had to undergo an eleventh cesarean, in spite of the urging of numerous doctors over the years to stop having children. And although the woman survived, she ended up in the intensive care unit after an emergency hysterectomy to stop the bleeding following a placental complication. Obviously, this was a highly unusual case, given the fertility rate in most developed countries and the increasingly later age at which women are having their first babies—just one or two cesarean births is far more common—but it does serve to illustrate that family planning is an important factor in minimizing the risk of abnormal placentation.

With today's radiology imaging technology, abnormal placental location and even an ingrown placenta can often be diagnosed or at least suspected with increasing accuracy. When doctors identify women who are at high risk for such complications, the treatment plan will be arranged accordingly. These treatments might include something called anticipatory embolization, which involves getting an interventional radiologist to thread a thin cannula through the femoral artery in the patient's groin all the way to the uterine arteries. These are then blocked prior to attempts to remove the placenta (but after delivery of the baby) by injecting some obstructing agent through the cannula. The uterine arteries are the main arteries through which most of the blood that circulates through the uterus and placenta is supplied, one on each side of the uterus. In pregnancy, these arteries become raging torrents of blood, and this is why obstetrical bleeding can be so catastrophic so quickly. Blocking these arteries with little balloons or more permanent material has the same effect as closing a valve in a water pipe: shutting it off. Fortunately, the uterus has enough other, smaller arteries to provide sufficient blood for the organ itself, but not enough for a baby, and therefore the embolization is done only after the baby is out.

Other options for minimizing bleeding risk involve special sutures to compress the uterus, surgically tying off some feeding arteries to the uterus, intrauterine compression balloons, medication that causes very strong uterine contractions, blood transfusions, and, if all else fails (or is not available), hysterectomy.

Placenta Previa (Low-Lying Placenta)

Placenta previa occurs when the placenta is located over the very lowest part of the uterus, close to the cervix and sometimes right across the inside opening of the cervix. The cervix needs to open for vaginal birth to occur, and this is not possible with the placenta stuck to the inside of this opening, covering it. If the cervix *does* manage to start opening, however, it might start tearing away from the placenta, causing severe bleeding. Also, the placenta can cause problems by partially or completely blocking the cervical opening. In cases where a previous cesarean had been done, placenta previa is sometimes associated with placenta accreta, since this area of the uterus is the thinnest and is also precisely where a cesarean scar will be located. The combination of placenta previa and accreta is an especially high-risk situation for bleeding if labor starts prior to the inevitable cesarean.

Abruptio Placentae

This is where the placenta tears away from the uterus prior to labor or birth, causing bleeding and possible fetal distress. It can occur at any time during pregnancy and is a common cause for an immediate cesarean section (even though the cesarean may have been planned for thirty-nine-plus weeks) due to the fear of imminent fetal death. The actual risk depends on the extent of the placental separation from its uterine attachment, which could be minimal, moderate, extensive, or complete—with the risk commensurate with the increasing degrees. What's important to realize, however, is that abruptio placentae is actually a risk with all pregnancies, not just those that follow a previous cesarean; any *increased* risk as a result of the previous cesarean is actually quite rare.

Who Is Most at Risk?

Some of the main risk factors associated with abruptio placentae include smoking, alcohol use, a history of previous abruption, hypertension in pregnancy, and, to a lesser degree, abnormal placentation problems associated with a previous cesarean birth.[30]

How Can the Risk Be Minimized?

Again, as before, the main way to minimize the risks of placenta problems as they pertain to planned cesarean birth is to limit the number of cesareans, and, therefore, to consciously plan and accept a smaller family. For women who have only one repeat cesarean birth, the absolute risk of all serious placental complications is low and reasonable. With two or more repeat surgeries, however, the risks go up exponentially, and at some point they become so high that all the benefits of planned cesarean births discussed throughout this book become overwhelmed by potentially serious, even life-threatening, risks.

Adhesions

All abdominal surgery carries the risk of postoperative adhesions, and these are a challenge for every surgeon. Adhesions basically consist of abdominal content that is stuck together. This often involves parts of bowel being stuck to each other, to other organs, or to the abdominal wall. Normally, the intra-abdominal organs are all lined by a moist, slippery layer that allows the organs (especially bowel loops) to move and slide over each other. Anything that causes inflammation, infection, or any injury to these moist layers (this could be as innocuous as drying out during surgery, the touch of a surgeon's hand, or compression from a swab or an instrument) could cause the layers to lose their integrity and to stick to each other or even merge together. The adhesions that most commonly occur after a planned cesarean include bladder adhesions forming onto the uterus, as the bladder is normally covering the lower part of the uterus. This, in turn, may increase the risk of bladder injury during a subsequent cesarean delivery or later on during a hysterectomy, should one be required.[31] Since adhesions can also sometimes cause bowel loops to be stuck together and to the abdominal wall, they increase the risk of a bowel injury during any future surgery in which abdominal penetration is required, no matter how that penetration is planned (either by open incision or laparoscopy). Fortunately, a planned cesarean is not likely to cause significant bowel adhesions, since the incision is made directly over the large uterus, which pushes the bowel up and out of the way. If properly and carefully managed, adhesions from a previous cesarean are rarely a big problem, in contrast to some other abdominal operations that require an incision higher up on the abdomen.

Other potential long-term problems with adhesions involve possible development of abdominal and pelvic pain and, more seriously, the risk of bowel obstruction.[32] The risk of small bowel obstruction after all types of cesarean delivery is five per ten thousand births.[33] A more common bowel-related complication after any abdominal surgery is something called ileus, a temporary paralysis of the small bowel leading to abdominal swelling and a delay in the ability to start eating and drinking. However, this is usually a nuisance issue, not life-threatening.

Concern is sometimes expressed that a planned cesarean might lead to fallopian tube or ovarian entrapment in adhesions, with the resultant fertility concerns. But medical studies are reassuring, showing no such association.[34]

Who Is Most at Risk?

Adhesion formations increase with the number of cesarean deliveries or any abdominal surgeries, with a number of studies showing statistically significant differences between patients with only one previous cesarean and those with two or more previous cesareans.[35] However, it is also important to remember that *all* surgery increases the risk of adhesions, so even if a woman has had only one or two cesareans but needs surgery for a completely different medical condition in the future (which is, of course, entirely unpredictable), the risk of injuries as a result of adhesions is still increased.

How Can the Risk Be Minimized?

Again, limiting family size and the number of surgeries is important, but there are also some ways surgeons can influence limiting the formation of adhesions: for example, using meticulous surgical technique to try to prevent bleeding as much as possible; minimizing infection through the use of prophylactic antibiotics; handling the bowel minimally and carefully;

making sure none of the tissues dry out; avoiding powdered gloves (since the talc in the powder on latex gloves can cause adhesions); and suturing only the necessary layers during closing, allowing others to be free to move and find their own orientation to heal together.[36] Unfortunately, however, adhesions cannot be eliminated completely.

Anesthesia

Overall, the risks of anesthesia for cesarean delivery are low. One large study in New York State found a complication rate associated with anesthesia procedures of only 0.46 percent, most of which were minor complications and overall led to only an average of one extra day in the hospital.[37] There are two main types of anesthesia: regional and general. Regional anesthesia involves local or regional blocking of nerve sensation or function (for instance, with an injection from the dentist or for excision of a small skin lesion). Injecting "freezing" into the spinal column affects nerves over a larger area, and the goal is usually to "freeze" the lower body up to the mid-chest. The epidural and spinal are examples of such regional anesthesia. In contrast to this, general anesthesia involves being put to sleep and is accomplished by a combination of putting the brain to sleep and ensuring that the body is not experiencing pain. During general anesthesia, which is sometimes necessary in some surgical procedures to provide the best possible conditions for the surgeon, patients usually need help with breathing, since general anesthesia affects the breathing centers of the brain.

General Anesthesia

Women planning a cesarean birth will occasionally express an interest in being "put to sleep" during the birth. These are often women with severe tokophobia (fear of labor and delivery) and no desire to experience the birth itself, but also women with a fear of needles (which regional anesthesia involves). However, general anesthesia is almost never used for planned cesarean birth, and for good medical reasons: namely, the risks of general anesthesia in late pregnancy are much higher than in the non-pregnant woman. For example, for the purposes of induction (putting the patient to sleep), a woman in late pregnancy is considered to always have a full stomach. In pregnancy, the hormones, as well as the pressure from the uterus, cause a significant delay in stomach emptying and also increase gastroesophageal reflux (a rise of stomach content containing a strongly acidic fluid into the esophagus). This condition is commonly known as acid reflux. During induction of general anesthesia, the risk of this fluid being inhaled is much higher than would otherwise be the case, and aspiration of stomach content into the lungs can lead to life-threatening complications. Furthermore, edema (fluid swelling) in the back of the mouth and the airway, combined with tissue friability (bleeding easily), increases the difficulty of passing the breathing tube into the airway and ensuring the patient's safety.

Since this situation can be easily prevented by avoiding general anesthesia and favoring regional anesthesia instead, most anesthetists will use general anesthesia only for the most serious and urgent emergency cesareans when there is simply no time for regional anesthesia. There are other reasons why doctors strongly discourage general anesthesia's use in planned cesareans, which are not as serious but nonetheless significant. These include the unnecessary effect on the baby's breathing that general anesthesia may have, and that the woman will take longer to come around, whereas with regional anesthesia she will feel less groggy and lethargic after surgery. There is also a remote but real possibility that anesthesia awareness (being awake during surgery) could occur. In our view, general anesthesia should be avoided for planned cesarean birth.

Regional Anesthesia
Postdural Puncture Headache (Spinal Headache)

The main difference between an epidural and a spinal is that only in a spinal is the dura layer (the tough outermost membrane enveloping the brain and spinal cord) punctured with a very thin needle. The anesthetic agent is then injected around the nerves and into the spinal fluid surrounding the spinal cord. This is in contrast to an epidural, in which the agent is injected on the outside of the dura and affects the nerves where they come out of the spinal column en route to the body part they're destined for. As a result of this closer, direct relationship of the spinal anesthetic and the spinal fluid, a much lower dosage of medication can be given, and through a thinner needle. As a consequence of the thinner needle, a leak of spinal fluid after spinal anesthesia is less common than after an epidural, with which the dura sac can be accidentally punctured. If it does happen, however, the result in both spinal and epidural could be the same: nausea and severe headaches, sometimes debilitating ones that are very dependent on posture and thought to be caused by decreased spinal fluid pressure in the spinal column and brain as a result of the leak. Since an upright position brings on these headaches, only lying down can provide relief. This situation can go on for up to a week.

Rates reported in studies vary so widely (depending on the wide range of techniques employed and the thickness and type of the needles used, for example) that the figures are unhelpful here (0.44–22 percent).[38] Anecdotally, Dr. Murphy can vividly remember developing a spinal headache as a medical student after having undergone an epidural a few days previously for a surgical intervention. The memory of the embarrassment of having to lie down on the floor in the middle of a medical ward, with his feet propped up against a wall, while the astonished professor, peers, and ward patients looked on will never leave him. However, if the problem is recognized early, the headache can be treated by performing a blood patch (injecting a bit of the patient's own blood) in the area, utilizing the normal clotting mechanism. Although not 100 percent successful, it is the best treatment available.

Subdural Hematoma/Abscess

Postdural puncture headaches, or pain in the back near the injection site that doesn't clear up or is getting worse, could be a sign of something more concerning. For instance, a blood collection in the area of the spinal cord or even the brain (spinal or cerebral hematoma) would need immediate surgical removal. An infection or abscess would need intense antibiotic treatment and can be life-threatening. And any headache that keeps getting worse, doesn't improve with treatment or lying down, or is associated with neurological signs in the lower limbs or bladder (such as weakness in the legs or incontinence of stool or urine) or with fever should be promptly investigated, as it may constitute an emergency situation.[39] This eventuality is fortunately rare and is most commonly treated with antibiotics (although very rarely surgical draining of an abscess is necessary), but it is nevertheless very serious, even possibly causing paralysis or death.

Hypotension

Low blood pressure can happen quickly in a pregnant woman for a variety of reasons; even something as simple as lying on her back can trigger a fall in blood pressure as a result of the heavy uterus lying on a big blood vessel. However, more significant decreases in blood pressure could be caused by epidural, or especially spinal, anesthesia as a result of opening up all the little veins in the lower part of the body. This happens because vascular tone is under the control of small nerves, causing the muscles of blood vessels in the body to relax or contract in a very precisely regulated way to keep blood pressure in a tight range. Paralyzing the nerves of the lower half of the body during a spinal anesthetic also affects these muscles, and the result is often a drop in blood pressure as blood pools in the dilated pelvic and leg veins. Of course, this is well established, and anesthetists have developed various ways to prevent and to treat it, ranging from certain IV fluids to drugs that cause the contraction of blood vessel muscles, thus raising the blood pressure.

Uncorrected and sustained significant blood pressure drops may threaten the health or life of an unborn baby due to decreased blood flow to the placenta, but also, if significant and prolonged enough, it may endanger the mother. Sudden blood pressure drops are more common with spinal anesthesia (which is the more commonly used regional anesthesia in a planned cesarean) than with epidurals (usually used during labor) because with a spinal, the block is much more rapid and complete. This is, of course, vital, since pain relief for cesarean surgery requires a much denser block, and while epidural blocks can be ratcheted up to sufficient levels when a cesarean becomes necessary (and can be just as good), in practice, most "mobile epidurals" for labor are much lighter, allowing the laboring woman to move and even walk around.

Nerve Injury and Paralysis

Neurological complications after epidural or spinal anesthesia are extremely rare, due to the anatomy of the spinal cord and the level of the procedure. In fact, spinals and epidurals are also sometimes blamed for previously unrecognized problems in the delivery or problems that are actually related to a preexisting medical condition (for instance, a bulging disc or severe migraines).[40]

Back Pain

Although this is a relatively common complaint, there are myriad factors that may be responsible other than the spinal or epidural anesthetic. One study from Germany reported that 0.8 percent of people complain about the onset of new back pain up to three months after receiving spinal anesthesia,[41] but it is important to note that this study involved a nonobstetric population; a large number of much older people were included, and their incidence of back pain would naturally be expected to be higher than that of younger people. That said, after pregnancy and birth (regardless of mode of delivery), back pain is a common problem due to pelvic laxity and spine curvature, and it may be impossible to figure out precisely what causes it in each case. A large US study found that 44 percent of women have back pain up to two months after delivery, regardless of whether they have an epidural.[42]

Cardiac Arrest

Cardiac arrest is a possible risk in almost all medical and surgical interventions. A large study from France, published in 1998, that assessed outcomes during surgical procedures reported rates of cardiac arrest of around six per ten thousand.[43] By 2002, decreased use of general anesthesia and further refinements in medical techniques and drugs lowered that risk to a reported 2.7 per ten thousand in the same country.[44] These were general populations, including elderly patients with heart conditions and other risk factors for cardiac and neurological complications or events, and therefore it is likely that any study of obstetrical patients would yield only better results. Indeed, another study published in 1998, this time from Australia, looked at 10,995 epidural anesthetics in obstetrical patients and found a rate of potentially life-threatening complications of just two per ten thousand). Furthermore, the maternal mortality in this study was in fact zero, and there was not a single incidence of severe neurological complications across all delivery types.[45]

A more recent, and very large, study from Canada, published in 2007, compared maternal mortality and serious morbidity, including that from cardiac arrest. The results are very telling in terms of risk. To begin with, a planned cesarean group with babies in a breech presentation was used as a surrogate for planned cesarean (since there were no other reliable data for identifying planned cesareans), and the outcomes of this group were compared with a planned vaginal delivery group in which the babies' position was cephalic (head down). Although the reported overall complication rate in the planned cesarean group was higher, no women died in this group, compared with forty-one deaths in the planned vaginal delivery group, and the risk of both uterine rupture and bleeding severe enough to require transfusion was significantly lower. In other words, although the percentage risk for complications was higher overall with a planned cesarean (including the need for an emergency hysterectomy), the actual incidence per thousand of each of these specific complications was extremely low. So low, in fact, that none were noted to reach statistical significance. And remember, these babies were breech and were therefore a more complicated delivery than a maternal request cesarean in a healthy pregnancy. The women with the absolute worst outcomes here were those in the planned vaginal delivery group who ended up with an emergency cesarean, which is in keeping with what we say repeatedly in this book. Their mortality rate was 9.7 deaths per one hundred thousand deliveries. So in fact this study (and many others like it), despite being cited by some natural-birth advocates to discredit planned cesareans, can be interpreted as highly reassuring for women who are considering a planned cesarean.[46]

Hematoma and Intracranial and Intraspinal Hemorrhage

Serious neurological complications such as these are very rare, also in the 0.6 percent range, but have the potential of devastating permanent effects. By taking cues from patients in the event that they feel any tingling or shooting pain during needle placement, anesthetists can lower this risk even further. And any persistent neurological symptoms, other than persistently improving postdural puncture headaches, should be investigated aggressively.

Failure of Spinal and Conversion to General Anesthesia

Spinal or epidural anesthesia might fail for a variety of reasons, including because the needle cannot be placed correctly; the right quality anesthetic block cannot be obtained; or the block simply fails completely, with the presumption that the anesthetic solution didn't end up in the correct position or concentration. These cases are usually converted into general anesthesia, which effectively means that the attempt at a spinal anesthetic is abandoned and a general anesthetic is given instead. Fortunately, this doesn't happen often. In fact, the chance that spinal anesthesia will need to be converted to a general anesthetic is reported to be about six out of every one thousand cases,[47] and even then, this figure relates to all general surgical cases, not just cesareans. It simply happens too infrequently for good numbers to be available in medical studies.

As for regional anesthesia failing altogether, or even just feeling insufficient during surgery, the risk is very small, but cases have been documented. If an epidural fails, the anesthetic dose can be increased through the catheter that's still in place into the spine, but if a spinal fails, the only option is conversion, as above.

Trapped Epidural Catheter

This is an exceedingly rare complication, which occurs if the epidural catheter gets a kink or a knot in it, and the only solution is surgical removal.[48]

High Block

This happens when the anesthetic block rises too high along the spinal cord and risks affecting a woman's breathing and other higher functions. The rate is low, and recent drug developments have made it even lower, but even before many of these improvements, the rate quoted in one Australian study was 0.07 percent, or around seven per ten thousand.[49]

Nausea, Vomiting, Shivering, and Itching

These are all common results of drugs, particularly the opioid component that is added to the anesthesia solution to provide longer-term pain relief once the actual block during surgery has worn off. Opioids are a group of strong analgesic medications (including codeine, oxycodone, morphine, Demerol®, and fentanyl), and the cause of most of their side effects is the histamine release from certain blood cells. Leaving the opioid out could prevent these problems in most women, but the trade-off would be a loss of the extra twelve to eighteen hours postoperatively of excellent pain relief without other medication or injections.

Nausea, vomiting, shivering, and itching are usually described as "nuisance" problems and not of too much concern medically. This is largely because if they do occur, there are very simple medications that can relieve them. But while patients' preference questionnaires have also clearly demonstrated that these rank quite low on the list of possible concerns,[50] these problems can nevertheless still result in quite an uncomfortable experience, particularly for women who were not expecting them. Pauline experienced severe nausea with her cesarean spinal anesthetic—far worse than her closest comparison of past episodes of car sickness—but the discomfort was short-lived because a counteracting drug was given intramuscularly (it can also be given intravenously), and it helped that she had prior knowledge that this was a possibility.

Uterine Rupture

The risk of uterine rupture during pregnancy—or, more specifically, during labor—is one more risk that increases after each subsequent cesarean, and it is frequently cited by critics of cesarean birth. But what's different about this particular risk is that it is almost exclusively related to future attempts of a *trial of labor*, so for women who have no desire to have a vaginal birth, and who will always choose a planned cesarean, it is very unlikely to happen if surgery precedes labor. This is fundamental to understand, especially since many women hear a list of cesarean risks that includes uterine rupture, and they have no idea that it relates to future attempts at *vaginal* birth, not cesarean.

That said, you may have read about the risks of a VBAC (vaginal birth after cesarean), which is considered to be a high-risk labor. This is because if uterine rupture occurs, both the mother's and the baby's lives are in serious danger. Having a repeat planned cesarean eliminates the risk of rupture almost completely (though there is always a small chance that rupture could still happen before labor), and this is why so many doctors and mothers favor it.

Rehospitalization

This is a potential risk for both mothers and babies. The risk of maternal readmission is about twice as high after a planned cesarean with no indication, compared to spontaneous vaginal delivery.[51] This risk is mostly related to wound complications and infection. On the other hand, however, there is no significant difference between the risk of rehospitalization after cesarean delivery and after instrumental vaginal delivery.[52] In terms of real risk, the same Canadian study that showed the similarity between hospitalization rates after cesarean and instrumental vaginal deliveries also showed that the real risk is one extra rehospitalization for every seventy-five cesarean deliveries. Importantly, this study looked at all cesareans and did not break it down into elective pre-labor versus emergency cesareans. Since we discuss in this book how much higher the complication rate is after an emergency cesarean, this crystallization of the real risk is actually highly reassuring.

Human Error

Some of these risks have already been discussed, but a few specific ones merit mention. These include the possibility of bowel or bladder injury during the abdominal opening phase, as well as ureter injury, usually during the suturing phase. The risk of bowel injury increases with every abdominal surgical procedure (of any kind) a patient has, and the risk of bladder injury increases with the number of cesareans. Both of these are mainly related to adhesions, which distort anatomy and change not only the position and mobility of organs but also their proximity to the baby's birth route. The bladder is located just below where the incision is made during a cesarean, and it is easy to cut into. Also, especially in cases in which a wider uterine incision is necessary to deliver the baby (sometimes if the baby is very large or lying in an awkward position), it is possible to catch and obstruct the ureter on one or even both sides when suturing the corners of the incision in the uterus. However, the delivery of a baby's head that is low down in the pelvis is a lot more difficult than one that is higher, so an emergency cesarean later in labor carries a significantly higher risk of this type of incision extension and, therefore, of the related complications (increased bleeding and increased bladder and ureter injuries) that can result.

Other issues include the competence and skill of the cesarean surgeon (and assistant) and the general quality of care in the maternity hospital. For example, there have been cases where foreign objects (for example, surgical instruments or cleaning gauze) have been left inside a woman's body, and certainly internationally, hospitals operate with a diverse range of guidelines and standards that might affect best evidence-based care (e.g., the administration of prophylactic antibiotics). In the United States, women are encouraged to carefully select their doctors, and many do just that.

Delayed Outcomes

Scar

Any surgical procedure will leave a scar. The nature of that scar will depend on where the incision was, how it was sutured or stapled, and whether an infection occurred, but to a large degree, the end result is also genetically determined, and a surgeon has no control over that. For example, although fortunately rare, some people form something called "keloid" whenever their skin surface is interrupted, which is basically a prominent scar with swelling and disfigurement. Keloid occurs only in humans and can occur up to a year after any skin injury. It can sometimes be quite dramatic and ugly, but there are ways to deal with it or to minimize it. Carefully tending to all bleeding, suturing with small, thin sutures, avoiding using too much tension on the incision edges, and preventing infection go a long way in minimizing this. If keloid develops, the scar can be treated with steroid injections or other medications that influence healing and local immune reactions, especially after the scar is "revised" by cutting it out and starting from scratch. With a bit of luck, it will not reform. Various products have claims of decreasing the visibility of scars, and there may be truth to some, including silicone dressings and vitamin A,[53] but some claims are exaggerated or fraudulent.

Skin Overhang

After any abdominal incision, the skin is attached to the underlying tissues through scar tissue that is not as freely able to slide as it was before. In the case of a transverse scar (one that goes from side to side above or in the pubic hair line—also called the "bikini incision"), the result might be a little roll of skin that slightly hangs over the scar, or at least appears more prominent. Although this is dependent on healing and also on the individual woman's BMI (body mass index), it is nevertheless quite common and leads to relatively frequent requests for a tummy tuck in the months or years after the birth.

Skin Sensation Loss

Any time the skin is incised, some small nerve branches are cut. After a cesarean, this is usually experienced as an area of loss or reduction of sensation around the incision. Even though this area of sensation loss usually shrinks and might even disappear completely, this can take a very long time and may never be complete. However, the same is true of the nerves affected during a vaginal birth with an episiotomy or perineal tearing.

Chronic Pain

Chronic pain is an infrequent but possible complication after any surgical or interventional procedure. Chronic pain is the result of changes in a patient's neurological system, with nerves continuing to send pain messages to the brain, or with the brain continuing to interpret messages from specific nerves as pain, even though no problem remains at the original site. A well-known example of this situation is phantom pain, the remaining sensation of pain in a limb that was amputated. Chronic pain is possible not only after cesarean surgery but equally or possibly more likely after a painful vaginal delivery.[54]

Bladder Overdistention

This is where the bladder is allowed to fill up with liquid beyond its normal capacity, mainly due to the effects of anesthesia, and the woman cannot feel that she needs to empty her bladder. While the bladder catheter is still in place, this is no problem, but it's important to be aware that while the sensation to void is temporarily disrupted, there is a danger that the bladder may overfill, thereby damaging its muscle and nerves. If this is not avoided or promptly corrected by timely recatheterization, it could lead to lifelong bladder complications—especially difficulties with emptying. It happens just as commonly after vaginal births, especially in cases where an epidural is used, but it is often overlooked as a potential risk with planned cesareans.

RISKS FOR THE BABY

One of the most interesting articles comparing the risks of morbidity and mortality of planned cesarean versus "expectant management" (i.e., planned vaginal delivery) was published in the journal *Seminars in Perinatology*, in 2006. A decision tree was constructed evaluating the outcomes of a hypothetical one million deliveries by planned cesarean section at thirty-nine weeks after uncomplicated pregnancies versus a comparable one million planned vaginal deliveries with ultimate delivery no later than forty-one weeks. A large number of possible complications, injuries, and events were evaluated and compared using event rates and probability assessments obtained from recognized and accepted peer-reviewed publications. These included problems such as inadvertent prematurity as a result of ultrasound error, neonatal death, respiratory problems (including various forms of possible respiratory distress), persistent pulmonary hypertension, cerebral palsy, intracranial hemorrhage, brachial plexus injury, facial nerve injury, sepsis, and fetal lacerations, among others.

The conclusion of this hypothetical study was clear: planned cesarean birth yielded the highest likelihood of a healthy baby. The study was then expanded to look at earlier gestational ages. Only if the planned cesarean was performed at or below an estimated thirty-seven weeks' gestation did the neonatal death of the cesarean group rise above that of the planned vaginal delivery group. And even though the planned cesarean group had lower overall mortality and morbidity from thirty-seven weeks onward, the respiratory risks, especially, could be lowered even more dramatically by postponing the cesarean until thirty-nine weeks.

In their final analysis, the study authors concluded, "The controversy over cesarean delivery by maternal request would more appropriately be addressed by focusing on the impact of mode of delivery on maternal health, rather than on neonatal health. Our data have implications for obstetricians who discuss therapeutic options with pregnant women, and would suggest that neonatal considerations should not be the primary basis for the decision for planned cesarean delivery."[55] In other words, they conclude there are no reasons involving fetal risks to argue against maternal request cesareans. Nevertheless, there *are* risks for babies that every mother should be aware of, and they are listed below.

Respiratory Distress

It is well accepted in medical circles that planned cesarean birth increases the possibility of certain causes of respiratory distress in the newborn, and some very large studies support this association. Infants delivered by planned cesarean are at higher risk for developing transient tachypnea, also called "wet lung syndrome" (where a baby's difficulty in breathing leads to fast, shallow breathing efforts), as well as persistent pulmonary hypertension (high blood pressure in the lungs), which interferes with the function of the lungs and the transition to efficient air breathing and gas exchange. These problems lead to higher rates of neonatal intensive care unit admissions and the need for artificial ventilation and prolonged hospital stays. Also, the treatment of one problem might lead to another, with increasing evidence that, for instance, oxygen treatment might be at least partially responsible for lung damage leading to eventual persistent pulmonary hypertension.[56]

Although sometimes resulting in a serious situation, most of the problems associated with respiratory distress are mild and temporary, with full recovery being the norm. Unfortunately, a small subset will go on to develop severe respiratory failure or even permanent chronic lung disease and death,[57] but these often tend to be the especially premature babies.

For all these reasons, respiratory distress is possibly the most frequently cited reason why planned cesarean birth in a healthy pregnancy is not ethical in the context of risks to the baby. However, there is a *huge* caveat that fits alongside all of the above examples of risk: the gestational age of the baby at birth. All these studies show little, if any, difference between the respiratory outcomes of vaginal and cesarean babies after thirty-nine weeks' gestation. Remember, women planning a cesarean birth are advised to wait until after the thirty-ninth gestational week to ensure lung development, so the vast majority of births that take place before this date are due to urgent health considerations of the mother and/or fetus.

On balance, the doctor decides that the risk of respiratory distress is less than a potentially worse outcome if the pregnancy is allowed to continue.

Who Is Most at Risk?

Essentially, every baby is at risk. After all, during birth, the fetus must essentially resuscitate itself by clearing its lungs of fluid after nine months of being completely submerged in fluid. And not only do the lungs have to be cleared, but the whole blood circulation system has to change suddenly, shunting blood away from a placental circulation and through the lungs. That said, we know babies born prematurely are at much greater risk. Even the difference of one or two gestational weeks can make a substantial difference in terms of respiratory health at birth. Every week before the thirty-ninth week of pregnancy that a baby is delivered increases the risk.

How Can the Risk Be Minimized?

In the simplest terms, delivery at thirty-nine-plus gestational weeks very effectively minimizes a baby's risk. In 2008, a large and widely reported study from Denmark concluded, "Compared with newborns delivered vaginally or by emergency cesarean sections, those delivered by elective cesarean section around term have an increased risk of overall and serious respiratory morbidity. The relative risk increased with decreasing gestational age." The inevitable criticism of "unnecessary" planned cesareans ensued, but the fact is that the percentage risk of *serious* respiratory morbidity was 0.1 percent for planned vaginal births and 0.2 percent for planned cesarean births, and for respiratory morbidity in general, it was 1.1 percent versus 2.1 percent.[58] As Pauline pointed out in a letter published on the *British Medical Journal* website, this "doubled risk should undoubtedly be taken into consideration by pregnant women — but in the context of other risks for the infant with planned vaginal delivery that have been recognized in other studies."[59] (See chapter 3, "The Safest Birth Choice for Your Baby," for more details). Similarly, in a large study carried out in Switzerland, it is mentioned almost in passing that there was no difference in the health of babies delivered by planned cesarean after thirty-nine weeks, compared with babies born by planned vaginal deliveries at the same gestation.[60]

There is also ongoing research about other ways to further mitigate the risk of respiratory distress—for example, injecting a woman with steroids a few days before her planned cesarean, as is routinely done for other premature deliveries.[61]

Fetal Injuries

This can be addressed by a simple statement: planned cesarean birth prevents serious fetal injuries in healthy pregnancies. There is a small risk of scalpel injury (occurring in a reported 0.74–1.5 percent of *all* cesarean births), but this is highly unlikely in a planned cesarean, and in fact, emergency cesarean and a laboring uterus have been identified as predominant risk factors in some studies—most notably, the 2004–05 NHS report of maternity statistics in England, which confirmed that of the estimated 0.9 percent of scalp injuries among 5,400 babies, "none" related to planned cesarean delivery.[62]

More serious cases of fetal injury during cesarean delivery have been described but are almost always associated with compounding factors, such as advanced labor (with a deeply stuck baby), breech presentation, and surgical inexperience, among others. For every case of an injury reported with a cesarean birth, however, the same can be found in cases of vaginal delivery.

For breech babies, although the debate continues and there are arguments about study designs, the only large prospective international study so far to look at the different outcomes between planned cesarean delivery of a breech baby at term versus planned vaginal delivery found *decreased* neonatal deaths and injuries in the cesarean group, with no increase in maternal complications. Incidentally, cesarean delivery was also found to be less costly than planned vaginal delivery in this study, but this issue is discussed further in chapter 11.

Gestational Age and Premature Birth

In an ideal world, premature birth should really not be a problem these days, and with today's accurate ultrasound technology and routine early-dating scans, gestational age is known more accurately than ever before. But of course, the ideal world doesn't exist, and there continue to be inadvertent—and, even worse, sometimes intended—planned deliveries of relatively premature babies.

Who Is Most at Risk?

Studies have found that between 30 and 50 percent of planned cesareans are done between thirty-seven and thirty-nine weeks, but while this period is clinically considered "at term," it is still before the recommended gestational age of thirty-nine-plus weeks and means that more babies are at greater risk. In one study from Alabama, researchers looked at the neonatal outcomes of 24,077 cesarean sections, of which 13,258 were planned, and of these, 35.8 percent were done prior to thirty-nine weeks. There was only one neonatal death, but it was clearly shown that a range of problems were more common in the earlier deliveries, including infections, the need for mechanical ventilation, low blood sugar levels, hospital stay for five or more days, and admission to NICU.[63]

This could happen as a result of dating mistakes, which are especially common in obstetrical units with fewer deliveries (and the associated reduction in ultrasound dating experience and expertise) or in situations when prenatal care is initiated late. However, unfortunately and tragically, prematurity in the context of a planned cesarean often means that the limits of safety are pushed with full knowledge of that fact.

How Can the Risk Be Minimized?

Unless premature delivery is urgently required due to a medical condition, we strongly recommend, in line with the vast majority of medical literature, that planned cesarean should not be done prior to thirty-nine weeks' gestation. If you're planning to get pregnant, keep a note of the date you menstruate each month so you can accurately tell your doctor what the last day of your period was, and when you are pregnant, visit your doctor as soon as possible to arrange a dating ultrasound scan. Early scans are far more accurate at measuring gestational age than later ones.

A HISTORICAL PERSPECTIVE OF RISK

Realize How Lucky You Are

Many people today have little concept of how lucky they are when they require surgery. Even a cursory read of the history of surgery or anesthesia will make any sane person want to fall to her knees and thank someone for the fact that she lives in these times of medical proficiency. Anesthesia is, for the most part, highly effective, and an understanding of the risks of blood-clotting disorders (thrombosis), bacteria, and hygiene, as well as the availability of effective antibiotics, make it very uncommon to develop any serious complications. The days of taking a swig of brandy, clenching a wooden block between your teeth, and having five people hold you down while you scream and fight as the surgeon hacks away are, thank goodness, long gone. So, too, are the days of doctors doing surgery with filthy hands full of fresh pus from other patients or corpses, having no understanding yet that this was causing the deaths of more than half of their patients.

Other than accounts from antiquity of the use of opioids and other herbal products for inducing unconsciousness (something that was not available to the masses), what we understand as modern anesthesia has a relatively short history. Until the early 1800s, mainstream surgeons believed patient pain was a healthy part of surgery, and there was little attention given to nullifying it. And even though the anesthetic properties of nitrous oxide (more commonly known as laughing gas, and still used widely during childbirth today) were known since 1799, it was initially mostly used for entertainment. Major breakthroughs in pain relief only came about when ether and chloroform were discovered and were demonstrated to be effective agents, and they were brought to wider public attention after Queen Victoria was given chloroform during the birth of Prince Leopold in 1853.[64] But even then, the use of anesthesia, and, specifically, anesthesia in childbirth, was not universally embraced; indeed, just weeks after the birth, a highly critical editorial of the queen's doctor was published. And when you consider the debate that continues to rage in some quarters over the questionable "necessity" of epidurals (as discussed in chapter 9, "The Politics of Birth"), it is clear that the tradition of wanting to deny women adequate pain relief during childbirth has not completely gone away, more than 150 years on.

Future Risk

When thinking about how very recent many of the things we take for granted during pregnancy and birth actually are (not just the basics of surgery, anesthesia, antibiotics, ultrasound, hygiene, and a vast array of medical treatments but also amazing advances in fetal laparoscopic surgery), and when placing this along a time line running the length of the human species' existence, we can only marvel at the cruelty of nature and the suffering that millions and millions of women and babies have gone through before us, many of them eventually dying in agony. It is simply incredible how we humans have achieved the possibility of escaping this cruelty—by our own ingenuity and by doggedly insisting on medical advances and progress. In this light, we believe the development of and access to cesarean delivery is perhaps the ultimate measure of humankind's partial escape from the ravages of nature. With this one intervention alone, we have managed to reduce the suffering, death, and injury of our species and to gain a small but important triumph over our evolutionary biological reality.

Today, we have sterile operating rooms, gowned and masked surgeons and nurses with sterile garments and gloves, anesthesia machines, monitors to measure every possible vital function, and replacement fluids for almost all contingencies. We have antibiotics that are effective against most organisms, and we have instruments, sutures, and medications all tested and proven effective and safe for use in the absolute majority of cases. However, this is not to say there are *no* dangers for pregnant women and their babies anymore; there most certainly are, even if they choose a planned cesarean birth. The risks associated with cesarean surgery are unequivocal, and just like almost every other surgical procedure, these risks increase with each repeat procedure. It is simply an interesting and informative exercise to put the oft-maligned maternal and neonatal mortality rates of our twenty-first-century relative comfort into some sobering historical context.

Unfortunately, there are a few dark clouds on the horizon, as it appears that neither nature nor evolution will allow our medical advancements to go unchallenged.

The most significant problem we face in the future is the emergence of multiple antibiotic-resistant bacteria, and this is mainly a result of the abuse (through overuse or, conversely, failure to complete a course) of antibiotics. Most people by now have heard of "superbugs" (which simply means, in this context, bacteria) that are very effectively resisting our efforts to kill them, but not everyone realizes these superbugs are entirely of our own creation. How? Because the antibiotics we take when ill are never specifically targeted at *only* the organism they are trying to fight. For example, let's say you have a urinary tract infection caused by a specific type of bacteria. Antibiotics are prescribed. This antibiotic will ideally be effective against the offending organisms, but it will also have an effect on other bacteria in your body.

This is because human beings have billions of bacteria on and inside their bodies; even every bowel movement we have consists of about 30 percent bacterial content. If you discontinue taking the prescribed antibiotics before *all* sensitive bacteria are killed, then the ones that are left alive will be less sensitive to that particular antibiotic than those that were killed off. Imagine this situation occurring a few times, and you can easily understand why the antibiotic will be less and less likely to work, until the remaining organisms are completely resistant to the antibiotic. In essence, that antibiotic will never work on you again. In addition, compounding the situation, even when the complete prescribed dose is taken, there are always a few bacteria that survive an antibiotic assault for a variety of reasons, including mutations. Basically, after the antibiotic treatment, the bacteria survivors have carte blanche and a clean slate to rapidly increase in numbers so that the overall balance of resistant versus sensitive organisms becomes more and more slanted toward resistant. And in spite of the ugly consequences for us as humans, this is a beautiful example of evolution at work.

It is also not a good idea to take antibiotics when there is no actual bacterial cause for the condition (a very common situation with colds and flu) because, since many common ailments are viral in origin, and viruses are completely insensitive to antibiotics, taking an antibiotic for a viral ailment makes no sense. Unfortunately, doctors sometimes feel pressured into prescribing antibiotics, even when they don't think they are required. Also, as a society, our internal bacterial cultures (which are essential for health) are continuously bombarded and abused by environmental exposure to antibiotics used in agricultural and animal husbandry in our incessant striving for higher production yields and a more sterile environment. Consequently, our abuse of antibiotics fuels ever faster growth of resistant bacteria.

In relation to thinking about a planned cesarean birth, and for that matter, a planned vaginal birth, we know that hospitals can often become infested with such resistant cultures of bacteria too. A large number of patients have been contaminated with MRSA (Methicillin-resistant *Staphylococcus aureus*), for example, during a hospital stay. Fortunately, hospitals are quite aware of this, and in almost all hospitals today, you will find hand-sanitizing alcohol dispensers every few meters — mostly to prevent healthcare workers from spreading these organisms.[65]

It's as though we have come full circle back to the "Aha!" moment when it was first realized by people like Ignaz Semmelweis and Alexander Gorden that the simple act of washing hands before delivering a baby could dramatically reduce the maternal death rate from puerperal sepsis (a very severe infection that could occur both during and after delivery, usually ending in maternal death). Ironically, these visionary obstetricians were vilified for their ideas but probably saved more women from a horrible death through their nineteenth-century message on the virtues of the simple act of hand washing than any other medical breakthrough, technologically advanced or not.[66]

Yet in spite of the threats to the future effectiveness of antibiotics, there is every hope the situation will improve. People are becoming more receptive to the idea that inappropriate use of antibiotics is dangerous and are more accepting of their family doctor's refusal to prescribe them unless absolutely necessary. Also, the pharmaceutical industry has a good record of developing new drugs. But whatever happens, the risk surrounding the future of antibiotics is not exclusive to women planning cesarean surgery; prophylactic antibiotics are common in vaginal births (for example, where Strep B is present), and, of course, where a vaginal birth plan has an emergency cesarean outcome.

SUMMARY

Perception of Surgical Risk

As a society, our acceptance of surgical procedures for various nonurgent situations has dramatically increased over the decades. Today, even some once-radical surgical procedures are accepted and supported, with very little second thought, as being an entirely personal choice, in spite of the known risks. Examples include various cosmetic procedures (such as breast enlargement/reduction, facial sculpting, and liposuction), gastric stapling for obesity, and interventions for many essentially nuisance issues, such as ablation or hysterectomy for heavy menstrual bleeding. Notably, this latter issue of menstruation is, like birth, a perfectly natural physiological process, endured with discomfort and even pain by women throughout the ages simply because they had no other choice. Yet today, when the option to do something about it is available, many choose that option.

For some conditions (for example, stress urinary incontinence), technological and scientific breakthroughs have meant a dramatic reduction in the invasiveness of surgical procedures, which in turn has led to a significantly increased uptake. As more and more women choose surgery for treatment, in many situations, it has become the default or preferred quick fix, even when natural alternatives are also available (for example, physiotherapy for stress urinary incontinence or strict dieting and exercise for obesity). However, with this increased demand for surgery, an acceptance of the inevitable possibility of complications must go hand in hand. And while the individual makeup of different women, coupled with the diversity of surgeon competence and hospital quality, can affect all risks and outcomes, it is interesting to note that in the United States, the rate of deaths after cosmetic surgery is equal to the country's overall maternal mortality rate (which includes *all* cesarean births), and higher than that of planned cesareans in Britain (the same comparison is unavailable for the United States, as its data on maternal deaths include all cesarean types combined).[67] Yet socially, disapproval of maternal request cesarean prevails.

Separation of Data

Obviously, there is no absolute guarantee of success when you have surgery or of a complication-free experience and recovery. Surgery is, by definition, a traumatic insult on the body. The fact is that the possibility of complications during and after surgery will always be a reality, and we simply cannot foresee the day when this will not be the case. However, there is also a risk involved in overstating or overemphasizing risks of surgical intervention and denying its benefits compared with the natural alternative. We believe that sometimes it's OK to take a risk in order to minimize another, especially given that when you compare a planned cesarean delivery group with a planned vaginal delivery group in healthy first-time mothers, it has been clearly shown that the chances of immediately life-threatening maternal complications are the same, but the risk of life-threatening complications for the baby is significantly reduced, and the long-term risk of complications for the mother is arguably lower too.[68]

The problem is that many studies reporting increased maternal risks with planned cesarean births have grouped *all* cesarean births together, including emergency cesareans and other high-risk cesareans (that may have been hastily planned due to medical or obstetrical indications), and then compared these with a group of successful, spontaneous vaginal births. Fortunately, the tendency to group all cesareans together in medical studies is happening less and less, but an acceptance that emergency cesarean outcomes should be applied to the planned vaginal birth group is proving to be a much slower process. Only when all birth data are appropriately separated and assessed, and the risks of planned cesareans are placed in context, will a clearer picture emerge.

Important Note

Although in this chapter we do our best to cover most of the serious risks associated with planned cesarean birth, including some with low probability, we do not claim this to be an absolute or complete list of every risk possible. For example, there is ongoing debate about the length of time between pregnancies as a possible risk factor for future pregnancies, which is not discussed here. There are other issues, too, where there is either no consensus or very little data available, but as with all issues of risk, you should discuss them in an individualized context with your own doctor or midwife.

Chapter 14

The Day of Surgery:
What Happens, Step by Step

Fortune favors the mind that is prepared.
—Louis Pasteur, Lecture,
University of Lille, December 7, 1854[1]

For doctors and medical staff, the operating room in a hospital, with its bright lights, stainless steel surfaces, various machines, and myriad tubes in sight, is simply their natural working environment. But for many women, a cesarean birth might be their first foray into this medical and surgical world, and they may not be sure about exactly what is going to happen or how they might feel when it does. Therefore, this chapter aims to provide you with detailed information about what is likely to happen on the day of your surgery and immediately afterward. The specific timings, order of events, hospital routines, and surgical techniques that we describe are meant only as a general example and can obviously vary from country to country and hospital to hospital, but we hope this will provide a useful prompt during discussions between women and their doctors about what to expect with a cesarean birth.

06:00 ARRIVAL AT THE HOSPITAL

Ideally well rested and excited about welcoming your baby into the world, you may also be a little nervous about what lies ahead, which is perfectly normal. You have not eaten or drunk anything since midnight, as you are "nil by mouth" in preparation for surgery. You are first checked in with the main hospital administration and then admitted to your ward.

287

06:45 PREPARATION FOR THE OPERATING ROOM

You will be asked to undress completely and don a most fashionable and attractive hospital gown. This is the last chance for taking photographs of your bump! If you haven't already done so (usually the previous day or two before surgery), you will need to have your preoperative blood work carried out. This is for checking your hemoglobin count and for type matching your blood group in case you need a transfusion later. Your baby's heart rate will also be checked and notated. And you may be asked a number of general questions by a nurse who is logging your personal information either directly onto a computer or in the form of traditional paperwork. Next up is the insertion and start of your intravenous (IV) with normal saline, which will allow fluids and medication to be delivered into your body. This may be done by a nurse or your anesthetist and involves inserting a needle into your forearm. It is a fairly straightforward procedure, although sometimes there can be difficulty finding a large enough vein in pregnant women because there may be some generalized soft tissue swelling, called edema, that hides the veins. Depending on individual hospital procedure, you may have your catheter inserted before going into the operating room, and the best advice here is to relax and take a nice deep breath, and it will be in before you know it.

The anesthetist and/or anesthesia resident will visit you to discuss how and when your anesthesia (usually spinal) will be administered. This is a great opportunity to ask any questions you may have and receive reassurances to calm your nerves if the anesthesia administration is something that worries you.

Your doctor/obstetrician (who is also your surgeon today) may visit too, if time allows in her morning schedule. Ideally, this will be the same person you have been meeting with throughout your pregnancy, or at least a member of the same obstetric practice, and again, it is your opportunity to ask last-minute questions. Perhaps you've made special arrangements, such as for music to be played during the birth to help you relax. Take this time to find out if everything has been set up, but keep in mind that as with all plans, there may be some hiccups on the day (ranging from something as simple as a broken CD player to something as unexpected as the postponement of your surgery until later in the day). Finally, your husband or partner will be provided with a rather fetching set of scrubs to put on in place of his clothes so that he can accompany you into the operating room.

07:15 ARRIVAL IN THE OPERATING ROOM

You will either walk into the operating room or be wheeled in on a gurney. You should be introduced to your nurses and the surgical assistant (two doctors will be operating). Then something called "surgical time out" occurs. This is a World Health Organization–mandated time of reflection in the operating room to check who the patient is, who the operating room team consists of, what the patient is there for, and whether there are any specific concerns (for instance, allergies or medical risks) that are particular to that individual patient. This procedure was developed mainly as an attempt to avoid wrong-site surgery or missing something of importance during the preparation for the actual procedure. Your name will be checked and any allergies confirmed or ruled out. Your blood type and blood antibody screen results will also be checked, and any concerns with anesthesia, obstetrical, or pediatric service will be discussed.

07:15 ADMINISTRATION OF ANTIBIOTICS

It has been unequivocally proven that the administration of a broad-spectrum antibiotic decreases the risk of infective complications post-surgery. The specific antibiotic you'll receive will depend on local antibiotic resistance in the area where you live or on the hospital, but it will most likely be a cephalosporin, a class of antibiotic with a broad spectrum and wide application in obstetrics and general surgery. As we discuss in more detail in chapter 13, "The Risks of Planning a Cesarean," current thinking makes it likely you will be given the antibiotic before the cesarean, either by the nurse just before transfer to the operating room or by the anesthetist shortly after arriving, rather than after delivery of the baby.

07:30 SPINAL ANESTHETIC

You will be asked to sit on the operating table (or helped onto it) with your legs dangling down on one side. A blood pressure cuff will be placed on your arm, and your IV is already running for preloading. The IV preloading is a volume of fluid being infused to help prevent the drop in blood pressure that might otherwise happen as a result of a sudden opening of peripheral blood vessels (in this case, in the legs) when their nerves are suddenly paralyzed by the anesthetic. You will be asked to bend forward and relax, making an outward curve with your spine. You may be given a supporting pillow on your abdomen, or you may be encouraged to put your arms around the shoulders of a supporting and comforting nurse and lean forward. At this point, you may feel a little chilly, but this could also be nerves, so try to relax, and try to remember that it'll all be over in a few minutes.

The anesthetist will ask you to call out if you feel a sharp pain at any point during the spinal procedure, especially one that shoots down your leg, since this will indicate that a nerve root was touched and the needle position needs to be slightly changed before continuing (try not to worry; this is not a usual occurrence). The anesthetist will then begin cleaning your lower back to ensure sterility. He will inject a small amount of local anesthetic agent (or "local freezing") into the skin of your lower back, and you may feel some pressure from his probing fingers as they feel along the vertebrae and intervertebral spaces. The freezing stings slightly, but for no more than a few seconds. Then you'll feel a dull pressure and slight ache as the thin spinal needle is inserted.

When satisfied with the needle position and seeing a few drops of spinal fluid escaping through the needle, the anesthetist injects the local anesthetic agent, combined with a small dose of an opioid (usually morphine for longer action but sometimes shorter-acting analogs like fentanyl or sufentanyl). After the needle is removed, you will be kept upright for a few moments to prevent the anesthetic agent from blocking higher spinal areas (gravity keeps it low in the spinal column until all of it has bound to receptors and therefore is not able to migrate higher) and asked to report any warm or heavy sensations in your lower body and legs. Next, you will be laid down on your back and slightly to your left, with your right side supported by a triangular sponge, pillow, or towel (each hospital will do this differently) to prevent the heavy uterus from obstructing the inferior vena cava (the large vein that takes blood from the lower body and legs back up to the heart). In some cases, the lateral tilt is simply achieved by adjusting the tilt of the bed, or in the case of electric beds, pushing a button to make it happen automatically.

Every pregnant woman is aware of the danger of lying flat on her back, and this is also true on the operating table. Any decrease in blood flow though the inferior vena cava, which can be caused by the uterus lying on it, for instance, could lead to a significant drop in blood pressure for you and could also negatively affect the baby. If your blood pressure does drop at this point, you might feel a sudden onset of nausea and dizziness; if so, you should tell your anesthetist. He may have already noticed the change, but either way, he will increase the IV flow rate and may give you some medication, which will cause a contraction in small blood vessels throughout your body and rapidly restore your blood pressure. You will feel much better almost immediately, and this contraction is not in any way dangerous for your baby—whereas an uncorrected rapid fall in blood pressure might be, if left untreated.

Your vital signs (blood pressure, heart rate, and oxygen content of your blood) are being checked constantly by monitors on your finger, around your upper arm, and on the skin over your heart. You will be given an oxygen mask to increase your blood oxygen content; this fits loosely, and there is no smell. Or as an alternative, the anesthetist might choose small nasal prongs to deliver oxygen into your nostrils. If you are prone to feelings of claustrophobia, make sure you discuss this with the anesthetist beforehand, since the nasal prongs might be a better choice for you.

07:45 PREPARATION FOR SURGERY

While the surgeon and surgical assistant are being gloved and gowned with the help of the scrub-in nurse, another nurse usually cleans your abdomen with an antiseptic solution. The specific solution used is dependent on local preference and possible allergies. You are cleaned from chest to upper legs, and in some hospitals, the catheter will be inserted in your bladder at this point (rather than earlier) because waiting until the anesthetic is in place has the benefit that you will not feel a thing. It is unlikely that your pubic hair will be shaved, since this has been found to increase infection; more commonly, the hair might just be clipped nearer the top. While all this is going on, the pediatric team arrives and checks the pediatric resuscitation equipment. A neonatal resuscitation table is in the operating room, already warmed and ready to accept your new baby.

DAD/PARTNER'S ROLE

At this point, the father of the baby is usually called in (if he has requested to be present) and takes his rightful and proud place beside your bed, next to your head, where he is out of the surgical team's way but fully engaged in the process and supporting you. Some less squeamish dads-to-be like to watch the surgical procedure and even take photos or videos (as Pauline's husband did), but most don't, and of course, some hospital policies do not allow this anyway. You may simply appreciate your husband or partner holding your hand and telling you what's happening over the top of the curtain in front of you.

08:00 SURGERY COMMENCES

The leading surgeon will most likely be on your right-hand side if she is right-handed and on your left-hand side if she is left-handed, but this is not a rule. By now you will be draped in paper or cloth drapes and will not be able to see down below, since the drape is clipped to the IV pole on the one side of the bed and a bed extension on the other, forming a screen in front of you. Some surgeons allow this to be removed so that the baby can be handed to you for immediate skin-to-skin contact when it is born (this is referred to by some as a "natural cesarean"), but others advise that it's not worth the risk of infection (for you or your baby). Therefore, if this is something that is important to you, you will need to discuss the risks and benefits with your doctor well in advance of the day of surgery and bear in mind that there may be an official hospital policy on this practice.

The surgeon will ask you whether you can feel anything. What she is actually doing is pinching your belly with a sharp instrument where the cut is going to be made, to confirm the spinal anesthetic has been effective. Once the surgeon is satisfied the anesthetic is working, the first cut will be made.

Skin

The majority of (and almost all planned) cesarean incisions are made from side to side (transversely) across your lower abdomen, just below the pubic hair line and about three centimeters above your pubic bone. This is called a Pfannenstiel incision, or the so-called bikini incision. This incision has cosmetic benefits over a vertical incision since the scar will be mostly hidden by pubic hair and your bikini or panties, even when the rest of the abdomen is exposed. The name is in recognition of a German gynecologist, Hermann Johannes Pfannenstiel, who popularized this incision in the year 1900 mainly in an attempt to reduce the number of incisional hernias that were occurring with vertical incisions. Very occasionally, there is still the need for a classical cesarean today—for example, in cases when fetal death is imminent (the vertical incision is quicker) or when the patient already has a vertical scar from a previous abdominal surgery (so there will be only one scar rather than an inverted T scar, which often doesn't heal very easily at the junction).

Subcutaneous Layers

Below the skin but above the abdominal muscles, there are two main layers that have to be incised or separated. These include fat and fascia. The fat layer will usually simply be opened with fingers or, if necessary, cut by scalpel or electrocautery. Electrocautery is simply the effect on tissue of an electrical current induced in a needlelike metal tip, which can then be used to cauterize (seal with burning) or cut tissue. The fascia layer (also called the rectus sheath) is a very important layer, which the surgeon encounters next. The fascia layer is a major structural support layer and is also the main protection against abdominal wall herniation. Any defect of more than a centimeter in the fascia after abdominal surgery will possibly lead to a hernia, and the repercussions of this can range from being a cosmetic nuisance to causing discomfort or pain to causing a life-threatening bowel obstruction and strangulation. The fascia layer covers the abdominal muscles, and after it is incised in the same transverse orientation as the skin incision, the edges of the cut fascia are lifted up and separated from the underlying muscles. This is usually accomplished by gently pushing the muscles down while the fascia is lifted up, but some cutting or electrocautery is usually also necessary. There are also small blood vessels in this area that need to be cauterized, since any bleeding here after the procedure might lead to a hematoma (blood collection) in the space created.

Muscles

Next, the surgeon must get past your abdominal muscles. Many people have the misconception that the abdominal muscles are cut during a cesarean birth. You will often hear people explain away their "mummy tummy" as a result of the muscles having been cut and therefore weakened. In fact, no abdominal muscle is actually cut in the sense of transecting it. Rather, it is pushed aside. In the midline of the abdomen, there are really only two muscles, one on each side, called the rectus abdominal muscles. These muscles run from the lower ribs to the pubic bone and form the six-pack in well-trained athletes, with the indentations of the six-pack formed by fascia bundles visible through the skin when the muscle is large from training and the subcutaneous fat layer very thin. Fascia layers surround the muscles completely and are pinched together every few centimeters, forming the indentations. To access the abdominal cavity, all the surgeon has to do is find the area between the muscles, or pull the muscles both over to one side and find the edge on one side, where again there is only fascia, and incise that. It might help to imagine an animal being skinned: it is often necessary to cut the meat away from the skin, and yet neither the meat nor the skin is actually cut. This is the only "cutting" that is done.

After going through the fascia between or alongside the rectus muscles, the only layer left is the parietal peritoneum. This is a very thin, shiny layer with no structural integrity but an important role covering and protecting the intra-abdominal organs, almost like plastic wrap protecting your lunch. Your surgeon will carefully open the peritoneum, knowing that your bowel is directly underneath this layer and also aware that if you had any previous abdominal surgery, you may have bowel stuck underneath this thin layer.

Preparing to Open the Uterus

After opening the peritoneal layer, the surgeon will extend the incision to create an opening big enough to deliver your baby through. This is done by cutting the peritoneum toward the pubic bone and stretching the rectus muscles apart. This stretching undoubtedly injures some of the muscle fibers, but the damage is negligible compared to what it would be if your muscle were actually cut. Next, a retractor is placed through the incision.

This retractor is held by the assistant and is specially designed to protect the bladder and keep the incision open enough for the surgeon to be able to access the uterus. The next decision is whether to open a thin layer on the lower uterus and pull the bladder farther down (this is called creating a "bladder flap") or to simply cut this layer during the same incision used to open the uterus. This layer is the visceral peritoneum, a continuation of the peritoneum surrounding the pelvic organs. These days, most surgeons choose to cut the peritoneum but not pull the bladder down.

The next important step is to identify the lower segment of your uterus. Simplistically, your uterus consists of a thicker "upper" and a thinner "lower" segment. Most cesareans—and certainly almost all planned cesareans—are done by cutting the thinner lower segment in the same transverse orientation as the skin incision (a vertical uterine incision, although indicated in exceptional medical situations, has significant implications for future pregnancies but is beyond the scope of this book). Usually the first incision is made as a partial-thickness incision to prevent injuring your baby, who is lying underneath. The middle part of the partial-thickness incision is then completed with some blunt instrument (for instance, a grasper or some kind of clamp) or by carefully cutting until the uterus is just entered. The surgeon will then insert her two index fingers into the small opening and spread them in the direction of the partial-thickness incision, thereby completing the creation of a larger opening.

Not only does this method minimize the possibility of injuring your baby with the scalpel but it also reduces the risk of injury to some of the large blood vessels that run along the edges of your lower uterus. Simply cutting right across the lower segment would inevitably cut these vessels and could lead to immediate, significant bleeding. Not only would this bleeding create some urgency to complete the procedure, but it could also increase the risk of other injuries during the haste of trying to stop the hemorrhage. For example, your surgeon might place sutures in a hurry, and because of decreased visualization, these sutures could potentially obstruct or damage the ureters (tubes taking urine from the kidneys to the bladder), which run close to this area, one on each side. Since your surgeon is well aware of this danger, however, she will spread the tissue rather than cut it, and the vessels will stretch out of the way but most likely stay intact.

08:05 BIRTH OF YOUR BABY

Yes, you've read the time correctly. From the first incision to delivery of your baby, barely two or three minutes will pass. During these few minutes, you will experience a sensation of pulling, some heavy pressure on your stomach, or possibly nothing at all. Perhaps you will be listening to your choice of music or chatting with your husband/partner.

After opening the uterine wall, your surgeon will penetrate the amniotic sac by simply cutting it with the scalpel or by grabbing and tearing it with a surgical clamp. This will be accompanied by a gush of amniotic fluid, depending on how much fluid remains (the volume of amniotic fluid tends to decrease in late pregnancy). The surgeon will now reach in with her hand, carefully lift your baby's head out of the incision, and guide it through the opening in the uterus. Sometimes a baby's head might be a bit too far down in the birth canal to easily fit a hand around it, in which case, a soft vacuum cup might be used to lift the head up. After the delivery of your baby's head, its nose, mouth, and throat will be suctioned to get rid of any remaining amniotic fluid that might be inhaled with its first breath. Even though this seems counterintuitive, given that your baby's lungs are still full of fluid, this procedure is important in case there is any meconium inside the baby's nose, mouth, or throat. Meconium is a baby's first poop, a sterile (unless the membranes have been ruptured for a while) mixture of secretions and cells from its gastrointestinal tract. Babies tend to pass meconium in the uterus when stressed, but also sometimes for no reason, especially during late pregnancy, and the danger is that inhalation of this sticky, gummy material could cause respiratory complications and something called meconium aspiration syndrome.

After this suctioning, your baby's shoulders and arms will be carefully delivered, after which the rest of the body is pulled out. There may be some necessary tugging, turning, and twisting of your baby as it is pulled out, which may look rough if you play back the video later, but in comparison to the forces of vaginal delivery, this is no worse. At this point, the majority of babies will start breathing or even crying. If this is what happens with your baby, and there are no urgent problems, your surgeon may well show him/her to you by lowering the drape. Some may even give you your baby to hold on your chest (again, you should have discussed all these possibilities with your doctor prior to this day) while the cord is cut (either by your surgeon or your husband/partner, depending on arrange-ments) and cord blood is collected from the placental side of the cut and clamped cord. Cord blood is routinely collected for a variety of reasons including testing your baby's blood group, and in some hospitals, you may be asked whether you'd like to donate your baby's cord blood for research or donation purposes (unless, of course, you've already arranged to have it collected for your own family's use). In a short while (or immediately, if your baby is born not breathing or crying strongly), the assistant surgeon will hand your baby off to the pediatric team, who will place him/her on a warm blanket under a heater and proceed with their assessment. Your husband/partner might be called over to inspect the baby if things are going well, and as soon as the team is happy with your baby's condition, he/she might be wrapped up in a warm blanket and handed to Dad to bring over to you. Often, a friendly nurse will offer to take a photograph of you all together if your husband/partner has a camera at hand.

08:10 DELIVERING THE PLACENTA

Your placenta is delivered by your surgeon by gentle traction on the umbilical cord while waiting for the natural contractions that follow; she can then squeeze it out after it releases. In some cases, the surgeon will need to insert her hand into the uterus to separate the placenta from the uterine wall, but usually this is not necessary. After removing the placenta, your surgeon will want to make sure your uterus is empty of any placental fragments, since if there is any bleeding a few days afterward, it is reas-suring to know that the uterus was empty, and no large placental pieces remained that might subsequently require removal through a D&C (dila-tion and curettage — basically, an excavation and scraping process), as can happen after vaginal birth. In cases in which there is bleeding after a cesarean but the surgeon knows the uterus is empty, it can be managed either by simply waiting it out or with antibiotics, depending on the clin-ical course. This determination is done by inspecting the placenta and also looking or feeling inside the uterus.

08:12 TIDYING UP, INSPECTING, AND CLOSING
(Concurrent with Anesthetist's Introduction of Antibiotic)

The longest part of the procedure now starts: the exit. This stage is critical for your future well-being, but it is relatively straightforward, and the steps are well defined. The first step is something we believe should always be done but nonetheless is often neglected; inspecting the ovaries. Dr. Murphy can recollect hearing during his career about a few cases of women who underwent cesarean deliveries (not necessarily planned) and died of or were diagnosed with ovarian cancer within a relatively short time after the birth; the presumption (and that is all it is) is that an earlier diagnosis might have yielded a different outcome. Since there is no risk and many potential benefits in at least *looking* at both ovaries and tubes, ideally this is something your surgeon will do.

The next important decision is whether to pull the uterus out through the skin incision for ease of suturing or to perform the suturing with the uterus still inside the abdomen. Dr. Murphy feels strongly that there is almost never a need to take the uterus out and that doing so can have significant potential negative implications—for instance, air embolism or drying of the uterine, ovarian, and fallopian tube surfaces, which might cause adhesion formation. If the uterus is lifted up through the incision, what happens in effect is that the uterus is lifted higher than your heart, and this creates a pressure gradient, which can increase the entry of air through open venous sinuses in the uterine cavity where the placenta was attached. Manual removal of the placenta, especially after lifting the uterus through the incision, increases this tendency. Although some entry of air into the venous circulation is common during a cesarean and other surgical procedures, the lungs can usually deal with it by filtering it out. But massive air entry can lead to shock and cardiovascular collapse. Since your surgeon knows this, however, your uterus should remain safely where it belongs, inside your abdomen, while the assistant is helping the surgeon see by performing appropriate retraction and aspiration of amniotic fluid and blood.

The suturing steps proceed in the following order:

Uterus
Visceral (seldom done) and parietal peritoneum (often not done)
Rectus sheath (fascia)
Subcutaneous tissue (optional)
Skin

Uterus

The uterine incision is sutured in one or two layers. There is much debate about whether one layer is enough or whether two is better. Clearly, if one layer doesn't provide sufficient hemostasis (absence of ongoing bleeding), a second is needed. The question is whether a second layer decreases the risk of uterine rupture during a future pregnancy or delivery. The evidence seems to point toward a higher risk of rupture if a one-layer suturing technique is used, so if a woman is planning a further pregnancy, two layers are recommended.[1]

Bladder Peritoneum

There is evidence that it is best not to suture this layer on the way out, so your surgeon will most likely leave it alone and allow the layers to find their most appropriate opposite sides and heal. Placing sutures could cause stretching forces and impede normal movement of the layers, with the end result of more adhesions.[2]

Cleaning Out the Abdominal Cavity

After the uterus is sutured and before the abdominal wall is closed, this is the last chance for your surgeon to look around the abdominal cavity and make sure that no foreign object has been left behind inside your body and that all amniotic fluid, blood, and meconium have been swabbed or sucked up and removed. You should be aware that during the cleaning process, you may feel rather like someone is kneading dough inside your stomach as your surgeon probes in and around. This shouldn't be painful, but some women do find it very uncomfortable.

Parietal Peritoneum

This is the layer that was carefully opened earlier to prevent bowel injuries. There was a time when it was considered unnecessary to suture this layer, and many obstetricians still don't, but although it is by no means absolutely proven, suturing this layer seems to be beneficial since this might lead to fewer adhesions.

Rectus Sheath/Fascia

It is crucial that this layer be sutured, and sutured well. A variety of suture materials might be appropriate, and your surgeon will have her own preference. All obstetricians and surgeons understand the crucial role of this layer of the abdomen in maintaining the integrity of the abdominal wall, and at this point in the procedure, your surgeon is undoubtedly busy suturing your fascia studiously. The nurses will count all instruments and swabs/sponges/gauzes after the rectus fascia has been closed (having previously counted them going in), and this is a crucial stage to prevent mistakes such as leaving instruments or objects behind in the abdominal cavity. The reason the count is postponed until now is that if it were done prior to closing the rectus sheath, there would be the possibility of a last-minute swab or clamp used and forgotten. After closure of the fascia, the abdomen is essentially closed, so this cannot occur. Of course, there is still an open wound, but this is merely a superficial one with defined edges and a base that is clearly visible, in contrast to the open abdominal cavity with all the bowel loops that can easily hide objects.

Subcutaneous Tissue

You might remember that at the beginning of the procedure, your surgeon separated this layer by simple finger spreading or quickly cutting through with a scalpel or electrocautery blade. This layer consists largely of fat and has no structural strength, so therefore the only reason to suture it is if the fat layer is very thick and not doing so would leave a relatively large potential cavity for the possible collection of blood or serum.

Skin

Since a scar on your skin is the only physical reminder of the entire procedure (other than your baby, of course), it is important that the aesthetics of the scar not be neglected. The fact is, though, that in the case of a Pfannenstiel incision, there is practically no difference in cosmetic outcome however the skin is put back together. Whether it is stapled or sutured with external stitches or with subcutaneous sutures, the eventual cosmetic result will depend on genetics, whether or not an infection occurs, and, yes, a bit of luck—not on what it looks like the first few days after the procedure. Your surgeon will thus close the incision with the method of her own choice or sometimes your personal preference, if you have one, and as final extra security, some doctors will place tape strips across the wound before covering it with a dressing.

After all the suturing is complete, your surgeon will begin clearing out any excess blood through your vagina. This surprises some women, and indeed many are probably never aware of it happening since they don't feel a thing due to the anesthesia. Your stomach will be pressed on and internal fluid pushed downward toward your vagina—rather like you might squeeze out the remains of a tube of toothpaste—while the doctor uses a surgical sponge to soak up the escaping blood and, finally, gives your vagina and upper legs a general wipe clean.

By this time, your baby may well be in your arms or in the arms of Dad, who is sitting next to you again. Or it could be that your baby has been taken to the nursery (tagged with a security wristband matching your own and possibly even with Dad in tow). Both options are to allow you time to lie back and relax while surgery is being completed.

08:30 RECOVERY ROOM, WARD, OR PRIVATE ROOM

In some hospitals, you may be moved into a recovery room and covered in warm blankets for a short period of time (approximately thirty to forty-five minutes), while your doctor makes notes about your surgery. Alternatively, you may be transferred from the operating room bed straight into your own bed on the ward or in a private room. This depends on the hospital and your doctor. You will still be paralyzed from the waist down and won't feel any pain, but you may decide at this point to try breastfeeding immediately, and as long as both you and the baby are healthy, there is no reason why you can't.

12:00 RETURN OF SENSATION

Although you will start feeling and moving your legs by this time, you'll still feel almost no pain. The opioid you received in your spinal will keep you completely or mostly pain-free for up to eighteen hours. You can feel the intermittent compression of your calves by the sequential compression device stockings (SCDs) that have been put on your legs, and your doctor may give you a blood thinner to prevent blood clotting if she thinks it's necessary (it's not always). You will still have your catheter and IV in place, and you may be allowed to begin oral intake, starting with some water. How soon you'll be allowed to eat varies from institution to institution, but the modern tendency is for a very quick restarting of a full diet.

18:00 FIRST WALK AND MEAL

By now, you should feel strong enough to get up and walk around, even if only tentatively and slowly, and you will certainly be encouraged to try to sit up and get out of bed (even the shortest distance, to sit in a nearby chair, is sufficient). Your IV has been replaced by a saline lock, which is to protect the access to the vein in case it is needed again later, but this will not affect your mobility at all, and you'll hardly know it's there. Your abdomen will feel uncomfortable, and maybe you will have some pain, but many women say they are surprised by how little pain they actually feel, even once all their sensation is back. Your catheter will have been removed earlier by a nurse, and all being well, you've urinated once already. Your nurse will have also scanned your bladder immediately after urination to make sure it does indeed empty well and to reduce your chances of developing an overdistended bladder.

Throughout the afternoon and evening, and indeed during the rest of your hospital stay, you will receive frequent visits from junior nurses who need to take your temperature and blood pressure at various intervals. In fact, frequent interruptions are common during the days and nights in the hospital (nurses administering painkillers and checking you and your baby, for example). Your dinner will be delivered, and depending on your doctor's orders, you should be able to eat a little and will most likely be allowed to drink fluids as you wish. Your baby is most likely in your room in a bassinet, and ideally, a friendly nurse will be available to help and advise you on topics such as breastfeeding, bottle feeding, burping, and changing your baby.

Dad may well be asleep in the chair.

Chapter 15

Tips on Preparing for and Recovering from a Cesarean

To wish to be well is a part of becoming well.
—Seneca (Roman dramatist, philosopher, and politician),
mid–first century CE

This chapter is a collection of tips from women who have had planned cesareans themselves, and while we do not mean to present it as an exhaustive list of everything you might want to think about or should know, we hope it provides useful insight into some aspects of preparing for and recovering from a cesarean that you might otherwise not have considered. Notably, some of these tips reflect negative aspects of a planned cesarean birth in relation to how it is perceived and supported by others, but we are confident this situation will improve in the future. These stories are all actual accounts, but some names have been changed to protect identities where requested, and some stories have been edited for length.

PREPARING FOR A CESAREAN

- There are a few factors that helped with the success of the whole process. First, I was in the best physical shape possible. I continued to do exercise up until the last month of my pregnancy and read a lot about exercises appropriate for after the cesarean. Everything went very well with the surgery, I had an easy recovery and little pain two weeks after the birth.

  Secondly, what helped was having my spouse's absolute support with the decision of having an elective cesarean right from the beginning of the pregnancy. (*Natalia, Colombia*)

- The best preparation I did was reading as much information on cesareans as I could and speaking to as many people as possible about it. This meant that nothing that happened on the day surprised me! I enjoyed the experience 100 percent! I would also advise women to speak to their partner and have them as informed as possible, too, because it can be very distressing for them otherwise. (*Rhonda, United Kingdom*)

- Things I was glad to have known beforehand are: how many people were present in the operating room and what their roles were, that I could take my camera in, that I would need lots of maternity pads, that I might pass big blood clots, that the spinal anesthesia might make me itch and feel unwell, and that I would have a urinary catheter in place for twenty-four hours.

  Things I wish I had known beforehand are: that my husband and baby wouldn't stay for the whole of the surgery, how woozy I'd feel during and after the procedure, that they wouldn't offer to lower the screen so I could see our baby being born, quite how much blood I'd pass afterward, being unable to move for what seemed like hours, and how little help I would receive from the ward staff. But most of all, I wish I'd known how people would treat me afterward—ranging from indifference at best, to complete disdain and scorn—and generally from otherwise lovely people, which made the comments even more hurtful. This, coupled with the complete battle I had to secure my cesarean and the guilt this engendered, led to my postnatal depression. I was aware that women who deliver a baby vaginally can feel an immense sense of achievement, but I hadn't registered the flip-side: the overwhelming sense of failure for not even attempting to do so. I'm sorry this may not sound very positive but I think forewarned is forearmed. (*Anon, United Kingdom*)

- Know what is going to happen and when. I was very happy knowing this, and I think most working women prefer some element of control. I had some very difficult decisions with the consultants at the hospital, as they appeared judgmental about my decision to have a planned cesarean. But my doctor was fantastic;

he encouraged me to stick to my guns and supported me throughout my pregnancy. I was adamant that I knew what was best for my body, although in the end, I developed gestational diabetes and placental praevia, which meant they agreed to the cesarean easily. (*Farhana, United Kingdom*)

- The most painful part of prepping for surgery is having your IV put in, and then they give you a nasty green liquid shot to drink [note: this is an antacid to counter stomach acid in case aspiration occurs, but it is not routinely given with spinal anesthesia]. (*Claudia, United States*)

- To make a long story short, my doctor, who approved my maternal request cesarean, was on vacation when my labor started (three days before surgery was scheduled at forty weeks), so a second doctor from the ob-gyn practice performed the cesarean. But before doing it, she was incredibly coercive trying to talk me out of it (while I was in pain from contractions), and she almost refused at the last minute. If anything similar happens to you, or if you feel you are/were disrespected by doctors or any hospital staff because of your decision, *write a letter* to the management. I did so, and I know for a fact that it opened a dialogue at the ob-gyn clinic about maternal request. I also tell new moms-to-be of my experience. Some (even those choosing vaginal) are not choosing that hospital or clinic because of my story. (*Kathrine, United States*)

- One useful tip someone gave me before I went into hospital was to take nighties instead of pyjamas because it's a bit trickier to wear PJ's with a catheter in! (*Sarah, United Kingdom*)

- My (elective) cesarean was fantastic, and my biggest tip would just be to enjoy every moment. It's a day you'll never forget, and it's a wonderful experience! My husband chose to trim my son's cord, which we discussed with my midwife before the big day. He felt included and really enjoyed being able to do something!

  Another tip would be to be totally organized with your reasons for choosing a cesarean, and make your feelings known as soon as possible when deciding to request one. I told my doctor how I felt with regard to my birth choice on my first visit after having a positive pregnancy test, and he passed this on to my midwife, so that by my first visit with her she was aware. At every point (GP doctor, midwife, senior midwife at hospital, and consultant), I had notes with me and was very clear on every point. (*Hannah, United Kingdom*)

- Ask your doctor, and if necessary, the hospital, what their policy on photographs and video is. My husband recorded our children's births, but we had to get permission to do so beforehand, and this made everything run more smoothly on the big day.

  If your birth is to be paid for by private health insurance, it's a good idea to find out the company's policy on "maternal request" ideally *before* you get pregnant, in order to avoid unexpected hospital bills when your baby is just weeks or even days old. You may be too tired and indeed vulnerable to deal with this then, and pregnancy is not an ideal time to feel stressed either, but unfortunately, this is a battle that many women are having—particularly in the United States but also in other countries—because many insurance companies do not understand the prophylactic nature of a planned cesarean birth. (*Pauline, United States*)

RECOVERING FROM A CESAREAN

- I was determined to get up and walk the next day, even if it was just a trip to the bathroom. I made myself get out of bed and walk. Then gradually I would walk a little bit farther each day, which I felt helped me recover quickly. Also, don't be shy in asking for painkillers! That assisted me in getting through the first week. (*Jessica, Australia*)
- Don't take too many painkillers—they can fool you into thinking you're more ready to do things than your body actually is. Having said that, get out of bed as soon as you can manage (even though it can be painful), and start moving about, even if somebody has to walk with you. It helps get your circulation going. After leaving hospital, *walk!* Walk as much as you can, everywhere. Don't run or rush or strain. Just walk at a leisurely pace. There's no better and gentler exercise. (*Siriol, United Kingdom*)
- I was extremely satisfied with the operation itself and the fact that I was up the next day and removed my dressing and had a shower etc. It took a few days' rest before I trusted my body to cope with a

normal day's work, but I felt normal and was happy with my scar. (*Farhana, United Kingdom*)

- It's about staying active. Getting up and going to the toilet helps you get used to your body faster! Don't be shy to ask for stronger painkillers if you want—they gave me paracetamol (acetaminophen) that did nothing. After I had asked for something stronger, I could deal with it faster and was up and about in twelve hours after my operation. I was cleared to leave the hospital twenty-four hours after my baby was born, and I was up and about and driving again after two weeks! Most importantly, don't believe the nonsense people tell you that you can't lift your baby or look after her. I did everything myself with very little help from my partner and mom! (*Rhonda, United Kingdom*)

- We found it helpful to show our little girl my wound so that she understood Mummy's tummy was sore. It helped her put it into context, and since it was covered with this air bubble protection, it wasn't scary for her to see—in fact, she asked to see. You have to use your judgment, but in our experience, it did help her to understand—in fact, she offered to kiss it better for me!

  Also, I was always quite self-conscious about the fact I had chosen a cesarean, and when it later turned out that my baby was breech, I had a legitimate reason, so I used that to avoid any awkwardness on the topic. However, I think it's very sad and judgmental of people who think women shouldn't be allowed to have a cesarean, when often there are personal circumstances that really do make this the best option for a couple, such as ours at the time. My husband was away working in Geneva long term, and after the poor care I had with my first baby, I was very concerned about what would happen if my husband wasn't there to support me. (*Sarah, United Kingdom*)

- The only way to handle the remarks other mothers may give you with regard to your birth choice is to say exactly that—it's *your* birth choice! Be firm, don't get into any long discussions (it takes too much of your valuable energy when you are pregnant and a new mum) and if pushed, simply let them know that you have your opinion about how they chose to give birth, too, but you respect them enough to know that whatever they chose was great for them, and who are you to question that? (*Hannah, United Kingdom*)

- I asked my doctor for a belly band/corset to help keep everything tight post-surgery and it also helps your muscles re-tighten [note: not exactly "re-tighten," but something like a corset may make you feel more comfortable]. As long as you take your medication, pain is very manageable, although you will still feel sore. Then after the first week, you will see a big improvement. (*Claudia, United States*)

- My doctor's advice was to wait until the first time I'd passed gas before I tucked into any food (to make sure my bowels were getting back to normal after surgery), and she was very strict about this (in a nice way). And although some of the nurses told me to eat sooner and I'd be just fine, I did as I was asked, and it made good sense to me, too, since it removed the pressure (excuse the pun) of "needing" to go to the bathroom for the first time and worrying whether it would be OK. To help get my bowels moving, my doctor gave me "bed exercises" to do, rather like post-surgery physiotherapy, which I did. Also, I had read studies before going into hospital that found chewing gum could help enhance the recovery of bowel function, but I must admit that as a non-gum chewer in regular life, I kept forgetting to do this. It might work for you though, so it's definitely worth a try!

  Again on the subject of "getting things moving," my top tip would be to bring a large bottle of prune juice into hospital and have it ready to drink at least one glass, if not two, every day after surgery. I learned the hard way (since I didn't know this after my first baby) that both the painkiller Percocet and breastfeeding are very dehydrating, and this does not help in facilitating ongoing bowel movements and can cause constipation. After my second baby, and having talked to two doctors with personal cesarean and constipation experience, I did not use Percocet at all, relying instead on regular painkillers such as ibuprofen and paracetemol, and I packed plenty of prune juice to complement my water intake!

  Another thing I packed were comfy, yet attractive underwear in order to feel back to normal again as quickly as possible after surgery. As it happened, I had to wear rather unattractive elastic string panties while in hospital, which just made my husband and I laugh, but from a practical point of view, they were great for protecting the wound dressing and then staples, and for holding a sanitary pad in place (something I thought I'd never see again after discovering tampons in the 1980s, let alone twice the size I remembered them!).

In terms of food, I asked my husband to bring in healthy food to the hospital while I was recovering with my second baby (Panera Bread, I salute you!). The catering first time round was superb, with high-quality, healthy food options to help aid recovery, but less than two years later and the result of a cost-cutting exercise (staff told me), the food was cheap and processed. So while I would agree with the importance of getting active after surgery (get up out of bed as soon as possible, and certainly within the first twenty-four hours, as this reduces all sorts of risks), I would add the importance of eating healthy food to assist your body's repair too.

Finally, after my second baby was born, I had a great deal of gas in my stomach, and one of the ward nurses suggested I drink some ginger ale to reduce the pain. But what she failed to add is (and looking back, it seems completely obvious, but it took my doctor to tell me later . . .) that the ginger ale must be flat. Just drop a spoonful of sugar into the can to achieve this and avoid making your gas pains even worse! (*Pauline, United States*)

- Accept medication after surgery, even if you aren't in that much pain yet. Because if you don't, you will have pain, and it will take away from enjoying your newborn! I accepted medication for only about one day (and after that, only ibuprofen) and really never felt any significant pain [note: it's important to remember that each person is different, and that not everyone receives the same regional anesthesia for surgery, which affects the longevity of postpartum pain relief].

  Wear loose-fitting sweat pants with a *wide* waistband (like the wide maternity clothing waistband) because you'll find that even sweats that have the typical narrow stretchy part will hit right at your incision, which is uncomfortable. Go for slow walks outside as soon as your doctor says it's okay. About three days after surgery, I walked my baby for about a mile. It gets the endorphins flowing again and the fresh air is great.

- *Accept help*! This goes for any new mom. Let mom-in-law come over to babysit so you can sleep, hire house cleaners for every other week, let Dad prepare dinner.

Recovery from a cesarean, as any other surgery, is hugely a matter of your attitude. For some it will be harder than others, but I have had other surgeries before (on my knee and shoulder) and breaks (broken collarbone, broken wrist), and the cesarean was actually the least painful with the shortest recovery. Yes, that surprised me too! If you think, "I will get better, I will do as much as I can, I will take the medications that I need," you will get better quicker. But on the flip side, *you are a new mom*! So you do have a right to "milk it!" "Honey, I am very tired, can you get the groceries?" and "Yes, a backrub really would be good for me right now."

When telling people about my choice, at first I tried to hide the fact that it was by request. Now I always say I had a "planned cesarean," and most people don't ask any further. For those that do, I respond with a brief explanation: "I chose it electively, with no medical indication. I feel it was the safest choice for my baby and my body, after reviewing the research." It usually opens up a short discussion after that—no one yet has seemed judgmental, but they are interested! I always tell people the truth. To people who know me, they know that I look deeply into every decision I make—I am a very friendly, athletic, educated person (that works in the healthcare field), not some Hollywood star. To me, it is helping spread the word that it is a valid choice to be respected! (*Kathrine, United States*)

- Women who have elective cesareans don't get the opportunity to discuss their experience. No one is interested, but they're happy to tell you over and over again about their labors. This is both socially and in formal postnatal groups (in one three-hour session, it turned out to be all about labor, for example). It was completely awful! I felt that I had no right to be there. However, I later fed back to the leader, who promised that for future sessions it would be about childbirth—not just the labor. (*Anon, United Kingdom*)

Chapter 16

Cesarean Birth Stories

*Because things are the way they are, things will not stay the
way they are.*

—Bertolt Brecht (1898–1956)

We invited women to contribute their own birth stories to this book, and we have chosen those below because they represent a wide range of experiences and reasons for choosing surgery. These stories are all actual accounts, but some names have been changed to protect identities where requested, and some stories have been edited for length. You may be reading this book while pregnant or thinking about becoming pregnant, in which case, reading about other women's birth experiences can often help prepare you for the unknown, but we also expect this chapter will be beneficial for women who have already had a planned cesarean birth and might have felt (or still feel) alone, misunderstood, or angry regarding their thoughts, hopes, expectations, and experiences before, during, and after the birth. Knowing there are other women with similar experiences may help you feel stronger, and if you are already confident in your birth choice, these stories will simply strengthen your self-assurance. For all other readers, we hope these stories will provide a useful insight into the thoughts and feelings of the "mythical" or "vain and selfish" women who request a cesarean birth.

- "Informed Choice and Informal Coercion": Katherine, thirty-two, United States, 2009
- "Natural Cesarean": Sarah, twenty-nine, United Kingdom, 2008
- "Worth the Wait": Johanna, twenty-nine, United Kingdom, 2006
- "So Much to Gain and Not Much Pain": Leesa, thirty-five, Australia, 2008

- "Hat Trick Support": Lauren, twenty-eight, United States, 2009
- "Once a Vaginal Birth, Never Again": Jackie, thirty-five, United Kingdom, 2004
- "Psychological Dread": Sandy, thirty-seven, United Kingdom, 2009
- "Birth Story: They All Lived Happily Ever After": Andrea, thirty-three, Canada, 2009
- "Too Panicked—and Too Old—to Push": Justine, thirty-five, United Kingdom, 2008
- "Prepregnancy Birth Plan": Anonymous, thirty-four, United Kingdom, 2008
- "A Welcome Breech": Pauline, thirty-four, United States, 2007
- "Exacerbating Anal Fissures": Emma, thirty-six, United Kingdom, 2009
- "Choice and Support": Catherine, thirty-eight, United Kingdom, 2009
- "Miscellaneous Birth Stories": Anonymous

INFORMED CHOICE AND INFORMAL COERCION

Katherine, age thirty-two at the birth, United States, 2009

As soon as I discovered I was pregnant, I began considering maternal request. My husband is from Brazil, which has a high rate of cesareans, and many women there plan for a cesarean as their choice. It's assumed that because it's Brazil, the women choose a cesarean because of vanity. However, we spoke with many women in Brazil, and the main reason for their choice is the differences that exist within the healthcare system. Even if you have money and have private medical insurance, once you are in labor, you are not guaranteed to have an obstetrician deliver your baby. Often, the nurse ends up doing it, which is very risky, so they plan a cesarean delivery to guarantee a doctor's presence.

Personally, I work in the healthcare field, and I believe in decisions made by research and data (good data). I work with many children who have brain or physical damage that was likely a result of vaginal birth. After exhaustive research, the data seems *very* clear to me that either: (a) the risks are different for each method—but no one birth is "safer" than the other, or (b) that if one *is* "safer"—it is cesarean delivery on maternal request; at least it is safer for the baby. To me, studies seem to bend over backward trying to prove that vaginal delivery is somehow safer by a mile. Nothing supports this, and I have truly come to the conclusion that people have some sort of fundamental moral belief that a baby should be born vaginally. It's almost like trying to convince a Catholic that God isn't real. No matter how much the research and facts point in the other opposite direction to their view, you will never convince them.

At my antenatal consultation, I found out that by some amazing grace, my *male* ob-gyn was okay with my request for an elective cesarean. He had no problem with it at all and felt that it should be my choice. The other doctors in his office, however, were against it (they rotate appointments near the end of pregnancy) and told me that if I was their patient, they would refer me elsewhere. Still, my cesarean was scheduled for my delivery date, and unfortunately, when I went into labor four days early, my doctor was on vacation. The doctor on call was shocked when she discovered that this was a maternal request cesarean, and she tried to talk me out of it. Meanwhile, my labor progressed very rapidly in the hospital, and the pain became unbearable as she continued to try to talk me out of it. Never taking my no as an answer. She told me that the anesthesiologist had two emergency cesareans to do, so I was "in line" after them, but she *refused* to call in the second anesthesiologist who was on call—despite the fact that at this point, I was fully dilated and wanted epidural pain relief for during my two hours of full labor pains. The doctor then became very coercive in trying to convince me not to have a cesarean. I was screaming in pain, and she was telling me horror stories of what would happen to me.

Finally, after the ob-gyn came in to me more than eight times trying to convince me out of it, I was given an epidural, brought into surgery, and strapped on to the operating table with the anesthesiologist poised to put the medication in again. In a completely unethical move, the doctor *again* tried to talk me out of having a cesarean. Seriously?! I was on the operating table. . . . Finally, they began surgery, but the ob-gyn talked loudly to the second doctor about my "terrible decision," so that I could hear. She treated me terribly during the surgery; she wouldn't talk to me or tell me what was happening, so I was scared to death. And when the baby came out, she didn't say a word or even show him to me before they took him away. I felt so "beaten" by the treatment of this doctor that I was in tears and couldn't even enjoy the moment of the arrival of my son.

Fortunately, I was very lucky to have a nurse who was very pro-maternal request care for me, and she provided the little support I needed for sticking with my decision despite the coercion. The nurse told me that the cord was wrapped twice around my baby's neck (his heart rate had been dropping during labor while waiting for the anesthesiologist, and I only had oxygen), and although vaginal delivery would probably have been fine, too, I knew that a cesarean guaranteed a safe delivery for my baby. My son is wonderful, and we are so blessed.

I have no idea why there is this feeling that you are doing something ethically wrong if you do not want a vaginal delivery. I felt I protected both my body *and* my baby. Women have a right to control their own body and need a right to cesarean choice. Truly, it is oppressive for women not to be given this choice, given current research, and more than ever after my experience, I am a huge advocate of allowing maternal request. I would also like to make the point that while I was allowed to be in excruciating pain for two hours because of a refusal to call an anesthesiologist, if it had been a man with a broken ankle—also not an "emergency"—I guarantee that an anesthesiologist would have been called immediately.

NATURAL CESAREAN

Sarah, age twenty-nine at the birth, United Kingdom, 2008

From the moment I fell pregnant, I decided that I wanted to give birth by planned cesarean. The main driving force behind this decision was a marked fear of vaginal childbirth and the inevitable aftereffects (pelvic floor damage, stress incontinence, perineal trauma). The baby's father was supportive of whatever decision I wanted to take about the birth, as were my family. I was born by elective cesarean as a result of breech presentation in the same operating room as my son. But at my first hospital appointment, when I told the midwife that I wanted a cesarean, she just raised her eyebrows at me and said, "We'll see about that." I then went straight to my family doctor to submit my request and go over my fears. He was fully supportive of my concerns and wrote to my obstetrician to request an appointment.

When I met with my obstetrician, I was incredibly nervous as I had read no end of stories about the struggle some women go through to get a planned cesarean. My fears were not so much associated with the act of giving birth itself but the aftereffects. I had written down my concerns and went through them every night in my head; I knew I had to state my case from an informed point of view to even be considered! But he agreed instantly, saying that the reasons I stated (pelvic floor, transmission of group B streptococcus during vaginal delivery, etc.) were perfectly viable, and he was happy to book me in! My heart fluttered, and I felt a sense of relief.

The response to my request was met without judgment from doctors but with judgment from the midwives. At all my regular antenatal checks with the midwife, I was questioned about my choice and told I should reconsider. The reasons were clearly stated on my notes, but I was still made to feel like I was doing something wrong. Even when I went into the hospital on the day of the birth, I was being questioned by my lead midwife as to why I chose this. During the surgery, the anesthetist told me how she had had an elective cesarean and that her recovery was fine. She also said I had done the right thing, as my son was in an awkward position for a natural delivery, with the cord wrapped round his neck. They had to turn Otis to get him out, and the surgeon commented that I would have ended up in there for an emergency cesarean anyway. During the surgery, I requested that the screen be lowered so I could see the birth, and I also asked for the baby to be given straight to me unless there were evident complications, but my midwife ignored both requests, and my partner had to go across the operating room to get the baby for me.

Post-surgery, I was under the care of a very cold, indifferent midwife, which wasn't the greatest of feelings. She ignored my pleas for more anti-sickness medication and just told me to drink water; she left me to be sick while I tried my best to get my son to latch on and enjoy him. Later, on the ward, the care was good, but they were so busy. If I could change one thing, it would be to have had someone (my mum or partner) to stay with me and help me all night long. I was discharged on day three with painkillers and took to bed at home with a very hungry little boy.

Looking back, I am thoroughly glad of my decision to request a cesarean. I must admit that the recovery was long, and I don't think my partner fully understood beforehand (he expected me to be more active than I could be). But although it is better for a baby to be more active with Mum, and only a natural delivery can offer this, I had great family support to help with my son and used homoeopathy and natural medicine to help along the way. Also, even though I had a cesarean, I follow a very natural, instinctive pattern of care. I have always carried my baby in a sling and co-sleep with him, and I am still breastfeeding at ten months and intend to long-term.

WORTH THE WAIT

Johanna, age twenty-nine at the birth, United Kingdom, 2006

I was thirty-five weeks pregnant with my first baby when I was finally told that I would be allowed to have a cesarean at my own request! Since becoming pregnant (planned), my fear of delivery had taken over, and I suffered from anxiety, two panic attacks, and resentment from people saying I was too posh to push. I have always had a fear of childbirth but didn't think it was different from any other person's fear and, prior to becoming pregnant, would have always considered the option of elective cesarean if I could have afforded private care. My reasons for this were to prevent any damage to my own body and sex life, pain, length of labor, loss of control (I suffer panic attacks when I know I am not in control), intervention, and the disgust and humiliation of childbirth. After being laughed at by a community midwife on telling her some of my fears, I was determined to be granted a cesarean.

I spoke with my family doctor and midwife who both agreed that I should be referred to speak with a counselor and then a consultant obstetrician, which I did. The counselor was brilliant, as I was aware that the problem was in my head, but she agreed that I was tokophobic and had a fear of fear, and would refer me to the consultant. Unfortunately, the consultant obstetrician was not very nice, and I had already built up my anxiety about meeting him, as he was the one who would be deciding if I could have a cesarean or not. He completely dismissed everything I told him regarding my fears and said he would make a decision in six weeks, as he wanted to change my mind. He arranged for me to see a psychosexual counselor again and also to visit the delivery suite.

After being told I would have to wait until I was thirty-six weeks before finding out if I would be allowed to have a cesarean, I felt I could not cope; I was so down and crying all the time. I saw my own doctor again and although I didn't want to do this, I asked for something to take my anxiety away. I felt as though I couldn't do anything else. But my doctor refused to give me any medication, as she believed, as I did, that I was not depressed, and my anxiety would disappear if I was allowed a cesarean, so she decided to speak with the consultant obstetrician on my behalf, as she was concerned about the effect of my anxiety on my baby. Then, after a meeting with the counselor, who told me that I had the worst case of fear she had seen, she wrote a letter to the consultant, detailing this. And the following week, she called to tell me that she'd spoken with the consultant in person too. After being bombarded by my doctor and counselor, he agreed to allow me to have a cesarean.

When I saw the consultant to confirm my cesarean, he apologized for bullying me and stated that he is the least strict consultant on allowing elective cesareans! He also said that he had been extra hard on me as his hospital was desperately trying to reduce the cesarean rate. Instead of being angry with this (which I would have been in any other circumstances), I was just so relieved not to have to deliver vaginally that I didn't say anything. At 38.5 weeks, I was finally feeling so positive towards the whole thing, and I just wish I hadn't had to go through all the unhappiness and waiting for this outcome. I never felt as though I had any choice during my pregnancy, and although I had some support, the general attitude to women who may feel like me is not at all helpful. I also feel that there may be some pregnant women who may not be as forceful or determined as me (although even I felt like giving up; I just couldn't) who may be forced into vaginal delivery against their wishes and end up with postnatal depression (as I do believe would have happened to me).

It was really nice to hear a man's point of view regarding this. My husband really supported my decision for a c-section. One thing I have done differently, I have announced that I am having a section whether people agree or not, yes, some have been quite rude, and I have had loads of people saying that I am too posh to push, though I tell them the real reason is that I am too scared to push, they still dismiss me as being silly. Hey, I am the one who fought for my section, if I can go against the system and win, then I can certainly ignore a few idiots who have not yet realized that it's now the twenty-first century.

Almost five years after giving birth, I still believe I made the right decision. I have not had any medical issues relating to my cesarean, and neither has my child. I just would have liked a little bit more support from health professionals and for them to accept that I had come to the conclusion, after thoroughly researching cesareans, that this was the best way for me to have my child. I hope that things have changed in the last five years and that in 2011 women are allowed to make the informed decision on how to give birth, without people judging them.

SO MUCH TO GAIN AND NOT MUCH PAIN

Leesa, age thirty-five at the birth, Australia, 2008

I first attended antenatal classes with a pregnant friend who had no partner and no car, and maybe because I wasn't pregnant, and was therefore thinking differently, I remember reading about episiotomy and thinking, "That's the final straw. If I ever get pregnant, I'm having a cesarean!" And then I did get pregnant, and I was faced with the real decision. I was pretty sure that I wanted a cesarean still because I also have really awful period pains, and I know that I can't even do three hours of that without crying out for drugs, and I also thought I would end up having a messy birth and possibly an emergency cesarean. I had waited ten years to get pregnant (naturally), and I didn't want to risk any complications. Most of my friends were discouraging and felt that a cesarean was gross, unnatural, and selfish. But two friends were encouraging; one had four babies—one vaginal birth and three cesarean births—and felt that the first one's delayed birth may have been related to his mild autism. And the other would have definitely had a cesarean if public health had allowed, and now, pregnant with her second baby, she is paying her own way in order to guarantee a cesarean.

Fortunately for me, having been paying for private health cover because I thought we might need fertility treatment, I was in a position to choose. My ob-gyn said it was my choice, and he was happy to do it if that's what I wanted. He looked pleased and later said that a cesarean was probably safer if they did stats. I was very happy with my choice, and our baby was born with an Apgar score of 9 then 10 [note: this is a measurement of the newborn baby's condition, developed by American obstetrician Virginia Apgar, and is in worldwide use today. A score of 9 and 10 indicates excellent health], which I think is due to his easy birth. He started sucking in the recovery room, and we have never had any trouble feeding; actually he hardly ever cried and is a calm and content baby. As for the pain, it never came close to my normal period pain. I am now pregnant again (my first is only nine months old and will be fourteen months at the birth); after waiting so long to get pregnant the first time, we didn't expect to be so lucky again, and while breastfeeding! I plan to have another cesarean.

Several women have quietly asked about my cesarean, usually after a bad birth experience, and asked to see my scar. One lady admitted she didn't know if she could deal with people judging her, and someone else said my husband would be more proud of me if I had a natural birth. On the contrary, my hubby was there the whole time making me laugh, and I really feel like we went through it together; he cried when the baby came out. He said that since we walk upright, our natural birth is not the same as an animal giving birth, and if men did it, they would all have a cesarean!

HAT TRICK SUPPORT: HUSBAND, DOCTOR, AND INSURANCE COMPANY

Lauren, age twenty-eight at the birth, United States, 2009

I have always been a very petite person. At twenty-seven years old when I became pregnant, I was eighty-seven pounds, five feet tall and healthy. I have always been "the skinny girl," I eat whatever I want (and I love food!) and am extremely lucky to have a very high metabolism. My husband and I wanted a baby more than anything, and we were ready and fearless for all to come, except for the birth. I was *terrified!* My aunt hemorrhaged on the delivery table with her daughter and flatlined twice; by God's miracle the doctors were able to save her. And my sister (same body type) tore so badly with the birth of her six-pound, three-ounce son, it took her eight weeks to recover. I researched natural births extensively, vaginal births with pain management, and elective cesareans. After many books and a few birth classes, I ultimately decided an elective cesarean was what was best for me and my son. I was so terrified of giving birth naturally even with medication, I would have anxiety attacks even thinking about it. I also believe it is much safer for the child to be delivered by cesarean, and I feel there is medical evidence supporting this. My doctor agreed to perform the elective surgery with only requesting I research my options prior so I would be making an educated decision.

I ended up going into labor at twenty-nine weeks. I was given magnesium and spent four days in the hospital, and my labor was successfully stopped. I then spent the next ten weeks on bed rest and terbutaline [asthma drug also used for suppressing labor] as my labor, would start again every five to seven days. In the end I made it to my scheduled day for surgery at thirty-nine weeks. My gorgeous son was born seven pounds, two ounces, twenty inches long, and healthy. My prayers were answered! The only hiccup we had is that I was unable to breastfeed due to his low blood sugar levels, although after my milk came in, I decided I would not have breastfed even if I had had the opportunity. We spent a total of three days in the hospital, and I recovered extremely well. I was off all pain medication within the first six days and had no problems with daily activities.

Looking back, I knew I was making the right decision despite all of the negative comments and "trash talk" I received. After the birth of my son, my doctor said my recovery would have definitely taken three to four additional weeks if I had had a vaginal birth. I would not change a thing about the day my son was born, and I am forever thankful that my doctor, husband, and insurance company supported me and my decision to do what was best for my body.

ONCE A VAGINAL BIRTH, NEVER AGAIN

Jackie, age thirty-five at the birth, United Kingdom, 2004

If I fall pregnant again, I would opt for a cesarean after what happened to our first and only child at his birth, and at present, we have a legal case pending against the hospital following our experience.

Our son was born eight days after his due date. I was told during my pregnancy that I would have a big baby, but I was never advised to have a cesarean. He weighed nine pounds, fourteen ounces when he was eventually born. My waters broke at 4.30 a.m. on the Friday morning, and I was admitted to the hospital at 6 a.m. I was progressing rapidly, even though the midwife that I had was very abrupt with me and told me that I wasn't in as much pain as I was making out. The same midwife then went to a pre-booked appointment elsewhere in the hospital at 9.15 a.m., and when another midwife arrived fifteen minutes later, she examined me and said that to her surprise — as I hadn't been in labor very long — I was fully dilated.

Our son eventually decided to crown at approximately 11.35 a.m. and it was then that the problems occurred. My contractions ceased, and I was being told to push even though it had no effect. Eventually, ten minutes later, the emergency bells were pushed and all hell broke loose. I was pushed and pulled from one end of the bed to the other. I literally had people on top of me trying to squeeze our baby out, while others tried to pull him out at the same time, and this is when the condition that he now has occurred. He finally arrived at 11.46 a.m. and wasn't breathing; there was no crying to be heard, and he had a very weak heartbeat.

It wasn't until the next day that we were told that our son had suffered a "shoulder dystocia" delivery, and that he had Erb's palsy. They assured us that within three months, his injury would disappear, but how wrong they were. Our son is nearly five years old now, and he still has a daily routine of physiotherapy and visits a professional physiotherapist once a month. He had an operation at five months old to try and rectify some of the problem, and he also has to attend a clinic in London on an annual basis. He does miss out on school, as he is full-time now, and although we do try and make appointments out of school time, this is not always possible.

Our son will be disabled for the rest of his life, and his condition in his right arm could worsen at any time causing more problems for him. There is no way I would give birth vaginally again, as I could not put another child of mine through what he has had to go through. A cesarean will be demanded next time I fall pregnant.

PSYCHOLOGICAL DREAD

Sandy, age thirty-seven at the birth, United Kingdom, 2009

I remember telling my parents when I was twelve years old that I wouldn't be having any children. They didn't question it then, and although I knew it was unusual among my group of friends, I didn't think much of it. It was only as I approached my mid-thirties that I started to question why I felt that I didn't want children. From a very early age, my mother (a trained midwife) had told me how much pain childbirth involved and how much she had suffered and was still suffering. Usually this was if I had misbehaved and she was angry with me, but I have come to realize that she suffered from postnatal depression, probably resulting from a horrific childbirth experience. To this day I can't imagine a vaginal childbirth and how it is physically possible; obviously I know logically that it is, but I could just never relate it to myself.

Last year, at the age of thirty-six, my husband and I decided that we would like to have a child. I blocked out all thoughts of how the baby would actually enter the world if I were to conceive, and three months later, a positive pregnancy test brought about a real mix of emotions. While I was happy that I had conceived so quickly, I was also filled with dread about how I would give birth. I searched the Internet looking for how I could request a cesarean and found some comfort that if the worse came to the worse, I may be able to borrow enough money to pay privately at a London hospital. This was how I found electivecesarean.com, and I researched how to approach the medical team at a public hospital through others' experiences.

When the time came for my first appointment, I was pleasantly surprised that my midwife did not dismiss my fears, and told me that I could speak to a consultant later in my pregnancy about electing for a cesarean. By the time I was fourteen weeks pregnant, I was distraught. I felt I couldn't enjoy my pregnancy without knowing that I could have a cesarean delivery. My midwife referred me to a consultant, and again, when the appointment arrived I was surprised that she was very happy to book the cesarean there and then and seemed to understand me perfectly. I'm sure that this isn't the experience at every British hospital.

The only negativity I encountered came from some of the ward staff after the birth. They would ask why I had a cesarean, and I would try to explain without having to go into all the ins and outs. I think that some of them thought I was mentally unstable. In terms of recovery, it's been longer than expected, but some of my friends who have given birth vaginally have taken even longer to recover. Either way—vaginally or by cesarean—I still think childbirth is very difficult, and women should be supported whatever they choose.

BIRTH STORY:
THEY ALL LIVED HAPPILY EVER AFTER

Andrea, age thirty-three at the birth, Canada, 2009

All my life, I have been immersed in story. As a very small child, I read stories, and as an adult, I wrote stories and taught others stories in university classrooms. Story has always been an integral aspect of my life, and so I knew how I wanted the story of my child's birth to unfold. Even before I was pregnant, I knew I wanted to have a cesarean. All the women in my family had had very difficult deliveries, I had done research on vaginal and cesarean birth, and I had spoken extensively to my girlfriends—some of whom had had vaginal deliveries, some cesareans—and my decision was clear: I wanted the ability to choose how I delivered my baby.

After discovering that I was pregnant, my family doctor informed me that I would be unable to choose a doctor to deliver my baby; instead, I would have to go to a maternity clinic where, as she put it, I'd be "like a football—whoever was available would be there to catch" me. This, regardless of my wanting a planned cesarean, was not my idea of an ideal birth plan. I wanted the experience to be seamless, full of the trust and intimacy one would associate with giving birth, and I was not comfortable with the idea of a rotating roster of doctors throughout my pregnancy and delivery. The idea of a cesarean versus a vaginal birth was never even approached. When I asked my doctor for more information on delivery options, she informed me that an elective cesarean was unethical. End of discussion. It shocked me that I could not choose to have a cesarean, and nor could I choose the doctor who would deliver my baby. Pregnancy and delivery are both incredibly intimate processes, and it seemed barbaric to assume that I, as the mother, would not have a voice in any of it. Surely, I thought, we had moved beyond the days of such limitation and closed-mindedness when it came to healthcare?

Fortunately, I had done previous research and read many articles regarding elective cesareans before my pregnancy, many featuring Dr. Magnus Murphy out of Calgary. So after the lack of response from my own doctor, I finally contacted Dr. Murphy, who was kind, receptive, and beyond helpful; he put me in touch with supportive doctors in my home province of BC, going above and beyond any sense of duty he might have had. And thank God he did. I met my new ob-gyn shortly after, without any assistance or introduction from my family doctor. After that, my experience was incredibly positive. Not only could I actively decide how I wanted to deliver my baby but I had a supportive and understanding doctor. I related my fears of delivery, as well as my knowledge of the long-term effects of childbirth on the body and my wish to avoid the issues of prolapse, inconti-nence, etc. We also talked at length about cesareans, both the positives and the potential negatives of a surgical procedure. Above all, my doctor empha-sized his support for my ability to choose—whether that choice was a nat-ural delivery or a cesarean. This spoke to the heart of the matter to me—the choices I should be able to actively make in regards to my own body. In the end, a cesarean was scheduled for the week before my due date.

While I was nervous about the actual surgery, any fears I might have had were quickly allayed, and it could not have gone any better. Everyone involved was reassuring, professional, and supportive, from the anesthesi-ologist to the nurses. And once it came to the moment of delivery, I had another reason to be incredibly thankful that I had been able to choose a planned cesarean, and that I was able to find a doctor who believed in my right to do so. My daughter had the umbilical cord wrapped tightly around her neck three times. There was a moment of horrible silence and quick, intense work, but the doctors were able to unwrap the cord and de-liver a beautiful, healthy baby girl. Had I delivered vaginally, it is almost certain this would not have been the case.

My recovery was much easier than I had anticipated. Yes, I was tender, but there was no real pain to speak of. I was careful with what I did and how I moved, but the incision healed quickly and well, and I was back doing pretty much anything I might have done pre-pregnancy within six weeks. I had seen friends take much longer to recover from lingering issues after natural childbirth and was pleased, once again, with my decision. When I spoke with other girlfriends who had not yet had children, inevitably they asked about my choices and my experience; I was honest in reminding them that it was a personal choice, in explaining what to expect, and also honest in recommending a planned cesarean wholeheartedly.

If I have any more children, I would absolutely plan another cesarean without a moment's hesitation. My experience was wonderful, giving me back a sense of power over my own body that can often be lost in the medical community, especially in the area of childbirth, and the reassurance that I was able to control the way in which I delivered my daughter—both essentials for a positive delivery experience. And while I know the idea of choosing a cesarean is still controversial, I'm not sure why it should be. I can elect if and when I want to become pregnant, and I can decide if I want to continue with the pregnancy or terminate, so if these options of choice are acceptable, why not the manner in which I bring a child into the world? I'm beyond grateful that I was able to make the decision that was right for me and my family, and that I was able to find doctors who also believed in a woman's right to choose. The end result is all that should be important in the discussion—I have a lovely, healthy, happy baby daughter, and I'm not at all sure that would have been the case had my choice been made for me.

One day, I will tell my daughter the story of her birth, complete with the obstacles, cast of characters, the pivotal plot points, and will most certainly end with that most beloved of all lines, "And they all lived happily ever after. The end."

TOO PANICKED—AND TOO OLD—TO PUSH

Justine, age thirty-five at the birth, United Kingdom, 2008

I am not sure why I am so scared and disturbed by natural childbirth. It could have been the very graphic video of a woman giving birth shown at school in a life-skills class or hearing my mother describe how both she and my brother nearly died during his birth. But the fear has also been compounded over the past few years as I hear countless horror stories from friends and family close to me who have gone through "natural" birth. (As an aside, I often smile at the term "natural" birth. Biologically, we are designed to have our first child optimally between fifteen to twenty years old. Thanks to contraceptives, and most significantly the pill, we are now pushing back the age of having this first child by fifteen years or so, through very "unnatural" means, so I do not believe it is "natural" to have a first baby at thirty, and I think this is why so many women have complications. You wouldn't leave a brand-new car in a garage for fifteen years, then take it on the longest, fastest journey it will ever go on and expect it to be a problem free journey, would you?)

So I knew I didn't like the idea of natural birth, but it wasn't until I was actually pregnant that I realized I was actually terrified of it. The pictures of natural birth in the pregnancy and birth book that they give out literally gave me a panic attack. Anyone talking about birth to me could invoke a similar response. I knew I had to do something about this, as I didn't want my poor little baby spending the next nine months soaking up the excessive levels of stress hormones that kept shooting around my body every time I thought of giving birth; the poor little thing would come out a nervous wreck!

At about eight to nine weeks, I spoke with my midwife about my concerns. Thankfully, she was a nonjudgmental, caring midwife (a rarity, I have since heard) and suggested that a little further into my pregnancy, I speak with an obstetrician at my registered hospital, and an appointment was booked for me at about twenty weeks. Having this appointment booked calmed me a little, but when it came to having any scans I still couldn't sit in the waiting room with the other pregnant woman because they would remind me of childbirth and that would panic me. I had to wait outside each time, and my husband would come and get me. I have since read about a condition called tokophobia—fear of childbirth. I am not sure how exactly this is diagnosed, but I think I may well have had it.

I was exceptionally anxious about the meeting with the obstetrician. I had heard stories of hospitals refusing point-blank to allow elective cesareans on nonmedical grounds, and I had also heard that women could be sent to psychiatrists for assessment before being offered the option. My husband and I had made enquiries about private cesareans, but at £10,000, I knew it would be a real financial stretch, so we were hoping that our local public hospital would agree on this occasion.

I am a scientist by training and have a PhD in genetic toxicology. Though of course this does not make me an expert in obstetrics, it did allow me to do a little bit of literature searching on the risks of the various forms of childbirth, and I understood that the best chance of my getting an elective cesarean was to demonstrate that I understood the risks associated with the surgery. What I found interesting from the research I did was that there is a strong correlation between the age of the mother and the risk of medical intervention being required. So much so, that a woman giving birth at thirty-five or above is very unlikely to be able to have a non-medically intervened birth. This being the case, you then have to weigh up the risks associated for the baby and mother for each of the medical interventions: episiotomy, forceps, vacuum, etc. (Another aside: At the antenatal classes I attended, the average age of the mums-to-be in our group was thirty-five. The information to us was based on "average" data from women giving birth aged around fifteen to forty. Though I didn't say anything, knowing what I did about the elevated level of risk for older mums, I felt that the class leaders actually misled the women in my group into thinking they had a good chance of having a "natural," non-medically intervened birth, rather than preparing them to make choices and understand the risks of the medical interventions. As it turned out, the stats I'd read were right. Only one out of the six women in our group was able to give birth naturally with no intervention. The rest had some kind of drama: the home birth woman was rushed to hospital, another woman had forceps and vacuum, and two had such a horrific time that they were offered counseling after the birth.)

So I attended my appointment with the obstetrician armed with a bag full of medical papers and ready to argue my case based on the fact that I was fully informed about the risks, etc. As luck would have it, the hospital I went to has one of the highest cesarean rates in the country, and the obstetrician I spoke with had no issues at all with my choice. He had had his own child delivered by elective cesarean at the hospital the year before because he said he didn't want to take the risk of a natural birth. He felt that modern cesareans are now as safe if not safer than natural birth and happily booked me in for my operation for thirty-nine weeks. My meeting with the obstetrician really did put my mind at rest that what I was doing was the right thing for the baby and me, and it allowed me to relax; for the first time, I started looking forward to the birth and having a baby.

The birth itself was a truly amazing experience. I was admitted at 8 a.m. and was of course very nervous about the surgery, but I knew exactly what to expect. I knew it would all be under control, and I knew what was happening at each step of the way. The surgeons, nurses, and anesthetist were all lovely. Everyone was calm and comforting and at 10:30 a.m., just twenty minutes after being taken into the operating room, my little boy was born and in my arms. The nurse took pictures, which we have on our wall now at home.

The one downside to having the elective cesarean is that because I hadn't been through a long labor, and because the painkillers were so effective, when I got home two days later, I felt so good that I didn't rest enough and pulled my stitches a little. I was literally doing the washing, going out walking, and shopping, etc. But even that said, I truly believe that for us, making the decision to have an elective cesarean was up there with one of the best decisions I have ever made in my life! (My final aside: I work for a tobacco company, and I can honestly say that in terms of negative reactions from people, my choosing to have a cesarean has evoked more emotion, harsh questioning and snide comments in a year than has my working for a tobacco company in ten years! Bizarrely, when in a room of women who have either had babies or are pregnant, the stories of horrendous births are all accepted and not questioned. No one seems to think that in blindly assuming "natural is best" that they may have put their babies or themselves at adverse risk. And when I speak of my very positive, safe, and happy birth experience, they don't want to know, so I rarely mention it now unless asked directly. Human nature is a funny thing.)

I am a passionate believer in dispelling the myths around the cesarean itself. The ones I love are "You can't hold your baby for two days," "You can barely lift or move for six weeks," and "You can't drive for eight weeks," etc. I also want to dispel the myth that women choose this option because they're "too posh to push"; I would have loved to have been so blasé about giving birth to have made that label appropriate, but the truth is, I was totally "too panicked to push!"

PREPREGNANCY BIRTH PLAN

Anonymous, age thirty-four at the birth, United Kingdom 2008

I have always had a fear of pregnancy and childbirth since I was very young, and this stemmed from the fact that I learned about where babies come from when I was about eleven years old and overheard my aunt talking about her horrific childbirth experience. When I got older, the phobia got worse because I knew that I would be getting close to a time when I would have to go through "the process" to have a child. Even seeing a pregnant woman would actually freak me out.

I eventually decided to do some research, thinking that the more I knew, the more I could tackle my fear. After endless research, I decided that a cesarean would probably be the best option for me. I mentioned this to my female family doctor and asked for details about having a cesarean, but she was not at all sympathetic to my fears. She treated me as if I was an idiot and basically said that I couldn't get one. I felt that her attitude was, "Look, if I've had to push a watermelon through a small hole, then so should you!" I ended up in tears and was put off having a baby. In fact my fear was so bad that I began to have irrational thoughts, such as thinking, "If I don't eat during pregnancy then maybe I would have a smaller baby and I might be able to go through with a vaginal birth." I even looked into surrogacy. I was genuinely prepared to get someone to have a baby for me. However, the procedure was very invasive, and I decided that since I was fit and healthy, compared to some women that can't have children, I shouldn't be so stupid with my fear.

A year later, I decided to speak to another doctor about my phobia, and he was extremely helpful and understanding, and referred me to [a] specialist obstetrician. After being assessed, they decided that I would not be calm enough to go through with a vaginal delivery, as they believed that I would endanger myself and my baby. So they agreed to give me a planned cesarean. Only then did I start to make baby plans. I know it sounds pathetic, but that is what a phobia is—an irrational fear. And the fear was so bad that I refused to get pregnant unless I knew what kind of birth I would be getting. I got pregnant soon after that and really enjoyed my pregnancy, which was what I wanted. My husband was very understanding of my fears and very supportive of my decision to have a cesarean.

Every time I went for a check-up, the midwives would ask me why I was having a planned cesarean, and I would always feel that their initial reactions were quite negative, but once I gave them the long, boring story of my phobia, they were very supportive and actually agreed that a cesarean is better. My cesarean was planned for the thirty-ninth week, which I wasn't too happy about, as I was scared that I would go into labor earlier than the planned date. But the obstetrician explained the dangers of having a cesarean earlier, as the baby would have breathing difficulties, and he assured me that even if I went into labor early, they would still deliver the baby by cesarean.

As it turned out, I went into labor a week before the planned section date. I was totally unaware that I was having contractions and decided to go into hospital to get checked out. I thought I was just having strong Braxton Hicks [pre-labor uterine contractions], so I got the shock of my life. I was very lucky at the time, because the labor ward was very quiet, and everyone around me (midwives, nurses, surgeon, anesthetists) took their time to explain what would happen, and everything was relaxed and not rushed. I was very nervous and had violent shakes while being prepared for the spinal block, but everyone joked around and tried to keep me calm. Once I was numb from the waist down, I was taken into the operating room and my husband was brought in. At this point, I was still shaking violently, and they were having trouble checking my blood pressure, although I was feeling quite high from the drugs, which was good. Then everything happened really quickly, and within a few minutes I could hear my baby cry! They took a few minutes to clean him up, and then he was passed to me. I have to say that I had a wonderful experience, and it was exactly the way I wanted it—calm and not frightened. My husband really enjoyed it too, although he would have still supported me if I had opted for a vaginal delivery. Afterward, I was wheeled back into the labor ward at the recovery section, and at that time there was a sudden rush of mums coming in to give birth. All I could hear was endless moans and screams from these mums all the way down the corridor. I just shivered and looked at my hubby in horror. There were also a couple of midwives in the hospital ward that were quite negative about my cesarean, and they were very abrupt to me when questioning my decision.

Personally, I don't think that a cesarean delivery is better than a vaginal delivery. I only think that it's best for me and that I definitely made the right decision. I had the most amazing, wonderful birth experience and pregnancy, and I have a healthy baby, all of which I didn't think would happen to me. I have also not been put off having a second child. I totally support mums that take the vaginal route and really admire them. I also feel really happy for them if it turns out well, but around 90 percent of mums that I spoke to that had a vaginal delivery, had an awful experience—either due to the pain, problems with the delivery, or the eventual disappointment of having an emergency cesarean. I just didn't want to experience a vaginal delivery, and I didn't want to end up having an emergency cesarean.

A WELCOME BREECH

Pauline, age thirty-four at the birth, United States, 2007

When I first began thinking about getting pregnant, I talked to two different doctors about my desire to plan a cesarean birth, and I was met with the same nonplussed expression by both of them, followed by the assurance that I would not be allowed this choice at either of the nearest two large public maternity hospitals where I lived (at that time) in England. Indeed one doctor proffered that my only option would be to pay privately in London. I had expected this to be the case, and I always imagine that had I remained in England, my pregnancy would have consisted of stress related to battling my way through to meeting with a supportive obstetrician (essentially fighting to get my birth choice agreed) or, more likely I think, stress related to how I was going to afford to pay for private hospital fees. I used to joke with my husband that we'd have to get a loan if necessary, and treat the payment like the new roof we'd needed some years earlier—a very costly and painful bill but also an essential and unavoidable one.

As it happened, when I did get pregnant, my husband was working for a US company, and we were living in New Jersey. I was able to phone around and find a recommended doctor in my area, and by the end of our discussion at my first antenatal appointment (at around six weeks' gestation), my ob-gyn assured me that my cesarean birth plan would be completely supported. She couldn't have been more positive and helpful, answering a million and one questions that I had along the way, and I was able to meet with her practice partner in due course, too, who would be delivering my baby if for any reason my own doctor was unavailable.

In fact the only stumbling block with regards my maternal request was financial; that is, whether or not my insurance company would pay for the surgery. If I'm honest, I buried my head in the sand a little and figured I'd cross that bridge when I came to it; I was just so happy to have secured my preferred birth plan. But in hindsight, I think I should have made inquiries. Plowing through stacks of bills and paperwork (as I soon learned is the norm in American health insurance) when the insurance company *is* paying the bulk of the costs was complicated enough, but it could have been much worse. Fortunately for me, it turned out that our baby girl was to be our lucky star and our saving grace, whichever country she had ended up being born in. Why? Because in the eighth month of my pregnancy, my doctor found her in a breech presentation (in her case, head up top and arms and legs wrapped around me) and she never moved position again. I now officially had an "obstetrical reason" for my cesarean, effectively removing all barriers to my planned positive and smooth birth experience.

I stayed in hospital for four nights after surgery, in my own private room, and I would happily have stayed another few. I was surrounded by a team of doctors (including pediatricians), nurses, and breastfeeding counselors and was able to ask questions and get advice about anything and everything. My own ob-gyn visited me and removed my stitches, and I visited her again in the week after returning home. I wouldn't say that I "enjoyed" the birth itself (aside from the obvious meeting our daughter, but that goes without saying), but neither did I set out to enjoy it. For my husband and I, we felt it was simply the safest way to bring our child into the world, and have had no regrets about our decision since.

EXACERBATING ANAL FISSURES

Emma, age thirty-six at the birth, United Kingdom, 2009

I delivered my first daughter vaginally in 2007; it was a long labor (thirty-six hours), but not traumatic, and I have never reflected on it with anything other than positive feelings. After about twenty-nine hours, I requested pain relief other than gas and air, and was persuaded to try pethidine [an opiate agent similar to morphine] (even though this was the only thing I had said I would rather not have) but then ended up with an epidural. After a couple of hours pushing, the midwife was concerned for my daughter, so I had an assisted delivery with episiotomy and vacuum. Like I say, no trauma about any of this, but unfortunately from that day on, I suffered extreme pain when passing stools. My immediate assumption was that it was piles resulting from the delivery, but after some months it was diagnosed as being anal fissures. Despite there apparently being no medical evidence that vaginal birth can result in anal fissures, I know they were caused by pushing during delivery.

The fissures were still very much a part of everyday life for me twenty months later, when I was seven months pregnant with my second child, taking laxatives several times a day to prevent pain and using ointments to try and allow them to heal. I had seen my doctor on numerous occasions, and tried all the available nonsurgical options to heal the fissures. I also saw two consultants on separate occasions to investigate possible surgical solutions and to discuss their risk of worsening during pregnancy and subsequent birth. Unfortunately I spent my whole second pregnancy anxious about how I would be able to have my second child without making this chronic condition worse, and as such was keen to be allowed to elect to have a cesarean. My feeling was that despite being major surgery, it was preferable to risking any worsening of the anal fissures, which were, and still are, impacting day to day life to some degree or another.

Thankfully, after much worrying and determination, I was lucky enough to be counseled by an extremely reasonable and understanding consultant who said he would support my decision whether it was to deliver naturally or via elective cesarean. I wish all health professionals were like him and would simply engage in rational and realistic dialogue with women who are looking to make this choice. I certainly didn't see it as an easy option, and having now had the operation, I know that it isn't, but five weeks after having my son by elective cesarean I can certainly say it was the right decision. I firmly believe that women should have the choice, as long as we are aware of the risks associated with both natural birth and cesarean. We are capable of making an informed decision based on this information, and it should be our decision to make. Too much health advice and guidance is based on costs and targets and not clinical evidence or patient needs, and I am sure this is often the case for cesareans in Britain.

CHOICE AND SUPPORT

Catherine, age thirty-eight at the birth, United Kingdom, 2009

I recently had a planned elective cesarean at my request in a public hospital; my son Freddie is my first child. I think it's probably pretty unusual, but I didn't find any real push back with my request once I had spoken to the consultant obstetrician regarding my options and concerns. I was referred by the midwife to discuss the option of an elective cesarean at my request, since this is not something that is automatically offered.

My cesarean was performed at a London hospital, and my son was born at 10:44 a.m. I was in hospital only twenty-eight hours before being discharged and have had a very quick and straightforward recovery. Again, not sure if I'm lucky, as most of the people I speak to seem to be pretty amazed that I was up and about the next morning and home by the evening. It's less than three weeks since my operation, and I have almost fully recovered with only a slight twinge when I get out of bed and some discomfort if I walk for long periods. However, certainly nothing that impedes my daily activities or ability to breastfeed and look after my newborn.

I absolutely believe that it should be the woman's right to choose the delivery method. I spoke to two obstetricians regarding my concerns on natural birth, specifically, the potential for brain damage and other serious injuries caused during vaginal delivery. They both concurred that a cesarean is ultimately safer for the baby if performed after thirty-nine weeks, as opposed to a vaginal delivery, which is safer for the mother. I think the risks involved in a vaginal delivery are underplayed by medical professionals and, in particular, midwives. My main reason for wanting a cesarean was to allow me to deliver my baby in the safest way possible and to have as much control over the process as I could. Also, that I took all the risk associated with the birth and not my baby. I did not want to venture into the unknown and put the life of my baby and family in the lap of the gods. It also seems that women have very little control over the birth once they are in labor. Decisions are made by midwives and doctors and can include serious surgical or chemical interventions at any point.

Being able to choose my delivery option made my pregnancy a lot less tense as I was able to make plans and felt that I had control of my situation. However, I think the hospital I gave birth in is probably more progressive in their attitude to choice. Many other women I've spoken to mentioned that a cesarean was not even something they were able to discuss further. I'm not sure if these requests are being blocked by midwives or obstetricians. I suspect that the midwifery profession is protecting its own interests rather than those of pregnant women.

I'm not sure if many people thought my decision was wrong; most of the comments from friends and colleagues were pretty positive, and they could see it was the right decision for me. "It's got to come out one way or another" seemed to be the general consensus. My mum and mother-in-law had the biggest reservations, but I think this is generational and more to do with a fear of surgery. However, since the birth, most people are now convinced that I made the right decision. Especially as my sister was also pregnant at the same time but decided on a natural birth. Her waters broke at thirty-six weeks, and she was in labor for five days before being induced the day before my cesarean. She has not had a particularly easy recovery, so I would have to disagree with the widely supported idea that natural birth is easier to recover from. Maybe physically, if there are no serious tears, but the mental stress and exhaustion is another area that is greatly underplayed by medics.

I was booked in for the cesarean at thirty-nine weeks, and our experience at the hospital was fantastic. They were incredibly efficient, we were introduced to all the medical staff before the op, and they made sure we were aware of each step of the process. It is a pretty daunting procedure if you've never had surgery—I had not. However, the team was great, we were able to play our choice of music in the operating room, and the process was pretty relaxed and very quick. Baby Freddie was born in five minutes, and it was all over in forty-five minutes. My partner was by my side and took video and pictures of the birth. He was also still able to cut the cord and pass the baby to me. It was an amazing experience for both of us.

I would definitely recommend a cesarean as a choice for any woman. I would add that it is important to have a positive attitude, and once the decision to have a cesarean has been made, go with it, try to relax in the operating room, and look after yourself before and after the surgery.

MISCELLANEOUS BIRTH STORIES

United States

I see no magic surrounding a vaginal birth, and I refuse to allow intervention via vacuum or forceps, and I want to avoid an emergency cesarean at all costs. An elective cesarean is just common sense to me; safe and controlled.

United Kingdom

I'm not convinced by the arguments that vaginal delivery is better, due to my experiences as a student doctor on a labor ward, and my concern about the lack of research into long-term psychiatric conditions from complications during vaginal or emergency cesarean birth.

Netherlands

I think it's contradictory that in many European countries abortion is allowed, even at the twenty-second week, but women cannot decide if they will have a cesarean or not. To me, that's ridiculous, especially when you do it in order to avoid the possible complications presented in a natural birth.

United Kingdom

My consultant is currently pushing me to have a vaginal delivery, but I have just had a thirty-two-week scan and been told the baby will be over nine pounds at term. With my current prolapses, I am very concerned about further damage to my pelvic floor (my first child was only seven pounds, six ounces) and intend to discuss a cesarean with my consultant at my next appointment next week.

United Kingdom

My sister had large babies and now suffers incontinence because of third-degree tearing. No one in the NHS so far has taken my concerns seriously, in spite of my baby also showing signs of being very large, so I am paying to go private.

France

My first baby was a vaginal delivery; my second baby was emergency cesarean due to fetal distress. I am awaiting my third baby and want an elective repeat cesarean, but I'm frustrated since my doctor has said I have no justification for it. I am really confused about this since it seems most women are pressured toward an elective repeat cesarean and not VBAC.

United Kingdom

I want a cesarean partly for medical reasons, but the doctor I've seen has been horrible about it and really dismissive. I also don't want the damage to my vagina, etc. or trauma to my body. I feel trapped and petrified I will be forced to have a vaginal delivery. I'm desperate for some help about how to get an elective cesarean even if I have to pay.

United Kingdom

I think most of the vaginal delivery aspects worry me! The damage it does to my body that will indirectly affect my sex life. The feeling of lost control is, at the moment, my biggest worry! I have no control with what is happening to my own body, and the fact that I have to beg and bargain to get an elective cesarean; it drives me insane! I should have a choice of what happens to my body, and the idea of no control over what happens to me is so bad that I am currently worried I might be suffering from depression because of it.

United States

I am a health professional requesting a first-time elective cesarean because I don't believe I can have the type of vaginal delivery I want in a hospital setting, and I am unwilling to have my baby in any other setting.

United States

I had an elective cesarean in July 2006. My doctor was supportive of my choice. It was a very good experience. I experienced pain for about five days, but it was manageable, and I have a very low pain tolerance. I was glad to get the extra time in the hospital, as having the nurses around to take care of the baby was great! This gave us extra time to learn how to care for the baby and to get lots of help with breastfeeding. I am very happy with my decision to have a cesarean and would not change my mind if I had it to do over again. I hope people will change their attitudes toward cesareans or at least keep their opinions to themselves—the only downside to the whole experience was people's bad attitudes and negativity toward my choice of having a cesarean.

United Kingdom

Terrified of the thought of having a natural delivery, I knew exactly how I wanted to give birth. From my very first visit to my consultant I knew when the delivery date and time was, and my husband and I happily prepared for the day. A textbook pregnancy and a perfect cesarean delivery provided us with the most amazing experience with very kind medical staff who did not consider my decision for a cesarean at all strange and shared our joy as our beautiful baby boy arrived. My experience over the nine months was probably near perfect due to me being lucky enough to go private. My husband supported my decision for a cesarean from the very beginning, but having had a very negative response early on from NHS doctors and my previous gynecologist when I mentioned my terror of natural childbirth (and the suggestion that I should see a counselor!), we decided to take the major step of pursuing private care. The cost was in fact the equivalent of hiring a private midwife who is guaranteed to stay with you through labor to delivery—not too much, we felt, but certainly it was the best investment we have ever made. Our obstetrician was very happy to carry out a cesarean. Every visit to him was a joy, as I had no fear of what was ahead, and if this is the one child we have in our lives then we are so very glad we did it this way. I am making a fantastic recovery—I really only had two days of pain in the hospital, and this was softened by very good medication. It was the best decision I made, and I would do it all again exactly the same.

Chapter 17

Informed Choice: Necessary, Complex, and Challenging

> *There are many truths of which the full meaning cannot be*
> *realized until personal experience has brought it home.*
> —John Stuart Mill, *On Liberty*, 1859

AN IDEAL WORLD...

Woman says: "I'm pregnant. I'd like to discuss my birth options, please."

Doctor or midwife says: "No problem. Here are comprehensive lists of the risks and benefits of planning a vaginal birth and the risks and benefits of planning a cesarean birth. We also need to factor in issues related to your own personal health situation, family history, and genetic makeup: namely, a, b, and c, as these can exacerbate the risks of x, y, and z. We can then further discuss any personal preferences or fears you may have and find the best birth plan for you. Obviously, the plan must be flexible enough to allow for any unforeseen complication that may occur between now and the actual birth, and again, we can explore the different options available to you if this should happen."

Hospital, government, and/or insurance provider policy says: "We support all reasonable and valid informed birth choices equally, and our goal is to facilitate the best physical and psychological health outcome for each mother and baby."

341

THE REAL WORLD . . .

Objectivity, subjectivity, autonomy, ideology, politics, fiscal reality, and local staffing constraints all present themselves and, indeed, frequently collide within the walls of many a prenatal consultation room. But why, you might ask, especially when the concept of "informed choice" or "informed decision" seems to be so well supported in maternity care? For example:

- While still reserving professional judgment and individualized care, the "clinician's role should be to provide the best evidence-based counseling possible to the pregnant woman and to respect her autonomy and decision-making capabilities when considering route of delivery."[1]
- "Obstetricians have an obligation to reconsider their assumptions about the relative merits of different delivery options and to convey the evidence to their patients in a clear and unbiased manner. Women have a right to consider the evidence and weigh the potential risks and benefits, and thereby participate more equally in the decisions concerning their pregnancy and mode of delivery."[2]

The problem is that medical professionals don't all agree about the information that should be provided to women deciding on a birth plan, and in some cases, they are not aware of the most up-to-date research themselves. This can be because once someone holds an opinion about which birth method is safest, there is a natural tendency to focus more on research reports that sustain that view and less on those that might challenge it. We know from chapter 5, "Doctors Who Support Cesarean Choice," for example, that medical professionals are capable of allowing their personal and professional experiences to influence their communication with pregnant women, and chapter 6, "Protecting Your Pelvic Floor," explores just one area of the disagreement that exists in relation to current evidence for the risks and benefits of different birth types. Unfortunately, a discussion about the pelvic floor is almost never had, partly because of a lack of time, partly because of the fear of opening Pandora's box to questions that have no easy answers, and partly because of a severe lack of knowledge even in some medical, nursing, and midwifery circles (although since evidence for a causal association between vaginal delivery and pelvic floor problems is increasing daily, this situation should change). And when financial, political, and ideological pressures are added into the mix with the aim of encouraging or discouraging one birth type over another, it is easy to see how polluted the informational process can become.

LANGUAGE OF CHOICE

It's worth remembering that the notion of patient autonomy and joint decision making is a relatively new one in medical history. Traditionally, when a woman asked the advice of a doctor or midwife, she had little choice but to follow the advice given. And in the context of cesarean birth, there was just no such thing as maternal request or an alternative to vaginal birth. When you think about it, cesarean birth (and in particular, elective or planned cesarean birth) is as groundbreaking in the evolution of humans as something like the development of antibiotics for the number of lives saved. And just as antibiotics have intrinsic risks and benefits, so, too, does surgical delivery.

There is also a language that has to be built up around surgical delivery, and this takes time to settle into accepted and implicit parlance — mostly because the world must understand what something actually *is* before being able to truly define and discuss it. In the case of maternal request cesareans, this is especially true. For example, when we talk about "maternal request," it is implied that the request really should be granted, but, of course, a "request" can be denied and often is, because the doctor is ethically opposed or is convinced it will do more harm than good. So another phrase is used: "cesarean on demand." This places the balance of authority back on the woman, and in a contemporary healthcare environment of "patient choice," if a woman demands to have a cesarean, it is therefore implied she will be given one, although again, there is a caveat. Compliance of the demand can often be dependent on a variety of factors, such as perceived fiscal constraints. For example, since maternal request cesareans are sometimes viewed as a drain on resources in public hospitals, compliance may be denied, whereas the opposite may be true in a private hospital, where the woman is paying the bills. Also, the professional judgment and opinion of the qualified and experienced physician concerned is a factor. For example, he might decide a woman is at significantly increased risk if a cesarean is performed. For instance, she may have an issue such as obesity, with its associations such as decreased glucose tolerance (a precursor and harbinger for future diabetes) and myriad other medical and health issues. And the nature of the problem may not be immediately obvious to her; in parts of the United States, for instance, obesity has been normalized by the sheer force of numbers.

Similarly, the classification of cesareans in general is interesting, particularly those that are not "emergencies" or "emergent" (there are a number of different classifications for cesareans that occur after labor has begun). When surgery is scheduled for a medical reason, this is most commonly known as the "elective" cesarean, and the term has ignited heated social debate over its use. Labeling a surgical birth "elective" implies the surgery has been chosen or at least agreed to voluntarily by a woman. In fact, maternal request cesareans are often referred to as "elective" too. As a result, women whose preference was a vaginal birth may be aggrieved by this term and prefer "planned cesarean," since it reduces any presumption of choice on the part of the mother.

And the list goes on.

The "unnecessary" cesarean, or "unnecesarean," as it is increasingly becoming known (note the advent of a whole new word), is laden with idiosyncrasy, and its meaning depends on your interpretation and perspective. Who decides if and when a cesarean is unnecessary? Is such a cesarean always unnecessary, even at the planning stage, or only in hindsight once the baby is out and doing well? Then there is the description of a cesarean with "no medical indication," "without medical reason," or "non-medically indicated," which is the exact same surgery as that referred to as a "prophylactic" cesarean. In effect, while one group of medical professionals will not agree to cesarean surgery unless a medical problem is imminently evident, another group of medical professionals are so convinced by the likelihood of injury with a trial of labor that they are willing to carry out preventive surgical measures.

Another interesting word in the context of informed choice is whether a woman has the "right" to have a cesarean birth. There has been much discussion about women's "right to refuse" an unwanted cesarean delivery, but, says the American College of Obstetricians and Gynecologists, "less clear is the right of patients to have a surgical procedure when the scientific evidence supporting it is incomplete, of poor quality, or totally lacking—a frequent scenario in medicine."[3] Of course, eight years on from this 2003 statement, further scientific evidence *has* become available, thus reopening the debate about rights.

Without doubt, the maternity world is on a steep language-learning curve. Doctors, midwives, women, and their partners are all in the process of educating themselves about what all these new terms mean, and trying to ensure their communication during prenatal consultations creates clarity and not confusion. Nevertheless, in some cases, problems may arise. Deciding when and how to incorporate women's preferences regarding birth choice is challenging for both obstetric providers and policy makers, and the "dangers of unfettered patient-preference-driven clinical decisions" are recognized.[4] For example, while we steadfastly believe a planned cesarean is a most natural birth choice, we would also concede that maternal request is contentious in its nature and fraught with caveats. For example, should a twenty-year-old woman who is planning to have at least five or six children be able to demand a cesarean birth? We think not. Similarly, should a woman whose baby is breech or macrosomic, or whose first birth was a cesarean (especially with a classical uterine incision), be able to demand a trial of labor at home? Again, we think not. Certainly, the risks are elevated, and any informed consent, or acquiescence to a patient's requests, needs to be tempered with this realization and the burden of professional responsibility.

THE "RIGHT" CESAREAN CANDIDATE

The decision to plan a cesarean birth is not a simple one, and, realistically, there is rarely enough time in a standard prenatal appointment to discuss everything in minute detail. Surgery involves coping with regional or general anesthesia; an operating room environment with masks, tubes, machines, and bright lights; possible nausea; an incision that will take time to heal and is vulnerable to injury and infection; post-birth pain medication; a visible, lasting scar; and, in the event of a second pregnancy, the same cycle of events but with the potential for increased morbidity, plus caring for two children during the recovery period. A woman's inclination to accept these risks is likely to depend on her individual health and her attitude toward risk. And for her doctor, there are many other questions to consider: Is the woman overweight or obese? Does she present with other medical conditions that increase her risk for adverse surgical outcomes? Is she planning a large family? Does she fully comprehend the potential for both planned vaginal birth and surgical morbidities, in this delivery and any future pregnancies? Does one set of risks weigh more heavily on her mind than the other? Are there any cultural or personal values or critical life experiences that need to be considered?[5] Is the desire for control important to her, or is she leaning more toward experiencing a natural course of events? Will she have support at home following the birth?

And while we don't presume that every woman will have done her homework, and we recognize there could be cases where a woman is a less than ideal candidate for planned surgery, working through ethical and practical dilemmas has always been a reality in medicine, and this is no different. We just don't believe the challenges involved in expanding access to maternal request cesareans are a good enough reason to deter or refuse those women who *are* good candidates for surgery, who have educated themselves, and who fully understand the risks involved in their perfectly legitimate birth plan.

BEHIND CLOSED DOORS

Despite doctors' assertions that increasing numbers of women are asking for a cesarean,[6] research to date has found little documented evidence of a deluge of maternal request, leading some to label the very concept a "myth."[7]

So who is right? From responses from the women who visit her website, Pauline agrees with the doctors who say maternal request *is* increasing, but she believes this is relatively unnoticed by medical literature because so many of these births take place in private hospitals, and in public hospitals, maternal request is not always classified as such. On top of this, there are still women who are so concerned about criticism from friends, family, and other women that they confess never actually admitting, if questioned, to having requested the cesarean. They feel more comfortable with presenting medical reasons or their doctor's advice to explain their surgery.

As you can imagine, this all makes maternal request a very difficult area to research. Another part of the problem is that the conversation that takes place between a doctor (or midwife) and a woman is very private, and so often, it's difficult to know for sure how the subject of cesarean birth is initiated or who makes the final decision. Clearly, if a woman walks into a doctor's office and demands a cesarean or says, "I've done my research, and I already know I would prefer a cesarean birth," then the choice is clearly her own, but if she merely requests information on the risks and benefits of a cesarean or asks about what might go wrong during a trial of labor (including her chances of needing emergency surgery), then her final decision on a birth plan will inevitably be influenced by what information her doctor presents and how it is presented.

UNPREDICTABILITY

Evidently, some women are left feeling as though the cesarean decision has been made for them without their true consent. But while stories abound worldwide of doctors encouraging and even forcing women who would prefer a vaginal birth to have an unnecessary cesarean, and while it goes without saying that we do not support *any* coercion of this kind, we are just as concerned about women who are being blindly encouraged and, yes, sometimes forced against their will into attempting a trial of labor. Just recently, a woman in North America corresponded with Pauline throughout her prenatal consultation process, during which she requested a cesarean and even had her request eventually agreed to. Devastatingly, however, on the day she was scheduled to have surgery, the birth was postponed until the following day, and then postponed again to the next day, until she finally went into labor and was told that not only was she unable to have her cesarean as promised but that no anesthetist was available to provide her with pain relief:

> It was not the calm, controlled birth that I had wanted and fought hard for. I would gladly trade the recuperation from a C-section from the experience I had. It was the most painful experience in my life, bar none—never before had I felt so out of control and powerless over what was happening. A woman who plans on a "natural birth" but winds up

with a C-section can find a wealth of support, a woman who plans on an "elective cesarean" but winds up with a 'natural birth," largely carries the burden on her own.

And the reaction of the doctor she visited some weeks later for treatment of a problem related to the birth? As she describes it, he was entirely lacking in empathy for what she had been through, and with no respect for her desired autonomy whatsoever, he simply commented that he was "happy" she didn't get a cesarean.

Unfortunately, although a planned cesarean is certainly more predictable than a planned vaginal birth, it is nonetheless true that a small percentage of cesarean birth plans will not result in the desired outcome. In the example here, this was due in part to a lack of resources in the hospital, but for some women, premature labor may reach such a late stage that by the time they arrive in the operating room, surgery is simply not advisable.

MODELS OF CARE

In 2008, the American College of Obstetricians and Gynecologists (ACOG) addressed the issue of informed consent and patient choice, which it says "are exemplified in the current debate regarding whether elective cesarean delivery should be offered as a birth option in normal pregnancy." The Committee on Ethics stated that "ethical evaluation is clouded by the limitations of data regarding relative short- and long-term risks and benefits of cesarean delivery versus vaginal delivery" and therefore no single ethical principle is sufficient for making the decision. But as part of its deliberations, ACOG outlined four different models of care that demonstrate the diverse range of potential relationships that can exist between a doctor and a patient, and we have included them here to illustrate what you might expect in your appointments with a doctor or midwife.

The Paternalistic Model

The "physician might only present information on the risks and benefits of a procedure that he or she thinks will lead the patient to make the 'right' decision (i.e. in this model, the physician-supported decision)," or the physician will simply inform the patient what course of action should be taken.

The Informative Model

[The] physician is a provider of objective and technical information regarding the patient's medical problem and its potential therapeutic solutions. The patient has complete control over surgical decision-making, and the physician's values are not discussed. . . . A serious drawback of this model is the physician's abandonment of the role of a caring partner and medical expert in the decision-making process. This model also assumes that patients have set values and are able to integrate the sometimes complex medical and surgical treatment decisions with those values. . . . This model may not be ideal for patient care in most situations because the physician's professional judgment generally is of considerable value to patients. In any case, it probably is impossible for a physician to counsel a patient with complete objectivity and without introducing some implied reference for one of many options.

The Interpretive Model

The "physician helps clarify and integrate her [the patient's] values into the decision-making process while acting as an information source regarding the technical aspects of any given medical procedure. . . . When implementing this model, the physician must be careful to help the patient clarify her values while not imposing his or her own values or beliefs on the patient."

The Deliberative Model

[The] physician's role is to guide the patient in taking the most admirable or moral (based on her values, needs, and fears) course of treatment or health-related action. It is similar to the interpretive model in that it includes a discussion of not only the medical benefits and risks but also the patient's individual priorities, values and fears. It goes beyond the interpretative model in that the physician must consciously communicate to the patient his or her health values; however, the physician should not use the moral discussion to dictate to the patient the best course of action.

Because of the potential for an unequal balance of power in the physician-patient relationship, great care should be taken in this model to avoid subjecting the patient to undue pressure.

Evidently, many women requesting planned cesareans with no medical indication have *not* received an ideal model of care (as described in chapter 16, "Cesarean Birth Stories," for example), with some doctors refusing to even discuss the option. Obviously, this situation is unacceptable, but we would add that there is also a danger of the pendulum swinging too far the other way, which would be equally unacceptable. That is, the traditional relationship could eventually be overturned to the point where doctors become mere technicians, expected to agree to patients' every demand, simply because our society, in the Internet age, has given everyone the tools to obtain information and a variety of opinions—the quality of which is often dubious. The danger here lies in the interpretation and assessment of this information deluge. Any denial of demand or attempt to influence a patient against her wishes could become a battle of wills, invoking quantity rather than quality of Internet opinions, and could ultimately be perceived as an attack on the patient's autonomy. This is not a good future for maternity care, either, and certainly not for the patients about whom the vast majority of medical professionals care deeply. However, the perfect answer to this challenge remains elusive.

ACOG concludes that "cesarean delivery on demand" best reflects the informative model, in which the physician simply describes options and provides the service chosen by the patient, but the phrase "elective cesarean delivery" is more suggestive of the deliberative and interpretative models, in which the physician and patient also discuss concerns, needs, and values. As such, "if the physician believes that cesarean delivery promotes the overall health and welfare of the woman and her fetus more than vaginal delivery, he or she is ethically justified in performing a cesarean delivery. Similarly if the physician believes that performing a cesarean delivery would be detrimental to the overall health and welfare of the woman and her fetus, he or she is ethically obliged to refrain from performing the surgery."[8]

In the same year, a review by American doctors concluded that for "a well informed patient, performing a cesarean delivery on maternal request is medically and ethically acceptable." However, while they conceded the acceptance of a request, they stressed that "it does not follow that obstetricians should routinely offer elective cesareans to all patients."[9] Our interpretation of these conclusions is that if a doctor believes the risk/benefit profile for a woman is more favorable with a cesarean birth, it would be unethical for her to suggest a trial of labor. But if a doctor does not believe a cesarean would be the safest option, she can decide not to perform it at all, to perform it on the grounds of patient autonomy, or to refer the woman to another doctor.

Given that the decisions regarding whether a planned cesarean is a good choice for an individual woman can become complicated, especially if there are other factors present (for instance, obesity or large family plans), attempts have been made to take some of the subjectivity out of the decision. One interesting approach tested by Canadian researchers involves the use of a "decision board" (basically, a formalized teaching tool that includes questions to test the level of a woman's increase in knowledge, at the same time analyzing the risks she is willing to accept) to facilitate the informed choice of different birth plans. Early research found the information conveyed to the patients through this method was helpful in their search for personal preferences, and although they are very preliminary, methods like this might help take personal biases and conflicts out of the picture.[10]

THE FUTURE

As we highlight in chapter 8, "Worldwide Cesarean Rates, Attitudes, and Experiences," an increased availability of choice in childbirth for women has meant that in some areas of the world, when women are provided with all the facts regarding the risks and benefits of different birth types, more, rather than fewer, women choose surgery. And this observation has been made by others too: "A culture of choice has been promoted in recent years, but contrary to the anticipated demand for less obstetric intervention by those promoting choice, there has been an increase in demand for delivery by cesarean section rather than the reverse."[11]

Our advice to women would be this: Educate yourselves. Read studies, talk to other women, and search for a doctor or midwife who is willing to really listen to you and respect your concerns. Be honest with yourself. Are you a good candidate for surgery? Are you sure you want a small family? Do you have support for when you come home? Be prepared to fight, be prepared to pay, and unfortunately for some, be prepared for changes to your birth plan to arise. That said, we see the situation for women who want to have a cesarean improving in the near future, and we hope this book will take some in the maternity world one step closer to understanding that not all cesareans are unwanted, negative birth experiences.

Chapter 18

The Evolution of Natural Birth and the Future of Cesarean Birth

In sorrow thou shalt bring forth children.

—Genesis 3:16

For centuries, the difficulty involved in human childbirth was seen simply as God's punishment for human sin. The terrible toll in dead, damaged, or suffering mothers and dead, brain-damaged, or birth-disabled children was accepted as a natural and even deserved cross that humanity must bear. It was just too bad that mainly mothers and babies paid the price.

In fact, difficult childbirth is a direct result of the relationship between the large head of the human fetus at term and the human female pelvic anatomy—and specifically, the unusually large and pointy bony prominences called the ischial spines (the "thorns" of the bones of the pelvis),[1] which can be quite faithfully described as "thorns in the flesh" for all the trouble they cause! All obstetricians and anthropologists know that these make childbirth difficult, even impossible at times;[2] their position, direction, and size could hardly have been designed in a worse way for enabling delivery. In fact, the inward orientation and size of the ischial spines almost negate all other positive evolutionary developments in childbirth, such as an elongation of the pubic bones and a widening of the pelvic inlet.[3] This is because, unfortunately, other than simply being a big bony obstacle, the ischial spines are at the absolute worst place for obstetrical ease—right in the middle of the pelvic canal and right where the descending fetus has to make a sharp turn of almost ninety degrees, then rotate through at least forty-five degrees to reach the pelvic outlet.

These are complicated, Houdini-like contortions the human fetus must go through to make it down the constricted and angulated passage that the

353

birth canal has become. And while this may be a natural and even marvelous physiological process most of the time, it can also lead to many complications during labor—for example, obstructed labor, fetal trauma, and maternal pelvic floor damage. Also, even though there is evidence some of our ancestors (e.g., the australopithecines), experienced a rotational birth in order to accommodate the passage of the fetus's shoulders also, the human fetus has to perform this unique set of acrobatics twice as it descends through the pelvis: once for its distinctly large head and again for its broad shoulders.[4] Therefore, from an obstetrical standpoint, the severe narrowing of the mid-pelvis caused by the ischial spines is one of the most significant problems with the human pelvic anatomy.

We know it was not a mythological act of reaching for and eating the apple that caused this otherwise inexplicably bad situation, so the question is "What, then?"

Simple: our upright posture.

Yes, the mere act of standing up and staying upright has had profound influences on the evolution of the pelvic floor and bony pelvis, involving almost every aspect of these structures, including orientation, measurements, size, and function.[5] In addition to making childbirth difficult, these changes have dramatically and irrevocably altered the function of certain structures. And there is no better example of this change in function, as well as the resultant vulnerability, than the pelvic floor. Not only is the pelvic floor vulnerable during vaginal birth, it has also been given the almost impossible task of countering gravity for an entire lifetime.

In the introductory statement of his paper titled "The Evolution of the Pelvic Floor of Primates," published in 1932, Herbert Elftman stated, "Man standing habitually erect, would be in constant danger of derangement of the viscera lodged in the pelvis, were it not for the presence of an adequate support of bones, muscles, and fascias."[6] Yet unfortunately, this "derangement" is exactly what happens to many, many women—today, as well as in centuries past.

A HISTORY LESSON

It is often said that few things are new under the sun. Certainly in medicine, we sometimes forget the wisdom of some of the late exceptional thinkers and the fact that we stand upon the shoulders of these intellectual giants of the past. The following excerpt is taken from the August 13, 1910, issue of the *British Medical Journal*, and we found it so striking that we decided to include it here, with full credit to the unknown author. As an introduction to the pelvic floor as an important structure for bodily integrity, it is particularly poignant given the understanding we now have of the effects of damage sustained during childbirth.

> Dr. R. H. Paramore, in his recent Hunterian Lectures on the Evolution of the Pelvic Floor, entered into the subject very minutely, and considered physiology and natural history as well as the bare morphology of muscles. He made little of the levator ani and coccygeus as tail movers and much of those muscles in relation to internal pressure. . . . Men, lions, and monkeys largely pass their lives in strife. The carnivora were from the first made to attack, not to flee. They depended on successful stalking and slaughter. Stalking required cunning, which stirred the higher psychical centres to greater activity. Slaughter necessitated the use of the fore limbs for striking purposes, and this in turn demanded a fixation, not only of the thorax, but of the whole body. The necessity to hold the breath entailed by such fixation called the muscles constricting the glottis into greater prominence; the simultaneous necessity to convert the soft and supple abdomen into a comparatively rigid mass determined the further development of the pubo-coccygeus and ilio-coccygeus, the preservation of which allowed a powerful and efficient vocalization, and eventually permitted the assumption of the erect attitude. In short, according to Dr. Paramore, the muscles of the pelvic floor were from their earliest type meant for a physiological end far higher than the wagging of tails, and hence, so far from their being degenerate in man, they are better developed than in many animals graced with lengthy caudal appendages.

And to understand why the pelvis and its various structures have undergone so many changes through the centuries, the following very simplified evolutionary tour, starting from the earliest beginnings of the pelvis, might be helpful to readers.

Life first developed in a marine environment in surroundings where the properties of the water were the same as that of the bodies of the organisms living in it, and they could thus be considered weightless. Only rudimentary support systems were required to keep their bodies together. In fish, for instance, the pelvis is very basic; it has no support function and no sphincter muscles. The earliest vertebrates that moved onto land were amphibians, and for the first time, some support became necessary to counteract gravity. The pelvis became marginally more complex. The development of air breathing required the bodily expansion of a rib cage and abdominal muscles, as well as a two-cavity body plan, which, in turn, led to an increased pressure gradient in the abdominal cavity that had to be countered by an increasingly sophisticated pelvic floor.

A complete escape from the marine environment subsequently led to evolutionary experimentation, but all forms were constrained by one over-arching dilemma: gravity. The effects of gravity underscore the differences between quadruped (walking on all fours) and bipedal (walking on two legs) animals—whether dinosaurs or mammals—with major differences between the two groups. The simplified explanation is that in quadrupeds, there is no need for the pelvic floor to have much of a support function; in fact, it doesn't have to be a floor at all. In some animals (dogs, for example), the pelvic cavity can be closed off when needed—such as when leaping or jumping—by pulling the tail tightly against the pelvic opening. Interestingly, the pelvic muscles of carnivorous animals (in which powerful explosive force is required to hunt) are generally more developed than those of herbivores, which have almost no pelvic floor at all and suffer from permanent fecal incontinence.

THE PELVIC FLOOR OF PRIMATES

Things get even more interesting, and enlightening, when we look at other primates, such as monkeys and the great apes. If we think in a logical, evolutionary way, these animals are not habitually erect, although they do frequently assume such a posture. Therefore, we might expect that their pelvises would show intermediary features between quadruped animals, with their very weak pelvic walls, and the pelvic floor of humans. And this is precisely true. Certain monkeys (like spider, macaque, and proboscis monkeys) and some lesser apes (like gibbons) have large fetal head sizes in relation to their pelvic size, and obstructed labor and even fetal death has been observed in these species.[7] These animals generally have very poor bladder and rectal control. But in contrast, for large apes, where the fetal head is smaller in relation to their pelvic size than it is in humans, this provides an altogether more spacious pelvis, and labor is usually relatively easier.

The first problems for humans probably started 2–2.5 million years ago with the origin of the genus *Homo* (our ancestors), when brain size almost tripled and the pelvis started to take on a more modern human shape. By about three hundred thousand years ago, brain size and pelvic features were basically identical to those of modern humans, and it is assumed that difficult childbirth and a very high mortality were a feature of daily life throughout this time.[8] Complicating things even further for human infants is the fact that compared with almost any other primate, they are born in a much more helpless state. Anthropologists and evolutionary scientists speculate that the possible reason for this is that as the human brain size increased, the only way to accommodate it and still allow for successful birth was to pull back delivery to an earlier stage of fetal development[9]—in effect, causing the human infant to be born an "extragestational fetus," or in other words, at a development stage when it would still reside happily inside the womb in other species.

And yet the main obstacle remained, and still remains, the inability of the human female pelvis to allow this broad-shouldered and large-headed fetus to pass through easily. In fact, in terms of evolution, the pelvis has continued to be a significant limiting factor to human head size (and therefore brain size), and the struggle between the two has settled into an uneasy truce, with the many benefits of a smaller, narrower pelvis (more efficient locomotion and better pelvic support) in direct competition with the absolute need of letting a sustainable percentage of fetuses through alive. Otherwise, our species would have come to an abrupt end.

Academically, this situation in which only "successful" fetuses survive is called "stabilizing selection," and it explains that babies that were heavier or lighter than average did not survive as well as babies of average weight. This effect continued in the human population for arguably one to two million years, until the twentieth century, when improved care for premature deliveries (at least in wealthier countries) and the availability of cesarean surgery for both small and large babies allowed more of them (and their mothers) to survive. But whereas the academic might see this as an interesting example of evolution in action, we take note of the human suffering that occurred throughout this time period and wonder: how many millions of babies and mothers died in the utmost agony while nature achieved this uneasy "stabilizing" balance? And in the future, how much suffering will be prevented by this single most humane operation — the cesarean?

SUPPORTED BIRTH

One other interesting development proceeding from the difficulty of human birth — and indirectly as a consequence of bipedal development — is the social adaptation of childbirth into a cultural, communal, and cooperative event during which laboring women are assisted with their delivery. In all other animals, including primates, delivery is a largely solitary event. Also, the human fetus is usually delivered facing away from its mother, and this fact, as well as the contortions of the fetus as it emerges, makes it very difficult for the human mother to assist with her own delivery — in contrast to most primates, where the fetus faces its mother, and she simply reaches down and pulls it out and toward her.[10] Fundamentally, it is most often true that at their most vulnerable moment — birth — humans truly need each other, and in a certain sense, it is profoundly human to be this helpless. Indeed, the human mother's need for support and assistance might have contributed to our development of socialization and given further impetus to human cognitive development.

We have only to be reminded that the chance of a mother dying in childbirth, even today, is as high as one in seven in some developing countries, and we can reflect on the incredible toll paid in the lives of mothers and babies. In the past, this terrible truth, being almost unbearable to face, led to mythological explanations as the only way to make sense of the situation. In *Maps of Meaning: The Architecture of Belief,* Jordan Peterson describes how mythology and belief become imperative to create, sustain, and protect groups of people against the fear of the unknown and the very real dangers that are "out there."[11] Thus, to explain the inexplicable, pain and suffering in childbirth came to be viewed as a curse on humanity and a sentence to be paid for our ancestors' sins — albeit, ironically, paid for mainly by women and innocent babies, as we noted at the beginning of this chapter.

In fact, if you think about it for a minute, it is an amazing testament to the power of human libido that humans continued to have sex throughout the ages, knowing any pregnancy (especially the first one) could lead to a very real chance of dying in agony, often after days of the most terrible suffering imaginable. In parts of Africa, there is a saying that a pregnant woman has one foot in the grave, which is why many women kiss their families good-bye when going into labor. And yet many people in the developed world today have a romantic and mythical idea of the "natural" birth of old and try to re-create a completely hypothetical "normal" delivery, while, at the same time, demanding safety and a perfect baby. Some rebel against the medicalization of childbirth, which they equate with a "processed" or "scientifically engineered" event that robs them of their individuality and the satisfaction of their own success. They consider it paradise lost, but they forget the hell we escaped. We wonder, though: if these natural-birth advocates could go back in time, or to a developing country, and witness a woman who has been in obstructed labor for days, the baby still inside her long dead, with no hope of a happy outcome and in imminent danger of dying herself, or a woman who has survived the birth but now lives with urinary and fecal incontinence, would they remain so cynical about the medical advancements available to them—or about our arguments for cesarean choice? Normal and natural delivery is *not* always wonderful. It is almost always painful, sometimes excruciatingly so, and it is always fraught with danger to both mother and baby, with the potential to affect the mother's body in ways that sometimes only become apparent long after the fact.

HUMAN SUCCESSES

It's funny, because in most areas of life, progress and change are not only accepted—they are expected and even demanded. Yet childbirth seems to be an odd exception. And ironically, whereas Alexander Fleming's discovery of penicillin is lauded as a miracle of medicine, all too often, the equally deserving cesarean—which has saved millions of babies from death, brain damage, and injuries and millions of women from certain death and serious injury—receives only begrudging respect. We believe the remarkable comparative safety of childbirth in most countries today can be unquestionably claimed as one of the greatest achievements of modern medicine. And furthermore, it is our opinion that cesarean delivery is one of the *most* humane developments in all of medicine and is possibly an evolutionary inevitability, regardless of choice, for many more pregnant women in the human species' future. It has probably saved more lives than any other surgery in contemporary history and has almost certainly relieved the most suffering of any surgical procedure. Indeed, we would go as far as to say that planned cesarean birth is one of the quintessential signs of human progress. It is a step into a confident future and a move away from the pain, suffering, and death of our evolutionary past. It is a way of gripping our humanity firmly in our own hands and refusing to be the powerless victims of evolution, the natural order, or some mythical god. To confidently declare, "I'm in charge of my body and my pregnancy and will not submit despairingly to the whims of Mother Nature."

But for now, on this subject at least, we leave the final word on all this to the Bard:

> Our remedies oft in ourselves do lie
> which we ascribe to heaven: the fated sky
> Gives us free scope; only doth backward pull
> Our slow designs when we ourselves are dull.
> —William Shakespeare, *All's Well That Ends Well*, 1623

Glossary

abruptio placenta	A potentially serious complication of pregnancy where the placental lining has separated from the uterus of the mother. Causes bleeding.
adhesions	The binding together of membranous surfaces, due to inflammation or injury.
amniotic fluid	The fluid surrounding a fetus within the gestational sac (amnion).
anal fissure	A crack or tear in the skin of the anal canal. May cause bleeding and/or pain from defecation.
anal incontinence	Incontinence of gas (flatus) or stool.
anesthesia	Insensitivity to pain, generally brought on with gas or drugs before surgery.
anesthetic	A substance that induces insensitivity to pain.
anesthetist	A medical specialist who administers anesthetics.
anterior	Nearer the front, especially in the front of the body. The opposite of posterior.
anthropology	The comparative study of human societies and cultures and their development.
anus	The opening through which solid waste matter leaves the body.
Apgar	Apgar score; a method to assess the health of newborns. Developed by Dr. Virginia Apgar.
asphyxia	Suffocation.
asphyxiation	Severe lack of oxygen—for example, choking. A fetus can be asphyxiated if it doesn't receive enough oxygen through the placenta.
atrophy	Wasting away, typically due to the degeneration of cells.
autonomy	Independence.
bias	Unfairly favoring one option over another.
bipedal	Using only two legs for walking.
birth plan	Detailed written plan of wishes, likes, and dislikes for labor and delivery.

bladder neck	Junction between the bladder and the urethra.
body mass index	Weight to height ratio, calculated by dividing one's weight in kilograms by the square of one's height in meters and used as an indicator of obesity and underweight.
brachial plexus palsy	Paralysis of the arm due to nerve injury. Same as Erb's palsy.
Braxton Hicks	Intermittent weak contractions of the uterus occurring during pregnancy.
cephalhematoma	Hemorrhage between the skull and the bone membranes of a newborn baby.
cesarean/c-section	A surgical procedure during which an incision is made through a mother's abdomen (laparotomy) and uterus (hysterotomy) to deliver one or more babies or, rarely, to remove a dead fetus.
chorioamnionitis	Inflammation of the fetal membranes due to a bacterial infection. It is most often associated with prolonged labor.
classical cesarean	A cesarean in which the incision in the uterus is made completely or partially in the thicker, upper part of the uterus.
coccygeus	A muscle of the pelvic floor located behind the levator ani and in front of the sacrospinous ligament.
connective tissue	The fibrous tissue that makes up bodily structures such as tendons.
continence	The ability to control the bladder and/or bowel.
dyspareunia	Difficult or painful sexual intercourse.
elective	An optional course of action or decision. In medicine, a treatment usually chosen by the patient rather than urgently necessary.
electrocautery	Using a needle or other instrument that is electrically heated to sear tissues (cautery).
embolism	Obstruction of an artery, typically by a clot of blood or an air bubble.
embolus	A blood clot, air bubble, piece of fatty deposit, or other object that has been carried in the bloodstream to lodge in a vessel and cause an embolism.

emergency cesarean	Cesarean section performed in an urgent manner for either maternal or fetal considerations.
encephalopathy	A disease in which the functioning of the brain is affected by some agent or condition.
endometritis	Inflammation of the endometrium.
episiotomy	A surgical cut made at the opening of the vagina during childbirth to aid a difficult delivery and to avoid rupture of tissues.
epithelial	The thin tissue forming the outer layer of a body's surface.
Erb's palsy	Paralysis of the arm caused by nerve injury, most commonly from shoulder dystocia during birth. Same as brachial plexus palsy.
evolution	The development and diversification of life over time.
fascia	Sheath of fibrous tissue enclosing a muscle or other organ.
fecal incontinence	The inability to control stool (but not gas).
feces	Waste material produced by the intestine. Feces are composed of bacteria, undigested food, and material produced from the intestines.
fertilization	The process by which male and female sex cells meet to produce a zygote.
fetus	The intrauterine unborn child.
fistula	An opening between two organs—for instance, between the bladder and the vagina, or the rectum and the vagina. In poor countries, the most common cause of fistula formation is obstructed labor.
flatus	Bowel gas.
forceps delivery	Delivery accomplished using a tongs-like instrument called obstetrical forceps.
gestation	Pregnancy.
Heisenberg's uncertainty principle	The belief that you cannot know the exact location and the velocity of a particle simultaneously. Heisenberg was a German mathematical physicist and philosopher who developed a system of quantum mechanics based on matrix algebra and won the Nobel Prize for Physics in 1932.

hematoma	Blood clot.
hemorrhage	Uncontrollable bleeding.
hypocontractile	Unable to contract strongly enough to do necessary tasks, as in a hypocontractile bladder.
hysterectomy	A surgical operation to remove all or part of the uterus.
ICU	Intensive care unit.
ideology	A system of ideas.
incidence	New occurrences of a disorder per year.
incontinence	Having no, or insufficient, control over urination or defecation.
induction of labor	Bringing on labor deliberately using drugs.
informed consent	An agreement based on the clearest possible understanding of the issues involved, as between a patient and a doctor.
instrumental delivery	Vaginal delivery facilitated or made possible by application and use of either forceps or vacuum (ventouse).
intermittent catheterization	Inserting a catheter into the bladder every few hours as needed to drain the bladder. This can be done by a healthcare worker or self.
intrapartum	During labor.
invasive	As in "invasive procedures"; procedures involving interference to change an outcome. It could also mean the penetration of a body cavity or the body surface with a device, needle, or blade, as in surgery.
ischial spines	The protrusions on the ischium that impede delivery.
ischium	The curved bone forming the base of each half of the pelvis.
IVF	In vitro fertilization. The egg is fertilized outside the woman's body, and then the zygote is transferred into her uterus.
Kegel exercises	Named after Dr. Arnold Kegel, exercises that consist of contracting and relaxing the muscles that form part of the pelvic floor (which some people colloquially call the "Kegel muscles").
laceration	Tear or deep cut, usually significant.

large for gesta-tional age (LGA)	Macrosomic; see macrosomia.
levator	A muscle whose contraction causes the raising of a part of the body.
levator ani	One of two broad, thin muscles that makes up most of the pelvis floor. In combination with the coccygeus muscle, it forms the pelvic diaphragm.
libido	Sexual desire.
macrosomia	Large for gestational age babies are those whose birth weight (or length or head circumference) lies above the ninetieth percentile for that gestational age.
medical indication	A medical reason for a treatment.
medicalize	To treat as a medical problem, especially unnecessarily.
midwife	A person (typically a woman) trained to assist women in childbirth. This person can be from a nursing background in some countries, but in North America, he/she usually is not.
morbidity	A diseased state, disability, or poor health due to any cause.
mortality	Death, dying.
mortality rate	The number of deaths in a given area or period or per population, from a particular cause.
multiparous	Having given birth two or more times. A multiparous woman might be referred to as a "multip."
mythology	Collection of myths from one tradition.
natural	Of nature; not caused by humans.
natural childbirth	A term normally used to indicate the natural order of childbirth as in the "natural" state. In reality, this would mean total noninterference by attendants. The term is used loosely, meaning different things to different people.
neonatal	Relating to newborn children, thus after delivery and up to twenty-eight days after birth.
NHS	National Health Service (United Kingdom).
obesity	Being very fat or overweight.
objectivity	Not being influenced by personal tastes and opinions.

obstetrical indication	A medical indication relating to a mother, fetus, or their interaction that requires a course of action (such as a cesarean).
opioid	An opium-like compound that binds to one or more of the opioid receptors of the body. Well-known examples include codeine, oxycodone, morphine, and Demerol®.
orgasm	Sexual climax.
parity	Number of previous live births.
pelvic cavity	The body cavity that is bounded by the bones of the pelvis and primarily contains reproductive organs, the bladder, and the rectum.
pelvic floor	The structure composed of muscle fibers of the levator ani, the coccygeus, and associated connective tissue, which span the area underneath the pelvis.
pelvic floor dysfunction	Disorders of the pelvic floor related to physiological or anatomical abnormalities. They include incontinence, prolapse, pain syndromes, and others.
pelvic floor exercises	Same as Kegel exercises. A treatment that requires repetitive active exercise of the levator muscles.
pelvis	In humans, the bony structure at the hips that supports internal organs and connects to the legs.
perinatal	Relating to the time immediately before and after birth. Usually denoting time up to seven days after birth.
perineum	The area between the anus and the vulva.
placenta accreta	A severe obstetric complication involving an abnormally deep attachment of the placenta, through the endometrium and into the myometrium (the middle layer of the uterine wall). There are three forms of placenta accreta, distinguishable by the depth of penetration.
placenta previa	A condition in which the placenta partially or wholly blocks the neck of the uterus, thus interfering with normal delivery of a baby.
postdural headache	See spinal headache.
posterior	Further back in position; of or nearer the rear or hind end.
postnatal	The period immediately after birth.

postnatal depression	Depression after birth.
postpartum	The period up to six weeks after delivery.
prematurity	Baby born before full-term gestation.
prenatal	The period immediately before and during pregnancy.
prevalence	Occurrence of a disorder in the general population.
primiparous	In the process of a first pregnancy. A primiparous woman can also be referred to as being "primipara" or "primip."
prognosis	Prediction of most likely future outcome.
prolapse	Slipping forward or down of one of the parts or organs of the body—for instance the uterus, bladder, or rectum.
prophylactic	A medicine or course of action used to prevent disease.
puborectalis	A hammock-like muscle that stretches from the pubic bone to the coccyx (tailbone), forming the floor of the pelvic cavity and supporting the pelvic organs. It is part of the levator ani group of muscles.
pudendal nerve	A large nerve branch of the sacral plexus that innervates the external genitalia of both sexes, as well as sphincters for the bladder and the rectum.
puerperal infection	Also called childbed fever, it usually starts as an infection in the womb but can develop into puerperal sepsis, which is a serious blood infection contracted by a woman during or shortly after childbirth, miscarriage, or abortion.
rectum	The last segment of the colon; the lowest part of the bowel found right before the anus.
rectus muscles	The vertical abdominal muscles. These are not cut but are spread apart during cesarean delivery.
rectus sheath	The fascia surrounding the rectus muscles.
regional anesthesia	Anesthesia affecting only a large part of the body, such as a limb.
sexual dysfunction	Difficulty experienced by an individual or a couple during any stage of a normal sexual activity, including desire, arousal, or orgasm.
shoulder dystocia	In childbirth, the very dangerous situation in which the infant's shoulders are unable to pass through the birth canal after the head has delivered.

sphincter	A ring of muscle surrounding and serving to guard or close an opening or tube, such as the anus.
spinal anesthetic	The anesthetic solution is injected into the spinal canal immediately surrounding the spinal column. No catheter is used, and the needle used is therefore thinner.
spinal fluid	Fluid surrounding the spinal column and brain.
spinal headache	Also called postdural puncture headache (PDPH). A headache that is a complication of puncture of the dura mater (one of the membranes that surround the brain and spinal cord). This occurs in spinal anesthesia and lumbar puncture and may, accidentally, occur in epidural anesthesia.
stillbirth	The birth of an infant who has died in the womb.
subdural	Between the dura mater and the arachnoid membrane of the brain and spinal cord.
subgaleal hematoma	Bleeding in the potential space between the scalp and the skull.
subjectivity	Being influenced by personal feelings, tastes, or opinions. The opposite of objectivity.
sudden infant death syndrome (SIDS)	The death of a seemingly healthy baby in its sleep, due to an apparent spontaneous cessation of breathing.
superior	Further above or out; higher in position.
surrogacy	The process of giving birth as a surrogate mother or of arranging such a birth.
surrogate	Substitute.
thromboembolism	Obstruction of a blood vessel by a blood clot that has become dislodged from another site in the circulation.
thrombophilia	The tendency to develop blood clots, caused by hereditary defects in blood clotting factors.
thrombosis	Blood clots.
tokophobia	Fear of childbirth.
trauma	Physical and/or psychological injury.
trial of labor	Allowing labor to proceed to see if it will be successful.
urethra	The structure carrying urine from the bladder to the outside.
urinary incontinence	Leaking or losing control of urine.

urogenital	The structures pertaining to the urological and genital systems. Usually used when discussing the urogenital opening (opening at the bottom of the pelvic cavity through which the aforementioned organ systems run).
urogenital atrophy	Shrinking, drying, and thinning of the vaginal epithelium, as well as changes in the support tissue of the urogenital area as a result of decreased estrogen levels. Usually associated with menopause.
urogenital hiatus	The opening between the muscles in the pelvic floor that allows the passage of the urethra, vagina, and rectum.
urogynecology	A surgical subspecialty of urology and gynecology dealing mostly with pelvic organ prolapse, urinary and fecal incontinence, and other pelvic floor disorders and pelvic medicine.
uterine prolapse	A condition in which the uterus has slipped (dropped) from its normal position, and the cervix is closer to the vaginal opening or may protrude.
uterus	The womb.
vagina	Also known as the birth canal. The genital opening of women, composed of smooth muscle and ending at the cervix.
voluntary control	Conscious control.

Notes

INTRODUCTION

1. O. Paul Humpstone, "Cesarean Section versus Spontaneous Delivery," *American Journal of Obstetrics and Gynecology* 1 (1920): 986–89.

2. H. A. Krone and J. Mattheus, "Maternal Mortality in Cesarean Section as Compared to Vaginal Delivery" [in German], *Fortschritte der Medizin* 93, no. 27 (September 25, 1975): 1266–68.

3. "Ethical Issues in Obstetrics and Gynecology by the FIGO Committee for the Study of Ethical Aspects of Human Reproduction and Women's Health," International Federation of Gynecology and Obstetrics, October 2009, http://www.figo.org/publications/miscellaneous_publications/ethical_guidelines (accessed January 19, 2011).

4. Stephen Robson and David Ellwood, "Should Obstetricians Support a 'Term Cephalic Trial'?" *Australian and New Zealand Journal of Obstetrics and Gynaecology* 43, no. 5 (October 2003): 341–43.

5. American College of Obstetricians and Gynecologists Office of Communications, "New ACOG Opinion Addresses Elective Cesarean Controversy," news release, October 31, 2003, http://www.acog.org/from_home/publications/press_releases/nr10-31-03-1.cfm (accessed February 24, 2011).

CHAPTER 3. THE SAFEST BIRTH CHOICE FOR YOUR BABY: PLANNED CESAREAN

1. Gary D. V. Hankins, Shannon M. Clark, and Mary B. Munn, "Cesarean Section on Request at 39 Weeks: Impact on Shoulder Dystocia, Fetal Trauma, Neonatal Encephalopathy, and Intrauterine Fetal Demise," *Seminars in Perinatology* 30, no. 5 (October 2006): 276–87.

2. Tim A. Bruckner, Yvonne W. Cheng, and Aaron B. Caughey, "Increased Neonatal Mortality among Normal-Weight Births beyond 41 Weeks of Gestation in California," *American Journal of Obstetrics and Gynecology* 199, no. 4 (October 2008): 421.1–7.

3. R. Joyce, R. Webb, and J. L. Peacock, "Associations between Perinatal Interventions and Hospital Stillbirth Rates and Neonatal Mortality," *Archives of Disease in Childhood. Fetal and Neonatal Edition* 89, no. 1 (January 2004): 51–56.

4. Virasakdi Chongsuvivatwong et al., "Maternal and Fetal Mortality and Complications Associated with Cesarean Section Deliveries in Teaching Hospitals in Asia," *Journal of Obstetrics and Gynaecology Research* 36, no. 1 (February 2010): 45–51.

5. Leanne S. Dahlgren et al., "Caesarean Section on Maternal Request: Risks and Benefits in Healthy Nulliparous Women and Their Infants," *Journal of Obstetrics and Gynaecology Canada* 31, no. 9 (September 2009): 808–17.

6. Charmaine K. Moczygemba et al., "Route of Delivery and Neonatal Birth Trauma," *American Journal of Obstetrics and Gynecology* 202, no. 4 (April 2010): 361.1–6.

7. Hankins, Clark, and Munn, "Cesarean Section on Request."

8. Ibid.

9. Jemel Bingham et al., "Recurrent Shoulder Dystocia: Q Review," *Obstetrical and Gynecological Survey* 65, no. 3 (March 2010): 183–88.

10. Sarah H. Poggi et al., "Intrapartum Risk Factors for Permanent Brachial Plexus Injury," *American Journal of Obstetrics and Gynecology* 189, no. 3 (September 2003): 725–29.

11. I. Z. MacKenzie et al., "Management of Shoulder Dystocia: Trends in Incidence and Maternal and Neonatal Morbidity," *Obstetrics and Gynecology* 110, no. 5 (November 2007): 1059–68; Magnus Christoffersson et al., "Shoulder Dystocia and Brachial Plexus Injury: A Case-Control Study," *Acta Obstetricia et Gynecologica Scandinavica* 82, no. 2 (February 2003): 147–51.

12. Shobha H. Mehta et al., "Shoulder Dystocia and the Next Delivery: Outcomes and Management," *Journal of Maternal-Fetal and Neonatal Medicine* 20, no. 10 (October 2007): 729–33.

13. Stergios K. Doumouchtsis and Sabaratnam Arulkumaran, "Are All Brachial Plexus Injuries Caused by Shoulder Dystocia?" *Obstetrical and Gynecological Survey* 64, no. 9 (September 2009): 615–23.

14. Fidelma O'Mahony et al., "Review of Singleton Fetal and Neonatal Deaths Associated with Cranial Trauma and Cephalic Delivery during a National Intrapartum-Related Confidential Enquiry," *BJOG: An International Journal of Obstetrics and Gynaecology* 112, no. 5 (May 2005): 619–26.

15. S. W. Wen et al., "Comparison of Maternal and Infant Outcomes between Vacuum Extraction and Forceps Deliveries," *American Journal of Epidemiology* 153, no. 2 (January 15, 2001): 103–07.

16. D. Towner et al., "Effect of Mode of Delivery in Nulliparous Women on Neonatal Intracranial Injury," *New England Journal of Medicine* 341, no. 23 (December 2, 1999): 1709–14.

17. Christopher B. Looney et al., "Intracranial Hemorrhage in Asympto-

matic Neonates: Prevalence on MR Images and Relationship to Obstetric and Neonatal Risk Factors," *Radiology* 242, no. 2 (February 2007): 535–41.

18. A. Shihadeh and W. Al-Najdawi, "Forceps or Vacuum Extraction: A Comparison of Maternal and Neonatal Morbidity," *Eastern Mediterranean Health Journal*, no. 1 (March 2001): 106–14.

19. L. M. Chadwick, P. J. Pemberton, and J. J. Kurinczuk, "Neonatal Sub-galeal Haematoma: Associated Risk Factors, Complications, and Outcome," *Journal of Paediatrics and Child Health* 32, no. 3 (June 1996): 228–32.

20. E. J. Geller et al., "Neonatal Outcomes Associated with Planned Vaginal versus Planned Primary Cesarean Delivery," *Journal of Perinatology: Official Journal of the California Perinatal Association* 30, no. 4 (April 2010): 258–64; C. Sunoo, T. S. Kosasa, and R. W. Hale, "Meconium Aspiration Syndrome without Evidence of Fetal Distress in Early Labor before Elective Cesarean Delivery," *Obstetrics and Gynecology* 73, no. 5 (May 1989): 707–709.

21. "Baby Died of Fractured Skull after Caesarean Section Delayed," *Telegraph*, November 19, 2009, http://www.telegraph.co.uk/news/uknews/6606245/Baby-died-of-fractured-skull-after-Caesarean-section-delayed.html (accessed October 18, 2010).

22. "Inquest Told Baby Suffered Head Injuries at Delivery." *Irish Times*, November 11, 2009, http://www.irishtimes.com/newspaper/ireland/2009/1121/1224259236904.html (accessed October 18, 2010).

23. "Liverpool Hospital Payout for Birth Paralysis Girl," BBC News Online, January 19, 2010, http://news.bbc.co.uk/2/hi/uk_news/england/merseyside/8467708.stm (accessed October 18, 2010).

24. "Newborn Wrongful Death Lawsuit Results in $1.85M over Vacuum Extraction," AboutLawsuits.com, August 3, 2009, http://www.aboutlawsuits.com/newborn-wrongful-death-lawsuit-over-vacuum-extraction-5199/ (accessed October 18, 2010).

25. Lois Rogers, "Babies Crippled as Midwives Bungle Births," Daily Mail Online, March 4, 2009, http://www.dailymail.co.uk/health/article-1158657/Babies-crippled-midwives-bungle-births.html (accessed October 18, 2010).

26. Jane Feinmann, "Forceps Left this Boy Brain Damaged. His Case Is Far from Unique. So Why *Are* They Still Used?" Daily Mail Online, October 19, 2010, http://www.dailymail.co.uk/health/article-1321674/Forceps-left-boy-brain-damaged-His-case-far-unique-So-ARE-used.html (accessed October 19, 2010).

27. "Couple's Heartbreak after Longed-for Baby Girl Dies after Doctors Use Forceps to Deliver Her," *Daily Record*, February 24, 2010, http://www.dailyrecord.co.uk/news/scottish-news/2010/02/24/couple-s-heartbreak-after-longed-for-baby-girl-dies-after-doctors-use-forceps-to-deliver-her-86908-22066219/ (accessed January 16, 2011).

28. Lucky Jain and Douglas C. Eaton, "Physiology of Fetal Lung Fluid Clearance and the Effect of Labor," *Seminars in Perinatology* 30, no. 1 (February 2006): 34–43.

29. Lucky Jain, "Alveolar Fluid Clearance in Developing Lungs and Its Role in Neonatal Transition," *Clinics in Perinatology* 26, no. 3 (September 1999): 585–99.

30. Lucky Jain and Golde G. Dudell, "Respiratory Transition in Infants Delivered by Cesarean Section," *Seminars in Perinatology* 30, no. 5 (October 2006): 296–304.

31. Freke A. Wilmink et al., "Neonatal Outcome following Elective Cesarean Section beyond 37 Weeks of Gestation: A 7-Year Retrospective Analysis of a National Registry," *American Journal of Obstetrics and Gynecology* 202, no. 3 (March 2010): 250.1–8; George A. Macones, "Elective Delivery before 39 Weeks: Reason for Caution," *American Journal of Obstetrics and Gynecology* 202, no. 3 (March 2010): 208.

32. Anne Kirkeby Hansen et al., "Elective Caesarean Section and Respiratory Morbidity in the Term and Near-Term Neonate," *Acta Obstetricia Et Gynecologica Scandinavica* 86, no. 4 (2007): 389–94.

33. Helen L. Tanger et al., "Less Neonatal Morbidity with Elective Caesarean Sections at Term: Local Guideline for Elective Caesarean Section Is Effective" [in Dutch], *Nederlands Tijdschrift Voor Geneeskunde* 154, no. 26 (2010): A1201; Steven L. Clark et al., "Reduction in Elective Delivery at [less than] 39 Weeks of Gestation: Comparative Effectiveness of 3 Approaches to Change and the Impact on Neonatal Intensive Care Admission and Stillbirth," *American Journal of Obstetrics and Gynecology* 203, no. 5 (July 7, 2010): 449; Michael C. Nicholl and Miriam A. Cattell, "Getting Evidence into Obstetric Practice: Appropriate Timing of Elective Caesarean Section," *Australian Health Review: A Publication of the Australian Hospital Association* 34, no. 1 (March 2010): 90–92.

34. Anthony Shanks et al., "Administration of Steroids after 34 Weeks of Gestation Enhances Fetal Lung Maturity Profiles," *American Journal of Obstetrics and Gynecology* 203, no. 1 (July 2010): 47.1–5.

35. Jagteshwar Grewal et al., "Risk of Cesarean Delivery When Second-Trimester Ultrasound Dating Disagrees with Definite Last Menstrual Period," *American Journal of Perinatology* 27, no. 7 (August 2010): 587–93.

36. B. O. Verburg et al., "New Charts for Ultrasound Dating of Pregnancy and Assessment of Fetal Growth: Longitudinal Data from a Population-Based Cohort Study," *Ultrasound in Obstetrics and Gynecology: The Official Journal of the International Society of Ultrasound in Obstetrics and Gynecology* 31, no. 4 (April 2008): 388–96.

37. Maria G. Dominguez-Bello et al., "Delivery Mode Shapes the Acquisition and Structure of the Initial Microbiota across Multiple Body Habitats in Newborns," *Proceedings of the National Academy of Sciences of the United States of America* 107, no. 26 (June 29, 2010): 11971–75.

CHAPTER 4. BIRTH SATISFACTION: CESAREAN RANKS HIGHEST

1. P. Husslein, "Elective Caesarean Section versus Vaginal Delivery: Whither the End of Traditional Obstetrics?" *Archives of Gynecology and Obstetrics* 265, no. 4 (November 2001): 169–74.

2. "Welcome to the Birth Trauma Association," Birth Trauma Association, 2007, http://www.birthtraumaassociation.org.uk/ (accessed February 22, 2011).

3. D. K. Creedy, I. M. Shochet, and J. Horsfall, "Childbirth and the Development of Acute Trauma Symptoms: Incidence and Contributing Factors," *Birth* 27, no. 2 (June 2000): 104–11.

4. "Women's Comments," Birth Trauma Canada, http://birthtraumacanada.org/6.html (accessed October 15, 2010).

5. A. Pantlen and A. Rohde, "Psychologic Effects of Traumatic Live Deliveries" [in German], *Zentralblatt für Gynäkologie* 123, no. 1 (January 2001): 42–47.

6. Stephen Robson et al., "Elective Caesarean Delivery at Maternal Request: A Preliminary Study of Motivations Influencing Women's Decision Making," *Australian and New Zealand Journal of Obstetrics and Gynaecology* 48, no. 4 (August 2008): 415–20.

7. Ingela Wiklund, Gunnar Edman, and Ellika Andolf, "Cesarean Section on Maternal Request: Reasons for the Request, Self-Estimated Health, Expectations, Experience of Birth, and Signs of Depression among First-Time Mothers," *Acta Obstetricia et Gynecologica Scandinavica* 86, no. 4 (2007): 451–56.

8. W. J. Graham et al., "An Investigation of Women's Involvement in the Decision to Deliver by Caesarean Section," *British Journal of Obstetrics and Gynaecology* 106, no. 3 (March 1999): 213–20; T. A. Mould et al., "Women's Involvement with the Decision Preceding Their Caesarean Section and Their Degree of Satisfaction," *British Journal of Obstetrics and Gynaecology* 103, no. 11 (November 1996): 1074–77; E. L. Ryding, K. Wijma, and B. Wijma, "Psychological Impact of Emergency Cesarean Section in Comparison with Elective Cesarean Section, Instrumental, and Normal Vaginal Delivery," *Journal of Psychosomatic Obstetrics and Gynaecology* 19, no. 3 (September 1998): 135–44; Behnaz Torkan et al., "Postnatal Quality of Life in Women after Normal Vaginal Delivery and Caesarean Section," *BMC Pregnancy and Childbirth* 9, no. 1 (2009): 4; Marianne Weiss, Jacqueline Fawcett, and Cynthia Aber, "Adaptation, Postpartum Concerns, and Learning Needs in the First Two Weeks after Caesarean Birth," *Journal of Clinical Nursing* 18, no. 21 (November 2009): 2938–48.

9. Joan L Blomquist et al., "Mothers' Satisfaction with Planned Vaginal and Planned Cesarean Birth," *American Journal of Perinatology* 28, no. 5 (May 2011): 383–88.

10. K. Hofberg and I. Brockington, "Tokophobia: An Unreasoning Dread of Childbirth: A Series of 26 Cases," *British Journal of Psychiatry: The Journal of Mental Science* 176 (January 2000): 83–85.

11. B. Areskog, N. Uddenberg, and B. Kjessler, "Experience of Delivery in Women with and without Antenatal Fear of Childbirth," *Gynecologic and Obstetric Investigation* 16, no. 1 (1983): 1–12.

12. Karen Nicholls and Susan Ayers, "Childbirth-Related Post-Traumatic Stress Disorder in Couples: A Qualitative Study," *British Journal of Health Psychology* 12, no. 4 (November 2007): 491–509; Z. Karaçam and K. Eroğlu, "Effects of Episiotomy on Bonding and Mothers' Health," *Journal of Advanced Nursing* 43 (August 2003): 384–94.

13. Cristie Glasheen, Gale A. Richardson, and Anthony Fabio, "A Systematic Review of the Effects of Postnatal Maternal Anxiety on Children," *Archives of Women's Mental Health* 13, no. 1 (February 2010): 61–74.

14. Edward Fottrell et al., "Risk of Psychological Distress following Severe Obstetric Complications in Benin: The Role of Economics, Physical Health, and Spousal Abuse," *British Journal of Psychiatry* 196, no. 1 (January1, 2010): 18–25.

15. Wiklund, Edman, and Andolf, "Cesarean Section on Maternal Request"; Annika Karlström et al., "Postoperative Pain after Cesarean Birth Affects Breastfeeding and Infant Care," *Journal of Obstetric, Gynecologic, and Neonatal Nursing* 36, no. 5 (October 2007): 430–40.

16. "Is It Possible to Breastfeed after a Cesarean Birth?" La Leche League International, October 13, 2006, http://www.llli.org/FAQ/cesarean.html (accessed February 22, 2011).

17. K. C. Evans et al., "Effect of Caesarean Section on Breast Milk Transfer to the Normal Term Newborn over the First Week of Life," *Archives of Disease in Childhood. Fetal and Neonatal Edition* 88, no. 5 (September 2003): 380–82; Heather J. Rowe-Murray and Jane R. W. Fisher, "Baby Friendly Hospital Practices: Cesarean Section Is a Persistent Barrier to Early Initiation of Breastfeeding," *Birth* 29, no. 2 (June 2002): 124–31; R. Pérez-Escamilla, I. Maulén-Radovan, and K. G. Dewey, "The Association between Caesarean Delivery and Breast-Feeding Outcomes among Mexican Women," *American Journal of Public Health* 86, no. 6 (June 1996): 832–36.

18. T. Tamminen et al., "The Influence of Perinatal Factors on Breast Feeding," *Acta Paediatrica Scandinavica* 72, no. 1 (January 1983): 9–12; V. Vestermark et al., "Influence of the Mode of Delivery on Initiation of Breast-Feeding," *European Journal of Obstetrics, Gynecology, and Reproductive Biology* 38, no. 1 (January 4, 1991): 33–38.

19. H. J. Rowe-Murray and J. R. Fisher, "Operative Intervention in Delivery Is Associated with Compromised Early Mother-Infant Interaction,"

BJOG: An International Journal of Obstetrics and Gynaecology 108, no. 10 (October 2001): 1068–75.

20. Emily Cook, "Women Who Have Caesareans 'Less Likely to Bond,'" *Daily Mail Online*, July 13, 2006, http://www.dailymail.co.uk/health/article-3952 18/Women-Caesareans-likely-bond.html (accessed February 24, 2011).

21. Man Wah Pang et al., "Impact of First Childbirth on Changes in Women's Preference for Mode of Delivery: Follow-Up of a Longitudinal Observational Study," *Birth* 35, no. 2 (June 2008): 121–28.

22. S. Avasarala and M. Mahendran, "A Survey of Women's Experiences following Instrumental Vaginal Delivery," *Journal of Obstetrics and Gynaecology* 29, no. 6 (2009): 504.

23. Stephen J. Robson et al., "Do Women's Perceptions of Care at the Time of Unexplained Stillbirth Influence Their Wishes for Management in Subsequent Pregnancy? An Internet-Based Empirical Study," *Journal of Obstetrics and Gynaecology Research* 36, no. 1 (February 2010): 108–14.

CHAPTER 5. DOCTORS WHO SUPPORT CESAREAN CHOICE

1. Elizabeth McClellan, "Rapid Responses to 'Elective Caesarean Section on Request': Women Should Have a Choice," *British Medical Journal*, December 10, 1999, http://www.bmj.com/content/318/7176/120/reply (accessed February 24, 2011).

2. R. Al-Mufti, A. McCarthy, and N. M. Fisk, "Obstetricians' Personal Choice and Mode of Delivery," *Lancet* 347, no. 9000 (February 24, 1996): 544.

3. American College of Obstetricians and Gynecologists Office of Communications, "Gallup Survey Reveals Women Ob-Gyns Benefit from 'Insider Knowledge,'" news release, December 9, 2003, http://www.acog.org/from_home/publications/press_releases/nr12-09-03-2.cfm (accessed February 24, 2011); Joseph R. Wax et al., "Patient Choice Cesarean: The Maine Experience," *Birth* 32, no. 3 (September 2005): 203–206; S. G. Gabbe and G. B. Holzman, "Obstetricians' Choice of Delivery," *Lancet* 357, no. 9257 (March 3, 2001): 722.

4. Gabbe and Holzman, "Obstetricians' Choice of Delivery."

5. Thomas Bergholt et al., "Danish Obstetricians' Personal Preference and General Attitude to Elective Cesarean Section on Maternal Request: A Nation-Wide Postal Survey," *Acta Obstetricia et Gynecologica Scandinavica* 83, no. 3 (March 2004): 26266.

6. P. McGurgan, S. Coulter-Smith, and P. J. O'Donovan, "A National Confidential Survey of Obstetricians' Personal Preferences Regarding Mode of

Delivery," *European Journal of Obstetrics, Gynecology, and Reproductive Biology* 97, no. 1 (July 2001): 17–19.

7. R. Land et al., "Personal Preferences of Obstetricians towards Childbirth," *Australian and New Zealand Journal of Obstetrics and Gynaecology* 41, no. 3 (August 2001): 249–52.

8. R. Al-Mufti, A. McCarthy, and N. M. Fisk, "Survey of Obstetricians' Personal Preference and Discretionary Practice," *European Journal of Obstetrics, Gynecology, and Reproductive Biology* 73, no. 1 (May 1997): 1–4; Katie M. Groom, Sara Paterson-Brown, and Nicholas M. Fisk, "Temporal and Geographical Variation in UK Obstetricians' Personal Preference regarding Mode of Delivery," *European Journal of Obstetrics, Gynecology, and Reproductive Biology* 100, no. 2 (January 10, 2002): 185–88.

9. T. S. Usha Kiran and N. S. Jayawickrama, "Who Is Responsible for the Rising Caesarean Section Rate?" *Journal of Obstetrics and Gynaecology: The Journal of the Institute of Obstetrics and Gynaecology* 22, no. 4 (July 2002): 363–65.

10. Vilhjalmur Finsen, Andreas Hopstock Storeheier, and Olaf Gjerløw Aasland, "Cesarean Section: Norwegian Women Do as Obstetricians Do — Not as Obstetricians Say," *Birth* 35, no. 2 (June 2008): 117–20.

11. R. Al-Mufti, A. McCarthy, and N. M. Fisk, "Survey of Obstetricians' Personal Preference and Discretionary Practice," *Acta Obstetricia Et Gynecologica Scandinavica* 83, no. 3 (March 2004): 262–66.

12. Scott A. Farrell, Thomas F. Baskett, and Karen D. Farrell, "The Choice of Elective Cesarean Delivery in Obstetrics: A Voluntary Survey of Canadian Health Care Professionals," *International Urogynecology Journal and Pelvic Floor Dysfunction* 16, no. 5 (October 2005): 378–83.

13. Sedigheh Hantoushzadeh et al., "Caesarean or Normal Vaginal Delivery: Overview of Physicians' Self-Preference and Suggestion to Patients," *Archives of Gynecology and Obstetrics* 280, no. 1 (July 2009): 33–37.

14. Bergholt et al., "Danish Obstetricians' Personal Preference."

15. Yves Jacquemyn, Fatima Ahankour, and Guy Martens, "Flemish Obstetricians' Personal Preference regarding Mode of Delivery and Attitude towards Caesarean Section on Demand," *European Journal of Obstetrics, Gynecology, and Reproductive Biology* 111, no. 2 (December 10, 2003): 164–66.

16. Christine MacDonald, Sheena B. Pinion, and Una M. MacLeod, "Scottish Female Obstetricians' Views on Elective Caesarean Section and Personal Choice for Delivery," *Journal of Obstetrics and Gynaecology: The Journal of the Institute of Obstetrics and Gynaecology* 22, no. 6 (November 2002): 586–89.

17. Wax et al., "Patient Choice Cesarean: The Maine Experience."

18. Joseph R. Wax et al., "Patient Choice Cesarean: An Evidence-Based Review," *Obstetrical and Gynecological Survey* 59, no. 8 (August 2004): 601–16.

19. Barbara A. Bettes et al., "Cesarean Delivery on Maternal Request: Obstetrician-Gynecologists' Knowledge, Perception, and Practice Patterns," *Obstetrics and Gynecology* 109, no. 1 (January 2007): 57–66.

20. American College of Obstetricians and Gynecologists Office of Communications, "Gallup Survey Reveals Women Ob-Gyns Benefit from 'Insider Knowledge,'" news release, December 9, 2003, http://www.acog.org/from_home/publications/press_releases/nr12-09-03-2.cfm (accessed February 24, 2011).

21. C. S. Cotzias, S. Paterson-Brown, and N. M. Fisk, "Obstetricians Say Yes to Maternal Request for Elective Caesarean Section: A Survey of Current Opinion," *European Journal of Obstetrics, Gynecology, and Reproductive Biology* 97, no. 1 (July 2001): 15–16; M Habiba et al., "Caesarean Section on Request: A Comparison of Obstetricians' Attitudes in Eight European Countries," *BJOG: An International Journal of Obstetrics and Gynaecology* 113, no. 6 (June 2006): 647–56; Anneke Kwee et al., "Caesarean Section on Request: A Survey in the Netherlands," *European Journal of Obstetrics, Gynecology, and Reproductive Biology* 113, no. 2 (April 15, 2004): 186–90; Patricia Faas-Fehervary et al., "Caesarean Section on Demand: Influence of Personal Birth Experience and Working Environment on Attitude of German Gynaecologists," *European Journal of Obstetrics, Gynecology, and Reproductive Biology* 122, no. 2 (October 1, 2005): 162–66; Land et al., "Personal Preferences of Obstetricians"; R. Gonen, A. Tamir, and S. Degani, "Obstetricians' Opinions regarding Patient Choice in Cesarean Delivery," *Obstetrics and Gynecology* 99, no. 4 (April 2002): 577–80.

22. Alfredo Mancuso, Antonio De Vivo, and Giusi Fanara, "Cesarean Section on Demand: Are There Differences Related to Obstetricians' Gender?" *Journal of Maternal-Fetal and Neonatal Medicine* 19, no. 5 (May 2006): 309–10; Chiara Ghetti, Benjamin K. S. Chan, and Jeanne-Marie Guise, "Physicians' Responses to Patient-Requested Cesarean Delivery," *Birth* 31, no. 4 (December 2004): 280–84.

23. Dorthe Fuglenes, Pål Oian, and Ivar Sønbø Kristiansen, "Obstetricians' Choice of Cesarean Delivery in Ambiguous Cases: Is It Influenced by Risk Attitude or Fear of Complaints and Litigation?" *American Journal of Obstetrics and Gynecology* 200, no. 1 (January 2009): 48.1–8.

24. Birgit Reime et al., "Do Maternity Care Provider Groups Have Different Attitudes towards Birth?" *BJOG: An International Journal of Obstetrics and Gynaecology* 111, no. 12 (December 2004): 1388–93.

25. C. E. Turner et al., "Vaginal Delivery Compared with Elective Caesarean Section: The Views of Pregnant Women and Clinicians," *BJOG: An International Journal of Obstetrics and Gynaecology* 115, no. 12 (November 2008): 1494–502.

26. Jennifer M. Wu, Andrew F. Hundley, and Anthony G. Visco, "Elective Primary Cesarean Delivery: Attitudes of Urogynecology and Maternal-Fetal Medicine Specialists," *Obstetrics and Gynecology* 105, no. 2 (February 2005): 301–306.

27. Parliament of Australia: Senate Community Affairs References Committee, *Rocking the Cradle: A Report into Childbirth Procedures* (Canberra: Senate Printing House, 1999), http://wopared.parl.net/senate/committee/clac_ctte/completed_inquiries/1999 -02/child_birth/report/index.htm (accessed February 24, 2011).

CHAPTER 6. PROTECTING YOUR PELVIC FLOOR

1. Asa Leijonhufvud et al., "Risks of Stress Urinary Incontinence and Pelvic Organ Prolapse Surgery in Relation to Mode of Childbirth," *American Journal of Obstetrics and Gynecology* 204, no. 1 (January 2011): 70.e1–7.

2. Arthur Block, *The Complete Murphy's Law* (London: Arrow Books, 1990), p. 126.

3. R. Al-Mufti, A. McCarthy, and N. M. Fisk, "Survey of Obstetricians' Personal Preference and Discretionary Practice," *European Journal of Obstetrics, Gynecology, and Reproductive Biology* 73, no. 1 (May 1997): 1–4; C. S. Cotzias, S. Paterson-Brown, and N. M. Fisk, "Obstetricians Say Yes to Maternal Request for Elective Caesarean Section: A Survey of Current Opinion," *European Journal of Obstetrics, Gynecology, and Reproductive Biology* 97, no. 1 (July 2001): 15–16; P. McGurgan, S. Coulter-Smith, and P. J. O'Donovan, "A National Confidential Survey of Obstetricians' Personal Preferences regarding Mode of Delivery," *European Journal of Obstetrics, Gynecology, and Reproductive Biology* 97, no. 1 (July 2001): 17–19.

4. "Women's Comments," Birth Trauma Canada, http://birthtraumacanada .org/6.html (accessed October 15, 2010).

5. Leigh East, *Caesarean Birth: A Positive Approach to Preparation and Recovery* (West Yorkshire: Tiskimo, 2011).

6. Ethicon Women's Health and Urology, "Survey Women about Pelvic Organ Prolapse and Most Say 'Who Knew?'" news release, April 30, 2007, http:// www.icrsurvey.com/Study.aspx?f=Ethicon_043007.htm (accessed December 9, 2010).

7. Helena Talasz et al., "Breathing with the Pelvic Floor? Correlation of Pelvic Floor Muscle Function and Expiratory Flows in Healthy Young Nulliparous Women," *International Urogynecology Journal and Pelvic Floor Dysfunction* 21, no. 4 (April 2010): 475–81.

8. Jane Elliott, "'My Natural Birth Wrecked My Body,'" BBC News Online, June 24, 2010, http://www.bbc.co.uk/news/10379831 (accessed February 24, 2011).

9. Hans Peter Dietz, Alec V. L. Gillespie, and Pramod Phadke, "Avulsion of the Pubovisceral Muscle Associated with Large Vaginal Tear after Normal Vaginal Delivery at Term," *Australian and New Zealand Journal of Obstetrics and Gynaecology* 47, no. 4 (August 2007): 341–44; Ka Lai Shek and Hans Peter Dietz, "Can Levator Avulsion Be Predicted Antenatally?" *American Journal of Obstetrics and Gynecology* 202, no. 6 (January 15, 2010): 586; Hans Peter Dietz and Valeria Lanzarone, "Levator Trauma after Vaginal Delivery," *Obstetrics and Gynecology* 106, no. 4 (October 2005): 707–12; Ladislav Krofta et al., "Pubococcygeus-Puborectalis Trauma after Forceps Delivery: Evaluation of the Levator Ani Muscle with 3D/4D Ultrasound," *International Urogynecology Journal and Pelvic Floor Dysfunction* 20, no. 10 (October 2009): 1175–81; Zeelha Abdool, Ka Lai Shek, and Hans Peter Dietz, "The Effect of Levator Avulsion on Hiatal Dimension and Function," *American Journal of Obstetrics and Gynecology* 201, no. 1 (July 2009): 89.e1–5; Virginia Branham et al., "Levator Ani Abnormality 6 Weeks after Delivery Persists at 6 Months," *American Journal of Obstetrics and Gynecology* 197, no. 1 (July 2007): 65.1–6.

10. John O. L. DeLancey et al., "Comparison of Levator Ani Muscle Defects and Function in Women with and without Pelvic Organ Prolapse," *Obstetrics and Gynecology* 109, no. 2 (February 2007): 295–302.

11. Ka Lai Shek and Hans Peter Dietz, "The Effect of Childbirth on Hiatal Dimensions," *Obstetrics and Gynecology* 113, no. 6 (June 2009): 1272–78.

12. Philip Toozs-Hobson et al., "The Effect of Mode of Delivery on Pelvic Floor Functional Anatomy," *International Urogynecology Journal and Pelvic Floor Dysfunction* 19, no. 3 (March 2008): 407–16; Jacobus Wijma et al., "Displacement and Recovery of the Vesical Neck Position during Pregnancy and after Childbirth," *Neurourology and Urodynamics* 26, no. 3 (2007): 372–76; J. P. Sartori et al., "Bladder Neck Mobility and Functional Evaluation of the Pelvic Floor in Primiparae according to the Type of Delivery," *Clinical and Experimental Obstetrics & Gynecology* 31, no. 2 (2004): 120–22.

13. Sebastien Novellas et al., "MR Features of the Levator Ani Muscle in the Immediate Postpartum following Cesarean Delivery," *International Urogynecology Journal and Pelvic Floor Dysfunction* 21, no. 5 (May 2010): 563–68.

14. Eva Reisinger and Wolfgang Stummvoll, "Visualization of the Endopelvic Fascia by Transrectal Three-Dimensional Ultrasound," *International Urogynecology Journal and Pelvic Floor Dysfunction* 17, no. 2 (February 2006): 165–69.

15. Dietz, Gillespie, and Phadke, "Avulsion of the Pubovisceral Muscle," pp. 341–44.

16. John O. L. Delancey, Norman F. Miller, and Mitchell B. Berger, "Surgical Approaches to Postobstetrical Perineal Body Defects (Rectovaginal Fistula and Chronic Third and Fourth-Degree Lacerations)," *Clinical Obstetrics and Gynecology* 53, no. 1 (March 2010): 134–44.

17. Omar Felipe Dueñas-García et al., "Bladder Rupture Caused by Post-partum Urinary Retention," *Obstetrics and Gynecology* 112, no. 2 (August 2008): 481–82; Roderick Teo et al., "Clinically Overt Postpartum Urinary Retention after Vaginal Delivery: A Retrospective Case-Control Study," *International Urogynecology Journal and Pelvic Floor Dysfunction* 18, no. 5 (May 2007): 521–24; Jörg Humburg, "Postpartum Urinary Retention—without Clinical Impact?" [in German], *Therapeutische Umschau* 65, no. 11 (November 2008): 681–85; W. J. Watson, "Prolonged Postpartum Urinary Retention," *Military Medicine* 156, no. 9 (September 1991): 502–503; Jörg Humburg et al., "Risk Factors in Prolonged Postpartum Urinary Retention: An Analysis of Six Cases," *Archives of Gynecology and Obstetrics* 283, no. 2 (December 19, 2009): 179–83.

18. Lior Lowenstein et al., "Can Stronger Pelvic Muscle Floor Improve Sexual Function?" *International Urogynecology Journal and Pelvic Floor Dysfunction* 21, no. 5 (May 2010): 553–56; Nevin Citak et al., "Postpartum Sexual Function of Women and the Effects of Early Pelvic Floor Muscle Exercises," *Acta Obstetricia et Gynecologica Scandinavica* 89, no. 6 (June 2010): 817–22.

19. Lowenstein et al., "Can Stronger Pelvic Muscle Floor?"; Megan O. Schimpf et al., "Does Vaginal Size Impact Sexual Activity and Function?" *International Urogynecology Journal and Pelvic Floor Dysfunction* 21, no. 4 (April 2010): 447–52.

20. DeLancey et al., "Comparison of Levator Ani."

21. Hans Peter Dietz and Lore Schierlitz, "Pelvic Floor Trauma in Childbirth: Myth or Reality?" *Australian and New Zealand Journal of Obstetrics and Gynaecology* 45, no. 1 (February 2005): 3–11.

22. James A. Ashton-Miller and John O. L. Delancey, "On the Biomechanics of Vaginal Birth and Common Sequelae," *Annual Review of Biomedical Engineering* 11 (2009): 163–76.

23. Hans Peter Dietz and Judy M. Simpson, "Does Delayed Child-Bearing Increase the Risk of Levator Injury in Labour?" *Australian and New Zealand Journal of Obstetrics and Gynaecology* 47, no. 6 (December 2007): 491–95.

24. S. Hunskaar et al., "The Prevalence of Urinary Incontinence in Women in Four European Countries," *BJU International* 93, no. 3 (February 2004): 324–30; Kim N. Danforth et al., "Risk Factors for Urinary Incontinence among Middle-Aged Women," *American Journal of Obstetrics and Gynecology* 194, no. 2 (February 2006): 339–45.

25. Maite Solans-Domènech, Emília Sánchez, and Montserrat Espuña-Pons, "Urinary and Anal Incontinence during Pregnancy and Postpartum: Incidence, Severity, and Risk Factors," *Obstetrics and Gynecology* 115, no. 3 (March 2010): 618–28.

26. S. A. Farrell, V. M. Allen, and T. F. Baskett, "Parturition and Urinary

Incontinence in Primiparas," *Obstetrics and Gynecology* 97, no. 3 (March 2001): 350–56.

27. Guri Rortveit et al., "Urinary Incontinence after Vaginal Delivery or Cesarean Section," *New England Journal of Medicine* 348, no. 10 (March 6, 2003): 900–907; Brian M. Casey et al., "Obstetric Antecedents for Postpartum Pelvic Floor Dysfunction," *American Journal of Obstetrics and Gynecology* 192, no. 5 (May 2005): 1655–62; Roger P. Goldberg et al., "Delivery Mode Is a Major Environmental Determinant of Stress Urinary Incontinence: Results of the Evanston-Northwestern Twin Sisters Study," *American Journal of Obstetrics and Gynecology* 193, no. 6 (December 2005): 2149–53.

28. Irene Diez-Itza et al., "Factors Involved in Stress Urinary Incontinence 1 Year after First Delivery," *International Urogynecology Journal and Pelvic Floor Dysfunction* 21, no. 4 (April 2010): 439–45.

29. S. J. Snooks et al., "Effect of Vaginal Delivery on the Pelvic Floor: A 5-Year Follow-Up," *British Journal of Surgery* 77, no. 12 (December 1990): 1358–60.

30. Sarah Hamilton Boyles et al., "Effect of Mode of Delivery on the Incidence of Urinary Incontinence in Primiparous Women," *Obstetrics and Gynecology* 113, no. 1 (January 2009): 134–41.

31. Hans Peter Dietz, "Levator Function before and after Childbirth," *Australian and New Zealand Journal of Obstetrics and Gynaecology* 44, no. 1 (February 2004): 19–23.

32. Esther M. J. Bols et al., "A Systematic Review of Etiological Factors for Postpartum Fecal Incontinence," *Acta Obstetricia et Gynecologica Scandinavica* 89, no. 3 (March 2010): 302–14.

33. Sari Räisänen et al., "The Increased Incidence of Obstetric Anal Sphincter Rupture: An Emerging Trend in Finland," *Preventive Medicine* 49, no. 6 (December 2009): 535–40.

34. Rainbow Y. T. Tin et al., "The Prevalence of Anal Incontinence in Post-Partum Women following Obstetrical Anal Sphincter Injury," *International Urogynecology Journal and Pelvic Floor Dysfunction* 21, no. 8 (April 27, 2010): 927–32.

35. Solans-Domènech, Sánchez, and Espuña-Pons, "Urinary and Anal Incontinence."

36. Victoria L. Handa et al., "Pelvic Organ Support among Primiparous Women in the First Year after Childbirth," *International Urogynecology Journal and Pelvic Floor Dysfunction* 20, no. 12 (December 2009): 1407–11.

37. Lieschen H. Quiroz et al., "Vaginal Parity and Pelvic Organ Prolapse," *Journal of Reproductive Medicine* 55, no. 3 (April 2010): 93–98; Christina Larsson, Karin Källen, and Ellika Andolf, "Cesarean Section and Risk of Pelvic Organ Prolapse: A Nested Case-Control Study," *American Journal of Obstetrics and Gynecology* 200, no. 3 (March 2009): 243.1–4.

38. S. E. Swift, T. Pound, and J. K. Dias, "Case-Control Study of Etiologic Factors in the Development of Severe Pelvic Organ Prolapse," *International Urogynecology Journal and Pelvic Floor Dysfunction* 12, no. 3 (2001): 187–92; Gunilla Tegerstedt et al., "Obstetric Risk Factors for Symptomatic Prolapse: A Population-Based Approach," *American Journal of Obstetrics and Gynecology* 194, no. 1 (January 2006): 75–81.

39. René Genadry, "A Urogynecologist's View of the Pelvic Floor Effects of Vaginal Delivery/Cesarean Section for the Urologist," *Current Urology Reports* 7, no. 5 (September 2006): 376–83; Hui Q. Pan et al., "Dual Simulated Childbirth Injury Delays Anatomic Recovery," *American Journal of Physiology: Renal Physiology* 296, no. 2 (February 2009): 277–83; Kuo-Cheng Lien et al., "Pudendal Nerve Stretch during Vaginal Birth: A 3D Computer Simulation," *American Journal of Obstetrics and Gynecology* 192, no. 5 (May 2005): 1669–76; T. Tetzschner et al., "Pudendal Nerve Function during Pregnancy and after Delivery," *International Urogynecology Journal and Pelvic Floor Dysfunction* 8, no. 2 (1997): 66–68; T. Tetzschner et al., "Delivery and Pudendal Nerve Function," *Acta Obstetricia et Gynecologica Scandinavica* 76, no. 4 (April 1997): 324–31.

40. Jennifer H. Johnson et al., "Immediate Maternal and Neonatal Effects of Forceps and Vacuum-Assisted Deliveries," *Obstetrics and Gynecology* 103, no. 3 (March 2004): 513–18.

41. Lucia M. Dolan and Paul Hilton, "Obstetric Risk Factors and Pelvic Floor Dysfunction 20 Years after First Delivery," *International Urogynecology Journal and Pelvic Floor Dysfunction* 21, no. 5 (May 2010): 535–44.

42. "Example NNTs: Obstetrics-Gynecology," Centre for Evidence-Based Medicine: Obstetrics-Gynecology, KT Clearinghouse, http://ktclearinghouse.ca/cebm/glossary/nnt/obgyn (accessed December 10, 2010).

43. Emily S. Lukacz et al., "Parity, Mode of Delivery, and Pelvic Floor Disorders," *Obstetrics and Gynecology* 107, no. 6 (June 2006): 1253–60.

CHAPTER 8. WORLDWIDE CESAREAN RATES, ATTITUDES, AND EXPERIENCES

Note: A small number of studies referred to in this chapter, which were originally presented in a foreign language, have been used with the authors' knowledge of their English (translated) abstract only.

1. Lucy Atkins, "'I Was So Completely Traumatised by the Fact that I Hadn't Given Birth,'" *Guardian*, March 23, 2004, http://www.guardian.co.uk/society2004/mar/23/health.lifeandhealth (accessed October 06, 2011).

2. "Appropriate Technology for Birth," *Lancet* 2, no. 8452 (August 24, 1985): 436–37.

3. Margaret C. Hogan et al., "Maternal Mortality for 181 Countries, 1980–2008: A Systematic Analysis of Progress towards Millennium Development Goal 5," *Lancet* 375, no. 9726 (May 8, 2010): 1609–23.

4. J. M. Belizán et al., "Rates and Implications of Caesarean Sections in Latin America: Ecological Study," *British Medical Journal (Clinical Research Ed.)* 319, no. 7222 (November 27, 1999): 1397–1400; Ana P. Betrán et al., "Rates of Caesarean Section: Analysis of Global, Regional, and National Estimates," *Paediatric and Perinatal Epidemiology* 21, no. 2 (March 2007): 98–113.

5. Department of Making Pregnancy Safer, "Egypt Country Profile," *Making Pregnancy Safer*, World Health Organization, 2008, http://www.who.int/making_pregnancy_safer/publications/en/ (accessed February 24, 2011).

6. Ana P. Betrán et al., "WHO Global Survey on Maternal and Perinatal Health in Latin America: Classifying Caesarean Sections," *Reproductive Health* 6 (2009): 18.

7. Mikkel Zahle Oestergaard et al., "Neonatal Mortality Levels for 193 Countries in 2009 with Trends since 1990: A Systematic Analysis of Progress, Projections, and Priorities," *PLoS Medicine* 8, no. 8 (August 2011): 1001080.

8. Ronald M. Cyr, "Myth of the Ideal Cesarean Section Rate: Commentary and Historic Perspective," *American Journal of Obstetrics and Gynecology* 194, no. 4 (April 2006): 932–36; Hans Peter Dietz and Michael J. Peek, "Will There Ever Be an End to the Caesarean Section Rate Debate?" *Australian and New Zealand Journal of Obstetrics and Gynaecology* 44, no. 2 (April 2004): 103–106; P. Rozenberg, "Evaluation of Cesarean Rate: A Necessary Progress in Modern Obstetrics" [in French], *Journal de Gynécologie, Obstétrique, et Biologie de la Reproduction* 33, no. 4 (June 2004): 279–89; M. S. Robson, "Can We Reduce the Caesarean Section Rate?" *Best Practice and Research: Clinical Obstetrics and Gynaecology* 15, no. 1 (February 2001): 179–94.

9. "NIH State-of-the-Science Conference Statement on Cesarean Delivery on Maternal Request," *National Institutes of Health Consensus and State-of-the-Science Statements* 23, no. 1 (March 27, 2006): 1–29.

10. Coalition for Childbirth Autonomy, "Birth Group, CCA, Calls on WHO to Re-Examine 'Outdated and Unsafe' 10–15% Recommended Cesarean Rate," news release, October 28, 2008, http://www.mmdnewswire.com/birth-group-cca-calls-on-who-to-re-examine-outdated-and-unsafe-10-15-recommended-cesarean-rate-4073.html (accessed January 16, 2011).

11. World Health Organization et al., *Monitoring Emergency Obstetric Care: A Handbook* (Geneva: WHO, 2009), http://www.who.int/reproductivehealth/publications/monitoring/9789241547734/en/index.html (accessed January 16, 2011).

12. Kitty Holland, "Caesarean Section: A Life-Saving Option," *Irish Times*, October 10, 2009, http://www.irishtimes.com/newspaper/health/2009/1006/1224 255974379.html (accessed January 16, 2011).

13. Coalition for Childbirth Autonomy, "WHO Admits: There Is No Evidence for Recommending a 10–15% Caesarean Limit," *Medical News Today*, October 29, 2009, http://www.medicalnewstoday.com/articles/169058.php (accessed February 24, 2011).

14. Ben C. P. Chan and Terence T. H. Lao, "The Impact of Maternal Height on Intrapartum Operative Delivery: A Reappraisal," *Journal of Obstetrics and Gynaecology Research* 35, no. 2 (April 2009): 307–14.

15. Nadav Schwartz et al., "Predictors of Severe Perineal Lacerations in Chinese Women," *Journal of Perinatal Medicine* 37, no. 2 (2009): 109–13.

16. T. Y. Leung et al., "Trends in Maternal Obesity and Associated Risks of Adverse Pregnancy Outcomes in a Population of Chinese Women," *BJOG: An International Journal of Obstetrics and Gynaecology* 115, no. 12 (November 2008): 1529–37.

17. Chung-Hey Chen and Shing-Yaw Wang, "Psychosocial Outcomes of Vaginal and Cesarean Births in Taiwanese Primiparas," *Research in Nursing & Health* 25, no. 6 (December 2002): 452–58.

18. Man Wah Pang et al., "Impact of First Childbirth on Changes in Women's Preference for Mode of Delivery: Follow-Up of a Longitudinal Observational Study," *Birth* 35, no. 2 (June 2008): 121–28.

19. W. W. Cai et al., "Increased Cesarean Section Rates and Emerging Patterns of Health Insurance in Shanghai, China," *American Journal of Public Health* 88, no. 5 (May 1998): 777–80.

20. Jonathan Watts, "Chinese Hospital Staff Face Attacks amid High Prices and Dubious Care," *Guardian*, May 12, 2007, http://www.guardian.co.uk/world/2007/may/12/china.jonathanwatts1 (accessed February 24, 2011).

21. Juan Liang et al., "Maternal Mortality in China, 1996–2005," *International Journal of Gynaecology and Obstetrics: The Official Organ of the International Federation of Gynaecology and Obstetrics* 110, no. 2 (May 12, 2010): 93–96.

22. Hong Qi et al., "Clinical Analysis of Maternal and Neonatal Outcomes in Uncomplicated Term Nulliparous after Different Routes of Delivery" [in Chinese], *Zhonghua Fu Chan Ke Za Zhi* 42, no. 12 (December 2007): 818–21.

23. Shi Wu Wen et al., "Determinants of Intrapartum Fetal Death in a Remote and Indigent Population in China," *Journal of Perinatology: Official Journal of the California Perinatal Association* 24, no. 2 (February 2004): 77–81.

24. W. C. Leung et al., "Unexpected Reduction in the Incidence of Birth Trauma and Birth Asphyxia Related to Instrumental Deliveries during the Study Period: Was This the Hawthorne Effect?" *BJOG: An International Journal of Obstet-*

rics and Gynaecology 110, no. 3 (March 2003): 319–22; W. C. Leung et al., "Continued Reduction in the Incidence of Birth Trauma and Birth Asphyxia Related to Instrumental Deliveries after the Study Period: Was This the Hawthorne Effect?" *European Journal of Obstetrics, Gynecology, and Reproductive Biology* 130, no. 2 (February 2007): 165–68.

25. Howard L. Minkoff and Richard Berkowitz, "The Myth of the Precious Baby," *Obstetrics and Gynecology* 106, no. 3 (September 2005): 607–609.

26. H. T. Li et al., "Caesarean Delivery on Maternal Request and Childhood Psychopathology: A Retrospective Cohort Study in China," *BJOG: An International Journal of Obstetrics and Gynaecology* 118, no. 1 (January 2011): 42–48.

27. Sufang Guo et al., "Delivery Settings and Caesarean Section Rates in China," *Bulletin of the World Health Organization* 85, no. 10 (October 2007): 755–62; Shu-yun Gao et al., "A Questionnaire Investigation on the Way of Delivery and Its Related Factors in 415 Women at Child Bearing Age in One Hospital" [in Chinese], *Zhonghua Liu Xing Bing Xue Za Zhi* 25, no. 9 (September 2004): 799–801; Herng-Ching Lin and Sudha Xirasagar, "Maternal Age and the Likelihood of a Maternal Request for Cesarean Delivery: A 5-Year Population-Based Study," *American Journal of Obstetrics and Gynecology* 192, no. 3 (March 2005): 848–55.

28. L. Y. Lee, E. Holroyd, and C. Y. Ng, "Exploring Factors Influencing Chinese Women's Decision to Have Elective Caesarean Surgery," *Midwifery* 17, no. 4 (December 2001): 314–22; Selina M. W. Pang et al., "Determinants of Preference for Elective Caesarean Section in Hong Kong Chinese Pregnant Women," *Hong Kong Medical Journal* 13, no. 2 (April 2007): 100–105; Guo et al., "Delivery Settings and Caesarean Section"; H. Guo, X. Zhou, and S. Li, "Analysis of Social Factors of Pregnant Women's Cesarean Section Demands" [in Chinese], *Zhonghua Yi Xue Za Zhi* 80, no. 9 (September 2000): 675–77.

29. Guo et al., "Delivery Settings and Caesarean Section."

30. Bin Wang et al., "National Survey on Midwifery Practice in Health Facilities in China" [in Chinese], *Zhonghua Fu Chan Ke Za Zhi* 42, no. 5 (May 2007): 305–308.

31. Ngai Fen Cheung, "Chinese Midwifery: The History and Modernity," *Midwifery* 25, no. 3 (June 2009): 228–41.

32. G. M. Leung et al., "Rates of Cesarean Births in Hong Kong: 1987–1999," *Birth* 28, no. 3 (September 2001): 166–72.

33. Wei-Hsing Liang et al., "Effect of Peer Review and Trial of Labor on Lowering Cesarean Section Rates," *Journal of the Chinese Medical Association: JCMA* 67, no. 6 (June 2004): 281–86.

34. Pisake Lumbiganon et al., "Method of Delivery and Pregnancy Outcomes in Asia: The WHO Global Survey on Maternal and Perinatal Health 2007–08," *Lancet* 375, no. 9713 (February 6, 2010): 490–99.

35. Esther Rosenberg, "Dutch Baby Death Rate Needs Improving," *NRC Handelsblad*, December 11, 2008, http://www.nrc.nl/international/Features/article2089864.ece/Dutch_baby_death_rate_needs_improving%5D (accessed February 24, 2011).

36. Therese A. Wiegers, "The Quality of Maternity Care Services as Experienced by Women in the Netherlands," *BMC Pregnancy and Childbirth* 9 (2009): 18.

37. Meagan Zimbeck, Ashna Mohangoo, and Jennifer Zeitlin, "The European Perinatal Health Report: Delivering Comparable Data for Examining Differences in Maternal and Infant Health," *European Journal of Obstetrics, Gynecology, and Reproductive Biology* 146, no. 2 (October 2009): 149–51.

38. Marc J. N. C. Keirse, "Perinatal Mortality in the Netherlands," *British Medical Journal (Clinical Research Ed.)* 338 (2009): b1491; A. D. Mohangoo et al., "Higher Perinatal Mortality in the Netherlands than in Other European Countries: The Peristat-II Study" [in Dutch], *Nederlands Tijdschrift Voor Geneeskunde* 152, no. 50 (December 13, 2008): 2718–27.

39. Annemieke C. C. Evers et al., "Mortality and Morbidity among Full-Term Neonates in a Neonatal Intensive Care Unit in the Utrecht Region, the Netherlands" [in Dutch], *Nederlands Tijdschrift Voor Geneeskunde* 154 (2010): 118.

40. L. Mascarenhas et al., "Dutch Model of Maternity Care: Dutch Model Limits Choice," *British Medical Journal (Clinical Research Ed.)* 308, no. 6924 (January 29, 1994): 342.

41. M. Eskes, D. van Alten, and P. E. Treffers, "The Wormerveer Study: Perinatal Mortality and Non-Optimal Management in a Practice of Independent Midwives," *European Journal of Obstetrics, Gynecology, and Reproductive Biology* 51, no. 2 (October 1993): 91–95.

42. Tony Sheldon, "Prompt Access to Expert Care Is among Advice to Reduce Perinatal Deaths in Netherlands," *British Medical Journal (Clinical Research Ed.)* 340 (January 15, 2010): 277; J. M. W. M. Merkus, "Obstetric Care in the Netherlands under Assessment Again" [in Dutch], *Nederlands Tijdschrift Voor Geneeskunde* 152, no. 50 (December 13, 2008): 2707–2708.

43. Wendy Christiaens, Anneleen Gouwy, and Piet Bracke, "Does a Referral from Home to Hospital Affect Satisfaction with Childbirth? A Cross-National Comparison," *BMC Health Services Research* 7 (2007): 109.

44. Annemieke C. C. Evers et al., "Perinatal Mortality and Severe Morbidity in Low and High Risk Term Pregnancies in the Netherlands: Prospective Cohort Study," *British Medical Journal* 341, no. 5639 (November 2, 2010), http://www.bmj.com/content/341/bmj.c5639.full (accessed October 11, 2011).

45. Min Su et al., "Planned Caesarean Section Decreases the Risk of Adverse Perinatal Outcome due to Both Labour and Delivery Complications in the Term Breech Trial," *BJOG: An International Journal of Obstetrics and Gynaecology* 111, no. 10 (October 2004): 1065–74.

46. Christine C. Rietberg, Patty M. Elferink-Stinkens, and Gerard H. A. Visser, "The Effect of the Term Breech Trial on Medical Intervention Behaviour and Neonatal Outcome in the Netherlands: An Analysis of 35,453 Term Breech Infants," *BJOG: An International Journal of Obstetrics and Gynaecology* 112, no. 2 (February 2005): 205–209; Joke M. Schutte et al., "Maternal Deaths after Elective Cesarean Section for Breech Presentation in the Netherlands," *Acta Obstetricia et Gynecologica Scandinavica* 86, no. 2 (2007): 240–43.

47. Freke A. Wilmink et al., "Neonatal Outcome following Elective Cesarean Section beyond 37 Weeks of Gestation: A 7-Year Retrospective Analysis of a National Registry," *American Journal of Obstetrics and Gynecology* 202, no. 3 (March 2010): 250.1–8.

48. Anneke Kwee et al., "Caesarean Section on Request: A Survey in the Netherlands," *European Journal of Obstetrics, Gynecology, and Reproductive Biology* 113, no. 2 (April 15, 2004): 186–90.

49. J. G. Nijhuis, "A Request for Caesarean Section without a Medical Indication Should Ultimately Be Granted" [in Dutch], *Nederlands Tijdschrift Voor Geneeskunde* 150, no. 14 (April 8, 2006): 788.

50. Leonie A. M. van der Hulst et al., "Dutch Women's Decision-Making in Pregnancy and Labour as Seen through the Eyes of Their Midwives," *Midwifery* 23, no. 3 (September 2007): 279–86.

51. Annika Karlström et al., "Cesarean Section without Medical Reason, 1997 to 2006: A Swedish Register Study," *Birth* 37, no. 1 (March 2010): 11–20.

52. Brady E. Hamilton, Joyce A. Martin, and Stephanie J. Ventura, "Births: Preliminary Data for 2008," *NVSS National Vital Statistics Reports* 58, no. 16 (April 2010); Joyce A. Martin et al., "Births: Final Data for 2008," *National Vital Statistics Reports* 59, no. 1 (December 2010).

53. US Department of Health and Human Services, *Healthy People 2010* (Washington, DC: US Government Printing Office, 2000), http://www.healthy people.gov/2010/Publications/ (accessed February 24, 2011).

54. Laura, "Introducing: 20% by 2020," *Born in Sarasota* (blog), April 30, 2010, http://borninsarasota.blogspot.com/2010/04/introducing-20-by-2020.html. (accessed February 24, 2011).

55. "Worst to First 2010," New Jersey Maternity Care, http://www.nj maternitycare.com/new_jersey_hospitals (accessed February 24, 2011).

56. HealthGrades, "Birth Complication Rates Vary Widely by Hospital," news release, June 30, 2010, http://www.healthgrades.com/business/news/press-releases/maternity-care-2010-carol.aspx (accessed February 9, 2011).

57. HealthGrades, "First-Time Preplanned 'Patient Choice' Cesarean Section Rates in the United States," HealthGrades, July 21, 2003, http://www.health grades.com/media/english/pdf/Patient_Choice_Csection_Study_July_2003.pdf

(accessed February 24, 2011); HealthGrades, "'Patient-Choice' C-Section Rate Rises 36%," news release, September 12, 2005, http://www.healthgrades.com/media/DMS/pdf/PatientChoiceStudy2005PressReleaseSept12.pdf (accessed February 24, 2011).

58. Barbara A. Bettes et al., "Cesarean Delivery on Maternal Request: Obstetrician-Gynecologists' Knowledge, Perception, and Practice Patterns," *Obstetrics and Gynecology* 109, no. 1 (January 2007): 57–66.

59. "NIH State-of-the-Science Conference Statement on Cesarean Delivery on Maternal Request," *National Institutes of Health Consensus and State-of-the-Science Statements* 23, no. 1 (March 27, 2006): 1–29.

60. J. Q. Xu et al., "Deaths: Final Data for 2007 (Leading Causes of Death)," *National Center for Health Statistics* 58, no. 19 (May 20, 2010), http://www.cdc.gov/nchs/products/nvsr.htm (accessed December 27, 2010).

61. Gopal K. Singh and Michael D. Kogan, "Persistent Socioeconomic Disparities in Infant, Neonatal, and Postneonatal Mortality Rates in the United States, 1969–2001," *Pediatrics* 119, no. 4 (April 2007): 928–39.

62. National Center for Health Statistics, "VitalStats: Perinatal Mortality," Centers for Disease Control and Prevention, http://www.cdc.gov/nchs/vitalstats.htm (accessed December 27, 2010).

63. Marian F. MacDorman and Sharon Kirmeyer, "Fetal and Perinatal Mortality, United States, 2005," *National Vital Statistics Reports* 57, no. 8 (January 28, 2009): 1–19; Marian F. MacDorman and Sharon Kirmeyer, "The Challenge of Fetal Mortality," *NCHS Data Brief* 16 (April 2009): 1–8.

64. Marian F. MacDorman and T. J. Mathews, "Behind International Rankings of Infant Mortality: How the United States Compares with Europe," *NCHS Data Brief* 23 (November 2009): 1–8.

65. Maternal and Child Health Bureau, "Child Health USA 2010: Maternal Mortality," US Department of Health and Human Services, Health Resources and Services Administration, 2010, http://www.mchb.hrsa.gov/chusa10/hstat/hsi/pages/205mm.html (accessed February 19, 2011).

66. Nathanael Johnson, "More Women Dying from Pregnancy Complications; State Holds on to Report," *California Watch*, February 2, 2010, http://californiawatch.org/health-and-welfare/more-women-dying-pregnancy-complications-state-holds-report (accessed February 24, 2011).

67. M. Lydon-Rochelle et al., "Cesarean Delivery and Postpartum Mortality among Primiparas in Washington State, 1987–1996(1)," *Obstetrics and Gynecology* 97, no. 2 (February 2001): 169–74.

68. Ina May Gaskin, "Maternal Death in the United States: A Problem Solved or a Problem Ignored?" *Journal of Perinatal Education* 17, no. 2 (2008): 9–13.

69. Roch Cantwell et al., "Saving Mothers' Lives: Reviewing Maternal

Deaths to Make Motherhood Safer: 2006–2008. The Eighth Report of the Confidential Enquiries into Maternal Deaths in the United Kingdom," *BJOG: An International Journal of Obstetrics and Gynaecology* 118, suppl. 1 (March 2011): 1–203.

70. G. Lewis, ed., "Saving Mothers' Lives: Reviewing Maternal Deaths to Make Motherhood Safer 2003–2005." The Confidential Enquiry into Maternal and Child Health (CEMACH)." The Seventh Report on Confidential Enquiries into Maternal Deaths in the United Kingdom (London: CEMACH).

71. Gwyneth Lewis, ed., "Why Mothers Die 2000–2002." The Sixth Report of the Confidential Enquiries into Maternal Deaths in the United Kingdom (London: CEMACH [RCOG]).

72. Anemona Hartocollis, "High Rate for Deaths of Pregnant Women in New York State," *New York Times*, June 18, 2010, http://www.nytimes.com/2010/06/19/nyregion/19obese.html (accessed February 24, 2011).

73. Confidential Enquiry into Maternal and Child Health, "Saving Mothers' Lives: Findings on the Causes of Maternal Deaths and the Care of Pregnant Women," news release, December 4, 2007, http://www.rcog.org.uk/news/cemach-release-saving-mothers-lives-findings-causes-maternal-deaths-and-care-pregnant-women (accessed February 24, 2011).

74. American College of Obstetricians and Gynecologists Office of Communications, "ACOG Issues Guidance to Ob-Gyns on Impact of Obesity during Pregnancy," news release, August 31, 2005, http://www.acog.org/from_home/publications/press_releases/nr08-31-05-2.cfm (accessed February 24, 2011).

75. Xu et al., "Deaths: Final Data."

76. Maternal and Child Health Bureau, *Women's Health USA 2009*, US Department of Health and Human Services, Health Resources and Services Administration, December 2009, http://mchb.hrsa.gov/whusa09/ (accessed February 24, 2011).

77. American College of Obstetricians and Gynecologists Office of Communications, "Female Ob-Gyns Name Obesity the Greatest Threat to Women's Health," news release, December 9, 2003, http://www.acog.org/from_home/publications/press_releases/nr12-09-03-1.cfm (accessed February 24, 2011).

78. American College of Obstetricians and Gynecologists Office of Communications, "ACOG Issues Guidance."

79. American College of Obstetricians and Gynecologists, "ACOG Committee Opinion Number 319, October 2005: The Role of Obstetrician-Gynecologist in the Assessment and Management of Obesity," *Obstetrics and Gynecology* 106, no. 4 (October 2005): 895–99; American College of Obstetricians and Gynecologists, "ACOG Practice Bulletin no. 105: Bariatric Surgery and Pregnancy," *Obstetrics and Gynecology* 113, no. 6 (June 2009): 1405–13.

80. Leonie K. Callaway et al., "The Prevalence and Impact of Overweight

and Obesity in an Australian Obstetric Population," *Medical Journal of Australia* 184, no. 2 (January 16, 2006): 56–59.

81. Amnesty International, "Deadly Delivery: The Maternal Health Care Crisis in the USA," *Amnesty International Secretariat*, March 2010, http://www .amnestyusa.org/dignity/pdf/DeadlyDeliverySummaryHiRes.pdf (accessed February 24, 2011).

82. Michelle Andrews, "Pregnant Women and New Mothers Will Get Benefits, Services under Health Care Law," *Kaiser Health News*, June 8, 2010, http:// www.kaiserhealthnews.org/Features/Insuring-Your-Health/Pregnant-Women -And-New-Mothers-Will-Get-Benefits-Services-Under-Health-Care-Law.aspx (accessed February 24, 2011).

83. O. Paul Humpstone, "Cesarean Section versus Spontaneous Delivery," *American Journal of Obstetrics and Gynecology* 1 (1920): 986–89.

84. American College of Obstetricians and Gynecologists Office of Communications, "Women's Access to Health Care Hurt by Medical Liability Crisis," news release, November 3, 2006, http://www.acog.org/from_home/publications/ press_releases/nr11-03-06.cfm (accessed February 24, 2011).

85. Thomas F. Heston, "Rapid Responses to Least Worst Solutions," *British Medical Journal*, April 21, 2002, http://www.bmj.com/content/324/7343/0.10 .extract/reply#bmj_el_21521 (accessed February 24, 2011).

86. American College of Obstetricians and Gynecologists Office of Communications, "New ACOG Opinion Addresses Elective Cesarean Controversy," news release, October 31, 2003, http://www.acog.org/from_home/publications/ press_releases/nr10-31-03-1.cfm (accessed February 24, 2011).

87. National Health Service, "NHS Maternity Statistics, England— 2009/10," NHS Information Centre for Health and Social Care, November 18, 2010, http://www.ic.nhs.uk/pubs/maternity0910 (accessed February 24, 2011).

88. National Collaborating Centre for Women's and Children's Health, "Caesarean Section: Clinical Guideline 13," NHS National Institute for Clinical Excellence, April 2004, http://guidance.nice.org.uk/nicemedia/live/10940/29334/29334 .pdf (accessed January 16, 2011).

89. Welsh Assembly Government, "Maternity Statistics: Method of Delivery, 1999–2009," *Llywodraeth Cymru*, February 10, 2010, http://wales.gov.uk/ topics/statistics/headlines/health2010/0210/?lang=en (accessed February 9, 2011).

90. National Health Service Scotland, "Births in Scottish Hospitals, Financial Year 2008/2009," ISD Scotland, August 31, 2010, http://www.isdscotland .org/isd/6364.html (accessed February 9, 2011).

91. "Child Health System (Northern Ireland)," Northern Ireland Department of Health, Social Services, and Public Safety, October 21, 2010.

92. National Perinatal Reporting System, "Perinatal Statistics Report 2008," Economic and Social Research Institute Health Research and Information Division, December 2010, http://www.esri.ie/health_information/nprs/nprs_reports/NPRS_AR_2008.pdf (accessed February 9, 2011).

93. NHS National Institute for Clinical Excellence, "NICE Weight Management in Pregnancy Guidance to Help Tackle Rise in Maternal Obesity," news release, March 23, 2010, http://www.nice.org.uk/newsroom/news/WeightManagementInPregnancyGuidance.jsp (accessed February 24, 2011).

94. Andrew Hough, "Women Giving Birth at Night More at Risk, Says Maternity Chief," *Telegraph*, January 1, 2011, http://www.telegraph.co.uk/health/healthnews/8234689/Women-giving-birth-at-night-more-at-risk-says-maternity-chief.html (accessed January 1, 2011).

95. National Collaborating Centre for Women's and Children's Health, "Cesarean Section: Clinical Guideline 13."

96. Pauline McDonagh Hull, "These Doctors View Cesarean Delivery as a Valid Choice," *Elective Cesarean Delivery* (blog), August 21, 2008, http://electivecesarean.blogspot.com/2008/08/these-doctors-view-cesarean-delivery-as.html (accessed October 10, 2011).

97. Ibid.

98. NHS National Institute for Clinical Excellence, "Guideline Consultation Comments Table: 23 May–22 June 2011," http://www.nice.org.uk/nicemedia/live/12156/56260/56260.pdf (accessed October 10, 2011).

99. NHS National Institute for Clinical Excellence, "Caesarean Section: Full Guideline DRAFT," September 2011, http://www.nice.org.uk/nicemedia/live/12156/56255/56255.pdf (accessed October 10, 2011).

100. National Collaborating Centre for Women's and Children's Health, "Caesarean Section (Update)," NHS National Institute for Clinical Excellence, November 2011 (in progress), http://guidance.nice.org.uk/CG/WaveR/97 (accessed February 24, 2011).

101. "Factsheet 3: Information on Claims 2009–10," NHS Litigation Authority, August 2010, http://www.nhsla.com/publications (accessed February 24, 2011).

102. NHS National Institute for Clinical Excellence, "Caesarean Section: Full Guideline DRAFT."

103. Lisa Smyth, "£3,500 C-Section Charge Proposal," *Belfast Telegraph*, September 29, 2011, http://www.belfasttelegraph.co.uk/woman/life/3500-csection-charge-proposal-16056600.html#idc-container (accessed October 10, 2011).

104. "Who We Are," National Childbirth Trust, http://www.nct.org.uk/about-us/who-we-are (accessed January 16, 2011).

105. Department of Health, "Changing Childbirth. Part I: Report of the

Expert Maternity Group. Part II: Survey of Good Communication Practice," Her Majesty's Stationery Office, 1993, http://www.dur.ac.uk/comparative.public health/healthfacts/hfacts5.htm (accessed January 16, 2011).

106. Maternity Care Working Party, "Making Normal Birth a Reality," Royal College of Obstetricians and Gynaecologists, November 1, 2007, http://www.rcog.org.uk/womens-health/clinical-guidance/making-normal-birth-reality (accessed January 9, 2011).

107. Ibid.

108. "Toolkit for Reducing Caesarean Section Rates," NHS Institute for Innovation and Improvement, November 27, 2009, http://www.library.nhs.uk/qipp/ViewResource.aspx?resID=330743 (accessed January 2, 2011).

109. Royal College of Obstetricians and Gynecologists, "Doctors Demand Radical Shake-Up of Women's Health Services Promoting Prevention rather than Interventions," news release, July 14, 2011, http://www.rcog.org.uk/news/rcog-release-doctors-demand-radical-shake-women%E2%80%99s-health-services-promoting-prevention-rather-i (accessed October 10, 2011).

110. Polly Stoker, "Women at Low Risk of Complications Should Be Able to Have All Their Antenatal Care in Midwife Led Units, Says College," *British Medical Journal (Clinical Research Ed.)* 343 (2011): d4524.

111. Maternity Care Working Party, "Making Normal Birth a Reality."

112. Canadian Institute for Health Information, "Caesarean Section: Proportion of Women Delivering Babies in Acute Care Hospital by Caesarean Section," Agency for Healthcare Research Quality, May 2010, http://qualitymeasures.ahrq.gov/content.aspx?id=15066 (accessed February 24, 2011).

113. Canadian Institute for Health Information, "Health Care in Canada 2010: Evidence of Progress, but Care Not Always Appropriate," news release, December 16, 2010, http://www.cihi.ca/cihi-ext-portal/internet/en/document/health+system+performance/indicators/performance/release_16dec10 (accessed February 9, 2011).

114. Raúl Andrés Mendoza-Sassi et al., "Risk Factors for Cesarean Section by Category of Health Service," *Revista de Saúde Pública* 44, no. 1 (February 2010): 80–89.

115. Cecilia McCallum, "Explaining Caesarean Section in Salvador da Bahia, Brazil," *Sociology of Health and Illness* 27, no. 2 (March 2005): 215–42.

116. Belizán et al., "Rates and Implications."

117. Katie Groom and Sara Paterson Brown; Luis G. A. Quadros; Christine Nuttall, "Letter: Caesarean Section Controversy," *British Medical Journal*, April 15, 2000, http://www.bmj.com/content/320/7241/1072.2.full (accessed February 24, 2011).

118. Simone G. Diniz and Alessandra S. Chacham, "'The Cut Above' and

'The Cut Below': The Abuse of Caesareans and Episiotomy in São Paulo, Brazil," *Reproductive Health Matters* 12, no. 23 (May 2004): 100–10.

119. Joseph E. Potter et al., "Women's Autonomy and Scheduled Cesarean Sections in Brazil: A Cautionary Tale," *Birth* 35, no. 1 (March 2008): 33–40.

120. Margareth Rocha Peixoto Giglio, Joel Alves Lamounier, and Otaliba Libânio de Morais Neto, "Obstetric Delivery and Risk of Neonatal Mortality in Goiânia in 2000, Brazil" [in Portuguese], *Revista de Saúde Pública* 39, no. 3 (June 2005): 350–57.

121. Zhuoyang Li, Paula Laws, and Elizabeth A. Sullivan, "Australia's Mothers and Babies 2008," Australian Institute of Health and Welfare, November 25, 2010, http://www.apo.org.au/research/australias-mothers-and-babies-2008 (accessed February 9, 2011).

122. Stephen J. Robson et al., "Estimating the Rate of Cesarean Section by Maternal Request: Anonymous Survey of Obstetricians in Australia," *Birth* 36, no. 3 (September 2009): 208–12.

123. "Perinatal Statistics in the Nordic Countries," National Institute for Health and Welfare, May 27, 2010, http://www.stakes.fi/EN/tilastot/statisticsby topic/reproduction/perinatalreproductionsummary.htm (accessed January 16, 2011).

124. HealthGrades, "First-Time Preplanned."

125. Sevim Songun, "Mothers Face Dilemma More Painful than Delivery Itself," *Hurriyet Daily News and Economic Review*, October 1, 2010, http://www .hurriyetdailynews.com/n.php?n=cesarean-or-normal-birth-a-dilemma-more -painful-than-delivery-itself-2010-10-01 (accessed January 16, 2011).

126. G. Koken et al., "Attitudes towards Mode of Delivery and Cesarean on Demand in Turkey," *International Journal of Gynaecology and Obstetrics* 99, no. 3 (December 2007): 233–35.

127. Women Deliver, "FIGO Launches Report on Maternal and Infant Deaths," news release, October 8, 2009, http://www.womendeliver.org/updates/ entry/figo-launches-report-on-maternal-and-infant-deaths/ (accessed February 24, 2011).

128. N. T. Moyo and J. Liljestrand, "Emergency Obstetric Care: Impact on Emerging Issues," *International Journal of Gynaecology and Obstetrics* 98, no. 2 (August 2007): 175–77; Carine Ronsmans, Sara Holtz, and Cynthia Stanton, "Socioeconomic Differentials in Caesarean Rates in Developing Countries: A Retrospective Analysis," *Lancet* 368, no. 9546 (October 28, 2006): 1516–23.

129. Humpstone, "Cesarean Section versus Spontaneous Delivery."

CHAPTER 9. THE POLITICS OF BIRTH

1. Susan P. Walker et al., "Cesarean Delivery or Vaginal Birth: A Survey of Patient and Clinician Thresholds," *Obstetrics and Gynecology* 109, no. 1 (January 2007): 67–72.

2. Pisake Lumbiganon et al., "Method of Delivery and Pregnancy Outcomes in Asia: The WHO Global Survey on Maternal and Perinatal Health 2007–08," *Lancet* 375, no. 9713 (February 6, 2010): 490–99.

3. Nigel Hawkes, "Funny Figures from WHO on Caesareans," Straight Statistics, January 26, 2010, http://www.straightstatistics.org/article/funny-figures-who-caesareans (accessed December 1, 2010); Nigel Hawkes, "A Bad Case of Bias against Caesareans," *Independent*, January 30, 2010, http://www.independent.co.uk/life-style/health-and-families/health-news/nigel-hawkes-a-bad-case-of-bias-against-caesareans-1883667.htm (accessed December 1, 2010).

4. Lumbiganon et al., "Method of Delivery."

5. Hawkes, "Bad Case of Bias."

6. Department of Error, *Lancet* 376, no. 9756 (December 4, 2010): 1902, http://www.thelancet.com/journals/lancet/article/PIIS0140-6736(10)62218-0/fulltext (accessed February 20, 2011).

7. "Appropriate Technology for Birth," *Lancet* 2, no. 8452 (August 24, 1985): 436–37.

8. Ibid.

9. World Health Organization et al., *Monitoring Emergency Obstetric Care: A Handbook* (Geneva: WHO, 2009), http://www.who.int/reproductivehealth/publications/monitoring/9789241547734/en/index.html (accessed November 27, 2010).

10. Catherine Deneux-Tharaux et al., "Postpartum Maternal Mortality and Cesarean Delivery," *Obstetrics and Gynecology* 108, no. 3 (September 2006): 541–48.

11. José Villar et al., "Caesarean Delivery Rates and Pregnancy Outcomes: The 2005 WHO Global Survey on Maternal and Perinatal Health in Latin America," *Lancet* 367, no. 9525 (June 3, 2006): 1819–29.

12. Marian F. MacDorman et al., "Infant and Neonatal Mortality for Primary Cesarean and Vaginal Births to Women with 'No Indicated Risk,' United States, 1998–2001 Birth Cohorts," *Birth* 33, no. 3 (September 2006): 175–82.

13. World Health Organization et al., *Monitoring Emergency Obstetric Care.*

14. Barbara A. Bettes et al., "Cesarean Delivery on Maternal Request: Obstetrician-Gynecologists' Knowledge, Perception, and Practice Patterns," *Obstetrics and Gynecology* 109, no. 1 (January 2007): 57–66.

15. Stephen J. Robson et al., "Estimating the Rate of Cesarean Section by Maternal Request: Anonymous Survey of Obstetricians in Australia," *Birth* 36, no. 3 (September 2009): 208–12.

16. Jun Zhang et al., "Cesarean Delivery on Maternal Request in Southeast China," *Obstetrics and Gynecology* 111, no. 5 (May 2008): 1077–82.

17. Fiona Bragg et al., "Variation in Rates of Caesarean Section among English NHS Trusts after Accounting for Maternal and Clinical Risk: Cross Sectional Study," *British Medical Journal (Clinical Research Ed.)* 341 (2010): 5065.

18. Robert L. Barbieri. "How Will We Know It When We've Got the Right Cesarean Rate?" *OBG Management* 20, no. 6 (June 2008).

19. Alastair MacLennan et al., "Who Will Deliver Our Grandchildren? Implications of Cerebral Palsy Litigation," *JAMA: The Journal of the American Medical Association* 294, no. 13 (October 5, 2005): 1688–90.

20. Francesca Monari et al., "Obstetricians' and Midwives' Attitudes toward Cesarean Section," *Birth* 35, no. 2 (June 2008): 129–35.

21. Nick Pisa, "Mother and Baby Fighting for Life after Doctors Get into Delivery Room Brawl," Daily Mail Online, August 30, 2010, http://www.daily mail.co.uk/news/article-1307158/Mother-baby-fighting-life-doctors-delivery -room-brawl.html#ixzz14cBDHAU5 (accessed November 8, 2010).

22. Michael C. Klein et al., "The Attitudes of Canadian Maternity Care Practitioners towards Labour and Birth: Many Differences but Important Similarities," *Journal of Obstetrics and Gynaecology Canada* 31, no. 9 (September 2009): 827–40.

23. Veronica Schmidt, "Dame Helen Mirren: 'Why I Never Had Children,'" Times Online, October 24, 2007, http://entertainment.timesonline.co.uk/tol/arts _and_entertainment/film/article2730124.ece (accessed February 20, 2011).

24. Anneke Kwee et al., "Caesarean Section on Request: A Survey in the Netherlands," *European Journal of Obstetrics, Gynecology, and Reproductive Biology* 113, no. 2 (April 15, 2004): 186–90.

25. "Assisted Birth (Forceps and Ventouse)," BabyCentre, February 2009, http://www.babycentre.co.uk/pregnancy/labourandbirth/labourcomplications/ assisteddelivery/ (accessed November 27, 2010).

26. "The Cesarean Section FAQ," Childbirth.org, 1999, http://www .childbirth.org/section/CSFAQ.html (accessed November 27, 2010).

27. Amayal Center for Health and Wellness Education, "Humanization of Birth: International Education Conference," news release, February 19, 2006, http:// www.prweb.com/releases/2006/2/prweb348767.htm (accessed November 14, 2010).

28. HealthGrades, "First-Time Preplanned 'Patient Choice' Cesarean Section Rates in the United States," HealthGrades, July 21, 2003, http://www.health grades.com/media/english/pdf/Patient_Choice_Csection_Study_July_2003.pdf (accessed November 8, 2010).

29. Julia Medew, "Caesarean Births a Better Option for Mothers?" *Age*, August 13, 2011, http://www.theage.com.au/national/caesarean-births-a-better-option-for -mothers-20110812-1ir24.html?from=age_sb (accessed October 10, 2011).

30. "Elective Caesarean—Positives and Negatives—Your Experiences Please, Not Emergencies," Mumsnet, November 10, 2010, http://www.mumsnet.com/Talk/childbirth/1080779-Elective-Caesarean-Positives-and-negatives-your-experiences-please-not-emerencies/AllOnOnePage (accessed November 27, 2010).

31. Coalition for Childbirth Autonomy, "Birth Group, CCA, Calls on WHO to Re-Examine 'Outdated and Unsafe' 10–15% Recommended Cesarean Rate," news release, October 29, 2008, http://www.mmdnewswire.com/birth-group-cca-calls-on-who-to-re-examine-outdated-and-unsafe-10-15-recommended-cesarean-rate-4073.html (accessed January 18, 2011).

32. Rebecca Smith, "Women Choosing Caesarean Have Low Death Rate," *Telegraph*, April 11, 2008, http://www.telegraph.co.uk/news/uknews/1584671/Women-choosing-caesarean-have-low-death-rate.html (accessed February 24, 2011).

33. Reuters Health, "Choosing C-Section May Not Prevent Incontinence," May 13, 2011, http://www.reuters.com/article/2011/05/13/us-c-section-incontinence-idUSTRE74C6JK20110513 (accessed October 10, 2011).

34. John Darnton, interview by Dave Davies, *Fresh Air*, NPR, August 4, 2008, http://www.npr.org/templates/story/story.php?storyId=93254258 (accessed October 10, 2011).

35. Associated Press, "Clash over Maternal Deaths Report Reveals Politics of Public Health," *USA Today*, April 15, 2010, http://www.usatoday.com/news/health/2010-04-15-maternal-deaths_N.htm (accessed February 24, 2011).

CHAPTER 10. BEFORE THEY SAY IT

1. "More Women Ask for Caesareans," *Times-Picayune*, August 5, 2004, http://www.nola.com/t-p/ (accessed February 24, 2011; article no longer available).

2. Roberta De Luca et al., "Incidence of Early Neonatal Mortality and Morbidity after Late-Preterm and Term Cesarean Delivery," *Pediatrics* 123, no. 6 (June 2009): 1064–71.

3. Freke A. Wilmink et al., "Neonatal Outcome following Elective Cesarean Section beyond 37 Weeks of Gestation: A 7-Year Retrospective Analysis of a National Registry," *American Journal of Obstetrics and Gynecology* 202, no. 3 (March 2010): 250.1–8.

4. Leanne S. Dahlgren et al., "Caesarean Section on Maternal Request: Risks and Benefits in Healthy Nulliparous Women and Their Infants," *Journal of Obstetrics and Gynaecology Canada* 31, no. 9 (September 2009): 808–17.

5. Shobha H. Mehta et al., "Shoulder Dystocia and the Next Delivery: Outcomes and Management," *Journal of Maternal-Fetal and Neonatal Medicine* 20, no. 10 (October 2007): 729–33; M. Baumert et al., "Epidemiology of Peri/Intraventricular Haemorrhage in Newborns at Term," *Journal of Physiology and Pharmacology* 59, suppl. 4 (September 2008): 67–75; Christopher B. Looney et al., "Intracranial Hemorrhage in Asymptomatic Neonates: Prevalence on MR Images and Relationship to Obstetric and Neonatal Risk Factors," *Radiology* 242, no. 2 (February 2007): 535–41; D. Towner et al., "Effect of Mode of Delivery in Nulliparous Women on Neonatal Intracranial Injury," *New England Journal of Medicine* 341, no. 23 (December 2, 1999): 1709–14.

6. Gordon C. S. Smith, Jill P. Pell, and Richard Dobbie, "Caesarean Section and Risk of Unexplained Stillbirth in Subsequent Pregnancy," *Lancet* 362, no. 9398 (November 29, 2003): 1779–84.

7. S. L. Wood et al., "The Risk of Unexplained Antepartum Stillbirth in Second Pregnancies following Caesarean Section in the First Pregnancy," *BJOG: An International Journal of Obstetrics and Gynaecology* 115, no. 6 (May 2008): 726–31.

8. R. Gray et al., "Caesarean Delivery and Risk of Stillbirth in Subsequent Pregnancy: A Retrospective Cohort Study in an English Population," *BJOG: An International Journal of Obstetrics and Gynaecology* 114, no. 3 (March 2007): 264–70.

9. Mert O. Bahtiyar et al., "Prior Cesarean Delivery Is Not Associated with an Increased Risk of Stillbirth in a Subsequent Pregnancy: Analysis of U.S. Perinatal Mortality Data, 1995–1997," *American Journal of Obstetrics and Gynecology* 195, no. 5 (November 2006): 1373–78.

10. Gary D. V. Hankins, Shannon M. Clark, and Mary B. Munn, "Cesarean Section on Request at 39 Weeks: Impact on Shoulder Dystocia, Fetal Trauma, Neonatal Encephalopathy, and Intrauterine Fetal Demise," *Seminars in Perinatology* 30, no. 5 (October 2006): 276–87.

11. Susan Y. Chu et al., "Maternal Obesity and Risk of Stillbirth: A Meta-analysis," *American Journal of Obstetrics and Gynecology* 197, no. 3 (September 2007): 223–28; Janni Kristensen et al., "Pre-Pregnancy Weight and the Risk of Stillbirth and Neonatal Death," *BJOG: An International Journal of Obstetrics and Gynaecology* 112, no. 4 (April 2005): 403–408.

12. Stas Vashevnik, Susan Walker, and Michael Permezel, "Stillbirths and Neonatal Deaths in Appropriate, Small, and Large Birthweight for Gestational Age Fetuses," *Australian and New Zealand Journal of Obstetrics and Gynaecology* 47, no. 4 (August 2007): 302–306.

13. Darios Getahun, Cande V. Ananth, and Wendy L. Kinzler, "Risk Factors for Antepartum and Intrapartum Stillbirth: A Population-Based Study," *American Journal of Obstetrics and Gynecology* 196, no. 6 (June 2007): 499–507; Pamela J. Surkan et al., "Previous Preterm and Small-for-Gestational-Age Births and the

Subsequent Risk of Stillbirth," *New England Journal of Medicine* 350, no. 8 (February 19, 2004): 777–85.

14. Olof Stephansson, Paul W. Dickman, and Sven Cnattingius, "The Influence of Interpregnancy Interval on the Subsequent Risk of Stillbirth and Early Neonatal Death," *Obstetrics and Gynecology* 102, no. 1 (July 2003): 101–108.

15. K. Wisborg et al., "Exposure to Tobacco Smoke in Utero and the Risk of Stillbirth and Death in the First Year of Life," *American Journal of Epidemiology* 154, no. 4 (August 15, 2001): 322–27.

16. Svein Rasmussen et al., "Prior Adverse Pregnancy Outcome and the Risk of Stillbirth," *Obstetrics and Gynecology* 114, no. 6 (December 2009): 1259–70.

17. R. Sutan et al., "The Risk Factors for Unexplained Antepartum Stillbirths in Scotland, 1994 to 2003," *Journal of Perinatology* 30, no. 5 (October 15, 2009): 311–18.

18. Katherine J. Stothard et al., "Maternal Overweight and Obesity and the Risk of Congenital Anomalies: a Systematic Review and Meta-Analysis," *JAMA: The Journal of the American Medical Association* 301, no. 6 (February 11, 2009): 636–50.

19. A. P. LaSala and A. S. Berkeley, "Primary Cesarean Section and Subsequent Fertility," *American Journal of Obstetrics and Gynecology* 157, no. 2 (August 1987): 379–83.

20. J. Jolly, J. Walker, and K. Bhabra, "Subsequent Obstetric Performance Related to Primary Mode of Delivery," *British Journal of Obstetrics and Gynaecology* 106, no. 3 (March 1999): 227–32.

21. Maureen Porter et al., "Does Caesarean Section Cause Infertility?" *Human Reproduction* 18, no. 10 (October 2003): 1983–86.

22. S. M. Collin, T. Marshall, and V. Filippi, "Caesarean Section and Subsequent Fertility in Sub-Saharan Africa," *BJOG: An International Journal of Obstetrics and Gynaecology* 113, no. 3 (March 2006): 276–83.

23. S. Bhattacharya et al., "Absence of Conception after Caesarean Section: Voluntary or Involuntary?" *BJOG: An International Journal of Obstetrics and Gynaecology* 113, no. 3 (March 2006): 268–75.

24. Anne Kjersti Daltveit et al., "Cesarean Delivery and Subsequent Pregnancies," *Obstetrics and Gynecology* 111, no. 6 (June 2008): 1327–34; J. J. H. Eijsink, L. van der Leeuw-Harmsen, and P. J. Q. van der Linden, "Pregnancy after Caesarean Section: Fewer or Later?" *Human Reproduction* 23, no. 3 (March 2008): 543–47; Mette C. Tollånes et al., "Reduced Fertility after Cesarean Delivery: A Maternal Choice," *Obstetrics and Gynecology* 110, no. 6 (December 2007): 1256–63; Engin Oral and Koray Elter, "The Impact of Cesarean Birth on Subsequent Fertility," *Current Opinion in Obstetrics & Gynecology* 19, no. 3 (June 2007): 238–43.

25. "NIH State-of-the-Science Conference Statement on Cesarean Delivery on Maternal Request," *National Institutes of Health Consensus and State-of-the-Science Statements* 23, no. 1 (March 27, 2006): 1–29.

26. F. W. Makoha et al., "Multiple Cesarean Section Morbidity," *International Journal of Gynaecology and Obstetrics* 87, no. 3 (December 2004): 227–32; Dilek Uygur et al., "Multiple Repeat Caesarean Section: Is It Safe?" *European Journal of Obstetrics, Gynecology, and Reproductive Biology* 119, no. 2 (April 1, 2005): 171–75.

27. Robert M. Silver et al., "Maternal Morbidity Associated with Multiple Repeat Cesarean Deliveries," *Obstetrics and Gynecology* 107, no. 6 (June 2006): 1226–32.

28. Nikki Lee, "Operative Delivery and Breastfeeding Success," *Birth* 31, no. 2 (June 2004): 159; author reply, 159.

29. La Leche League International, "Is It Possible to Breastfeed after a Cesarean Birth?" La Leche League International, October 13, 2006, http://www.llli.org/FAQ/cesarean.html (accessed February 22, 2011).

30. C. Roduit et al., "Asthma at 8 Years of Age in Children Born by Caesarean Section," *Thorax* 64, no. 2 (February 2009): 107–13; Johanna Metsälä et al., "Perinatal Factors and the Risk of Asthma in Childhood: A Population-Based Register Study in Finland," *American Journal of Epidemiology* 168, no. 2 (July 15, 2008): 170–78; American College of Obstetricians and Gynecologists, "ACOG Committee Opinion No. 386, November 2007: Cesarean Delivery on Maternal Request," *Obstetrics and Gynecology* 110, no. 5 (November 2007): 1209–12; S. Håkansson and K. Källén, "Caesarean Section Increases the Risk of Hospital Care in Childhood for Asthma and Gastroenteritis," *Clinical and Experimental Allergy* 33, no. 6 (June 2003): 757–64.

31. A. Maitra et al., "Mode of Delivery Is Not Associated with Asthma or Atopy in Childhood," Clinical and Experimental Allergy 34, no. 9 (September 2004): 1349–55; Young J. Juhn et al., "Mode of Delivery at Birth and Development of Asthma: A Population-Based Cohort Study," *Journal of Allergy and Clinical Immunology* 116, no. 3 (September 2005): 510–16.

32. Mette C. Tollånes et al., "Cesarean Section and Risk of Severe Childhood Asthma: A Population-Based Cohort Study," *Journal of Pediatrics* 153, no. 1 (July 2008): 112–16.

33. Anne Kirkeby Hansen et al., "Risk of Respiratory Morbidity in Term Infants Delivered by Elective Caesarean Section: Cohort Study," *British Medical Journal (Clinical Research Ed.)* 336, no. 7635 (January 12, 2008): 85–87.

34. Rebecca Smith, "Women Choosing Caesarean Have Low Death Rate," *Telegraph*, April 11, 2008, http://www.telegraph.co.uk/news/uknews/1584671/Women-choosing-caesarean-have-low-death-rate.html (accessed February 24, 2011).

35. Confidential Enquiry into Maternal and Child Health (CEMACH), "Saving Mothers' Lives: Findings on the Causes of Maternal Deaths and the Care of Pregnant Women," news release, December 4, 2007, http://www.rcog.org.uk/news/cemach-release-saving-mothers-lives-findings-causes-maternal-deaths-and-care-pregnant-women (accessed February 24, 2011).

36. Elizabeth J. Geller et al., "Maternal Outcomes Associated with Planned Vaginal versus Planned Primary Cesarean Delivery," *American Journal of Perinatology* 27, no. 9 (March 16, 2010).

37. Dahlgren et al., "Caesarean Section on Maternal Request."

38. Susan Ayers, "Thoughts and Emotions during Traumatic Birth: A Qualitative Study," *Birth* 34, no. 3 (September 2007): 253–63.

39. Stephen Robson et al., "Elective Caesarean Delivery at Maternal Request: A Preliminary Study of Motivations Influencing Women's Decision-Making," *Australian and New Zealand Journal of Obstetrics and Gynaecology* 48, no. 4 (August 2008): 415–20; T. A. Mould et al., "Women's Involvement with the Decision Preceding their Caesarean Section and their Degree of Satisfaction," *British Journal of Obstetrics and Gynaecology* 103, no. 11 (November 1996): 1074–77.

40. Lai Wa Law et al., "Randomised Trial of Assigned Mode of Delivery after a Previous Cesarean Section: Impact on Maternal Psychological Dynamics," *Journal of Maternal-Fetal and Neonatal Medicine* 23, no. 10 (October 2010): 1106–13; W. J. Graham et al., "An Investigation of Women's Involvement in the Decision to Deliver by Caesarean Section," *British Journal of Obstetrics and Gynaecology* 106, no. 3 (March 1999): 213–20; E. L. Ryding, B. Wijma, and K. Wijma, "Posttraumatic Stress Reactions after Emergency Cesarean Section," *Acta Obstetricia et Gynecologica Scandinavica* 76, no. 9 (October 1997): 856–61; K. Hofberg and I. Brockington, "Tokophobia: An Unreasoning Dread of Childbirth. A Series of 26 Cases," *British Journal of Psychiatry: The Journal of Mental Science* 176 (January 2000): 83–85.

41. Ingela Wiklund, Gunnar Edman, and Ellika Andolf, "Cesarean Section on Maternal Request: Reasons for the Request, Self-Estimated Health, Expectations, Experience of Birth, and Signs of Depression among First-Time Mothers," *Acta Obstetricia et Gynecologica Scandinavica* 86, no. 4 (2007): 451–56.

42. Gunhilde M. Buchsbaum et al., "Prevalence of Urinary Incontinence and Associated Risk Factors in a Cohort of Nuns," *Obstetrics and Gynecology* 100, no. 2 (August 2002): 226–29; Gunhilde M. Buchsbaum and Erin E. Duecy, "Incontinence and Pelvic Organ Prolapse in Parous/Nulliparous Pairs of Identical Twins," *Neurourology and Urodynamics* 27, no. 6 (2008): 496–98.

43. L. Elaine Waetjen et al., "Association between Menopausal Transition Stages and Developing Urinary Incontinence," *Obstetrics and Gynecology* 114, no. 5 (November 2009): 989–98.

44. Stephanie J. Brown et al., "Urinary Incontinence in Nulliparous Women

before and during Pregnancy: Prevalence, Incidence, and Associated Risk Factors," *International Urogynecology Journal and Pelvic Floor Dysfunction* 21, no. 2 (February 2010): 193–202.

45. Sandra A. Baydock et al., "Prevalence and Risk Factors for Urinary and Fecal Incontinence Four Months after Vaginal Delivery," *Journal of Obstetrics and Gynaecology Canada* 31, no. 1 (January 2009): 36–41; S. L. Wesnes et al., "The Effect of Urinary Incontinence Status during Pregnancy and Delivery Mode on Incontinence Postpartum: A Cohort Study," *BJOG: An International Journal of Obstetrics and Gynaecology* 116, no. 5 (April 2009): 700–707; Maite Solans-Domènech, Emília Sánchez, and Montserrat Espuña-Pons, "Urinary and Anal Incontinence during Pregnancy and Postpartum: Incidence, Severity, and Risk Factors," *Obstetrics and Gynecology* 115, no. 3 (March 2010): 618–28.

46. Eunmi Ham et al., "Risk Factors for Female Urinary Incontinence among Middle-Aged Korean Women," *Journal of Women's Health* 18, no. 11 (November 2009): 1801–1806; Rahmi Onur et al., "Prevalence and Risk Factors of Female Urinary Incontinence in Eastern Turkey," *International Journal of Urology* 16, no. 6 (June 2009): 566–69.

47. Jennifer M. Wu et al., "Forecasting the Prevalence of Pelvic Floor Disorders in U.S. Women: 2010 to 2050," *Obstetrics and Gynecology* 114, no. 6 (December 2009): 1278–83.

48. Hans Peter Dietz, Alec V. L. Gillespie, and Pramod Phadke, "Avulsion of the Pubovisceral Muscle Associated with Large Vaginal Tear after Normal Vaginal Delivery at Term," *Australian and New Zealand Journal of Obstetrics and Gynaecology* 47, no. 4 (August 2007): 341–44; Ka Lai Shek and Hans Peter Dietz, "Can Levator Avulsion Be Predicted Antenatally?" *American Journal of Obstetrics and Gynecology* 202, no. 6 (January 13, 2010): 586.e1–6; Hans Peter Dietz and P. D. Wilson, "Childbirth and Pelvic Floor Trauma," *Best Practice and Research, Clinical Obstetrics and Gynaecology* 19, no. 6 (December 2005): 913–24; Hans Peter Dietz and Valeria Lanzarone, "Levator Trauma after Vaginal Delivery," *Obstetrics and Gynecology* 106, no. 4 (October 2005): 707–12; Hans Peter Dietz, "Pelvic Floor Trauma following Vaginal Delivery," *Current Opinion in Obstetrics and Gynecology* 18, no. 5 (October 2006): 528–37; Ladislav Krofta et al., "Pubococcygeus-Puborectalis Trauma after Forceps Delivery: Evaluation of the Levator Ani Muscle with 3D/4D Ultrasound," *International Urogynecology Journal and Pelvic Floor Dysfunction* 20, no. 10 (October 2009): 1175–81; Ka Lai Shek and Hans Peter Dietz, "The Effect of Childbirth on Hiatal Dimensions," *Obstetrics and Gynecology* 113, no. 6 (June 2009): 1272–78; Zeelha Abdool, Ka Lai Shek, and Hans Peter Dietz, "The Effect of Levator Avulsion on Hiatal Dimension and Function," *American Journal of Obstetrics and Gynecology* 201, no. 1 (July 2009): 89.1–5.

49. Marta E. Heilbrun et al., "Correlation between Levator Ani Muscle

Injuries on Magnetic Resonance Imaging and Fecal Incontinence, Pelvic Organ Prolapse, and Urinary Incontinence in Primiparous Women," *American Journal of Obstetrics and Gynecology* 202, no. 5 (March 11, 2010): 488.e1–6; Esther M. J. Bols et al., "A Systematic Review of Etiological Factors for Postpartum Fecal Incontinence," *Acta Obstetricia et Gynecologica Scandinavica* 89, no. 3 (March 2010): 302–14.

50. Joseph R. Wax et al., "Patient Choice Cesarean: The Maine Experience," *Birth* 32, no. 3 (September 2005): 203–206.

51. Kai J. Buhling et al., "Rate of Dyspareunia after Delivery in Primiparae According to Mode of Delivery," *European Journal of Obstetrics, Gynecology, and Reproductive Biology* 124, no. 1 (January 1, 2006): 42–46.

52. Lior Lowenstein et al., "Can Stronger Pelvic Muscle Floor Improve Sexual Function?" *International Urogynecology Journal and Pelvic Floor Dysfunction* 21, no. 5 (May 2010): 553–56.

53. Katharina Klein et al., "Does the Mode of Delivery Influence Sexual Function after Childbirth?" *Journal of Women's Health* 18, no. 8 (August 2009): 1227–31.

54. Mohammad Reza Safarinejad, Ali Asgar Kolahi, and Ladan Hosseini, "The Effect of the Mode of Delivery on the Quality of Life, Sexual Function, and Sexual Satisfaction in Primiparous Women and Their Husbands," *Journal of Sexual Medicine* 6, no. 6 (June 2009): 1645–67.

55. M. Khajehei et al., "A Comparison of Sexual Outcomes in Primiparous Women Experiencing Vaginal and Caesarean Births," *Indian Journal of Community Medicine* 34, no. 2 (April 2009): 126–30.

56. Vahé A. Kazandjian et al., "Does a Cesarean Section Delivery Always Cost More than a Vaginal Delivery?" *Journal of Evaluation in Clinical Practice* 13, no. 1 (February 2007): 16–20.

57. Brent W. Bost, "Cesarean Delivery on Demand: What Will It Cost?" *American Journal of Obstetrics and Gynecology* 188, no. 6 (June 2003): 1418–23; W. A. Grobman, A. M. Peaceman, and M. L. Socol, "Cost-Effectiveness of Elective Cesarean Delivery after One Prior Low Transverse Cesarean," *Obstetrics and Gynecology* 95, no. 5 (May 2000): 745–51; S. L. Clark et al., "Is Vaginal Birth after Cesarean Less Expensive than Repeat Cesarean Delivery?" *American Journal of Obstetrics and Gynecology* 182, no. 3 (March 2000): 599–602; S. F. Murray, "Relation between Private Health Insurance and High Rates of Caesarean Section in Chile: Qualitative and Quantitative Study," *British Medical Journal (Clinical Research Ed.)* 321, no. 7275 (December 16, 2000): 1501–1505; Bruce R. Schackman, Kawai Oneda, and Sue J. Goldie, "The Cost-Effectiveness of Elective Cesarean Delivery to Prevent Hepatitis C Transmission in HIV-Coinfected Women," *International AIDS Society Journal* 18, no. 13 (September 3, 2004): 1827–34; John A. F. Zupancic, "The Economics of Elective Cesarean Section," *Clinics in Perinatology* 35, no. 3 (September 2008): 591–99, xii.

58. James Lumalcuri and Ralph W. Hale, "Medical Liability: An Ongoing Nemesis," *Obstetrics and Gynecology* 115, no. 2 (February 2010): 223–28.

59. Xiao Xu et al., "The Impact of Malpractice Burden on Michigan Obstetrician-Gynecologists' Career Satisfaction," *Women's Health Issues* 18, no. 4 (August 2008): 229–37; Xiao Xu et al., "The Effects of Medical Liability on Obstetric Care Supply in Michigan," *American Journal of Obstetrics and Gynecology* 198, no. 2 (February 2008): 205.1–9.

60. Lumalcuri and Hale, "Medical Liability."

61. Ibid.

62. Steven L. Clark, "Sleep Deprivation: Implications for Obstetric Practice in the United States," *American Journal of Obstetrics and Gynecology* 201, no. 2 (August 2009): 136.1–4.

63. Stephen J. Robson et al., "Estimating the Rate of Cesarean Section by Maternal Request," *Obstetrical and Gynecological Survey* 65, no. 1 (January 2010): 11–13.

64. Gordon C. S. Smith et al., "The Effect of Delaying Childbirth on Primary Cesarean Section Rates," *Public Library of Science (PLoS Medicine) Journal* 5, no. 7 (July 1, 2008): 144.

65. A. Herbst and K. Källén, "Influence of Mode of Delivery on Neonatal Mortality in the Second Twin, at and before Term," *BJOG: An International Journal of Obstetrics and Gynaecology* 115, no. 12 (November 2008): 1512–17.

66. Daniel W. Skupski et al., "Delivery Mode for the Extremely Premature Fetus: A Statement of the Prematurity Working Group of the World Association of Perinatal Medicine," *Journal of Perinatal Medicine* 37, no. 6 (2009): 583–86; Blair J. Wylie et al., "Method of Delivery and Neonatal Outcome in Very Low-Birthweight Vertex-Presenting Fetuses," *American Journal of Obstetrics and Gynecology* 198, no. 6 (June 2008): 640.1–7; J. Drife, "Mode of Delivery in the Early Preterm Infant (Less than 28 Weeks)," *BJOG: An International Journal of Obstetrics and Gynaecology* 113, suppl. 3 (December 2006): 81–85; Fetus and Newborn Committee, Canadian Paediatric Society and Maternal-Fetal Medicine Committee, Society of Obstetricians and Gynaecologists of Canada, "Management of the Woman with Threatened Birth of an Infant of Extremely Low Gestational Age," *CMAJ: Canadian Medical Association Journal* 151, no. 5 (September 1, 1994): 547–53.

67. H. Shelton Brown, "Lawsuit Activity, Defensive Medicine, and Small Area Variation: The Case of Cesarean Sections Revisited," *Health Economics, Policy, and Law* 2, no. 3 (July 2007): 285–96; Wayne R. Cohen and Barry S. Schifrin, "Medical Negligence Lawsuits Relating to Labor and Delivery," *Clinics in Perinatology* 34, no. 2 (June 2007): 345–60, vii–viii; Y. Tony Yang et al., "Relationship between Malpractice Litigation Pressure and Rates of Cesarean Section and Vaginal Birth after Cesarean Section," *Medical Care* 47, no. 2 (February 2009): 234–42; Lumalcuri and Hale, "Medical Liability."

68. Virasakdi Chongsuvivatwong et al., "Maternal and Fetal Mortality and Complications Associated with Cesarean Section Deliveries in Teaching Hospitals in Asia," *Journal of Obstetrics and Gynaecology Research* 36, no. 1 (February 2010): 45–51; Gary L. Darmstadt et al., "Reducing Stillbirths: Interventions during Labour," *Biomed Central (BMJ) Pregnancy and Childbirth* 9, suppl. 1 (2009): 6.

69. Geller et al., "Maternal Outcomes."

CHAPTER 11. CESAREANS COST LESS THAN YOU THINK

1. Maurice L. Druzin and Yasser Y. El-Sayed, "Cesarean Delivery on Maternal Request: Wise Use of Finite Resources? A View from the Trenches," *Seminars in Perinatology* 30, no. 5 (October 2006): 305–308.

2. National Collaborating Centre for Women's and Children's Health, "Caesarean Section: Clinical Guideline 13," NHS National Institute for Clinical Excellence, April 2004, http://www.nice.org.uk/nicemedia/pdf/CG013NICE guideline.pdf (accessed January 16, 2011).

3. "NIH State-of-the-Science Conference Statement on Cesarean Delivery on Maternal Request," *National Institutes of Health Consensus and State-of-the-Science Statements* 23, no. 1 (March 27, 2006): 1–29.

4. American College of Obstetricians and Gynecologists, "ACOG Committee Opinion No. 395. Surgery and Patient Choice," *Obstetrics and Gynecology* 111, no. 1 (January 2008): 243–47.

5. Brent W. Bost, "Cesarean Delivery on Demand: What Will It Cost?" *American Journal of Obstetrics and Gynecology* 188, no. 6 (June 2003): 1418–23.

6. Joanne Morrison and I. Z. MacKenzie, "Cesarean Section on Demand," *Seminars in Perinatology* 27, no. 1 (February 2003): 20–33.

7. Vahé A. Kazandjian et al., "Does a Cesarean Section Delivery Always Cost More than a Vaginal Delivery?" *Journal of Evaluation in Clinical Practice* 13, no. 1 (February 2007): 16–20.

8. Tsai-Ching Liu, Chin-Shyan Chen, and Herng-Ching Lin, "Does Elective Caesarean Section Increase Utilization of Postpartum Maternal Medical Care?" *Medical Care* 46, no. 4 (April 2008): 440–43.

9. Roberto Palencia et al., "The Costs of Planned Cesarean versus Planned Vaginal Birth in the Term Breech Trial," *CMAJ: Canadian Medical Association Journal* 174, no. 8 (April 11, 2006): 1109–13.

10. Patrick J. Culligan et al., "Elective Cesarean Section to Prevent Anal Incontinence and Brachial Plexus Injuries Associated with Macrosomia: A Deci-

sion Analysis," *International Urogynecology Journal and Pelvic Floor Dysfunction* 16, no. 1 (February 2005): 19–28.

11. National Collaborating Centre for Women's and Children's Health, "Cesarean Section: Clinical Guideline 13."

12. Ibid.

13. "Health Firm Stops Funding Caesareans," BBC News Online, November 2, 2002, http://news.bbc.co.uk/2/hi/health/2391843.stm (accessed November 19, 2010).

14. N. Heslehurst et al., "Obesity in Pregnancy: A Study of the Impact of Maternal Obesity on NHS Maternity Services," *BJOG: An International Journal of Obstetrics and Gynaecology* 114, no. 3 (March 2007): 334–42.

CHAPTER 12. CESAREAN FOR SEX: THE ULTIMATE BIRTH TABOO?

1. Lior Lowenstein et al., "Can Stronger Pelvic Muscle Floor Improve Sexual Function?" *International Urogynecology Journal and Pelvic Floor Dysfunction* 21, no. 5 (May 2010): 553–56; Nevin Citak et al., "Postpartum Sexual Function of Women and the Effects of Early Pelvic Floor Muscle Exercises," *Acta Obstetricia et Gynecologica Scandinavica* 89, no. 6 (June 2010): 817–22.

2. Sadettin Gungor et al., "Does Mode of Delivery Affect Sexual Functioning of the Man Partner?" *Journal of Sexual Medicine* 5, no. 1 (January 2008): 155–63.

3. C. M. Glazener, "Sexual Function after Childbirth: Women's Experiences, Persistent Morbidity, and Lack of Professional Recognition," *British Journal of Obstetrics and Gynaecology* 104, no. 3 (March 1997): 330–35.

4. Ingela Rådestad et al., "Tears in the Vagina, Perineum, Sphincter Ani, and Rectum and First Sexual Intercourse after Childbirth: A Nationwide Follow-up," *Birth* 35, no. 2 (2008): 98–106.

5. Zeelha Abdool, Ranee Thakar, and Abdul H Sultan, "Postpartum Female Sexual Function," *European Journal of Obstetrics, Gynecology, and Reproductive Biology* 145, no. 2 (August 2009): 133–37.

6. Kai J. Buhling et al., "Rate of Dyspareunia after Delivery in Primiparae according to Mode of Delivery," *European Journal of Obstetrics, Gynecology, and Reproductive Biology* 124, no. 1 (January 1, 2006): 42–46.

7. Linda Brubaker et al., "Sexual Function 6 Months after First Delivery," *Obstetrics and Gynecology* 111, no. 5 (May 2008): 1040–44.

8. Hanna Ejegård, Elsa Lena Ryding, and Berit Sjogren, "Sexuality after

Delivery with Episiotomy: A Long-Term Follow-Up," *Gynecologic and Obstetric Investigation* 66, no. 1 (2008): 1–7.

9. Amanda Williams, Sandy Herron-Marx, and Rebecca Knibb, "The Prevalence of Enduring Postnatal Perineal Morbidity and Its Relationship to Type of Birth and Birth Risk Factors," *Journal of Clinical Nursing* 16, no. 3 (March 2007): 549–61.

10. M. Khajehei et al., "A Comparison of Sexual Outcomes in Primiparous Women Experiencing Vaginal and Caesarean Births," *Indian Journal of Community Medicine* 34, no. 2 (April 2009): 126–30.

11. Nicola Dean et al., "Sexual Function, Delivery Mode History, Pelvic Floor Muscle Exercises, and Incontinence: A Cross-Sectional Study Six Years Post-Partum," *Australian and New Zealand Journal of Obstetrics and Gynaecology* 48, no. 3 (June 2008): 302–11.

12. Ahmed Shafik et al., "An Electrophysiologic Study of Female Ejaculation," *Journal of Sex and Marital Therapy* 35, no. 5 (October 2009): 337–46.

13. Margareta Nilsson et al., "How Do Urinary Incontinence and Urgency Affect Women's Sexual Life?" *Acta Obstetricia et Gynecologica Scandinavica* 90, no. 6 (June 2011): 621–28.

14. Victoria L. Handa et al., "Female Sexual Function and Pelvic Floor Disorders," *Obstetrics and Gynecology* 111, no. 5 (May 2008): 1045–52.

15. S. J. Lee and J. W. Park, "Follow-Up Evaluation of the Effect of Vaginal Delivery on the Pelvic Floor," *Diseases of the Colon and Rectum* 43, no. 11 (November 2000): 1550–55.

16. A. Griffiths et al., "Female Genital Tract Morbidity and Sexual Function following Vaginal Delivery or Lower Segment Caesarean Section," *Journal of Obstetrics and Gynaecology* 26, no. 7 (October 2006): 645–49.

17. Tara L. Hicks et al., "Postpartum Sexual Functioning and Method of Delivery: Summary of the Evidence," *Journal of Midwifery and Women's Health* 49, no. 5 (October 2004): 430–36.

18. Rebecca G. Rogers et al., "A Short Form of the Pelvic Organ Prolapse/Urinary Incontinence Sexual Questionnaire (PISQ-12)," *International Urogynecology Journal and Pelvic Floor Dysfunction* 14, no. 3 (August 2003): 164–68.

19. R. Rosen et al., "The Female Sexual Function Index (FSFI): A Multidimensional Self-Report Instrument for the Assessment of Female Sexual Function," *Journal of Sex and Marital Therapy* 26, no. 2 (June 2000): 191–208.

20. Leonard R. Derogatis et al., "The Female Sexual Distress Scale (FSDS): Initial Validation of a Standardized Scale for Assessment of Sexually Related Personal Distress in Women," *Journal of Sex and Marital Therapy* 28, no. 4 (September 2002): 317–30.

21. G. Barrett et al., "Women's Sexuality after Childbirth: A Pilot Study," *Archives of Sexual Behavior* 28, no. 2 (April 1999): 179–91.

22. Yvonne K. Fulbright, "Pregnant Women Have the Best Sex, Better Orgasms," Fox News, December 20, 2007, http://www.foxnews.com/story/0,2933,317693,00.html (accessed December 5, 2010).

23. "Women's Comments 5," Birth Trauma Canada, http://birthtraumacanada.org/38.html (accessed October 10, 2011).

24. "Does a Vasectomy Reduce a Man's Sexual Drive?" Vasectomy.com, http://www.vasectomy.com/ArticleDetail.asp?siteid=V&ArticleId=5 (accessed October 10, 2011).

25. Daisy Hsieh, "The Cesarean in Contemporary Taiwan," trans. Brent Heinrich, *Taiwan Panorama*, August 1996, http://www.sinorama.com.tw/ en/show _issue.php?id=199688508044E.TXT&cur_page=1&distype=text&table=2&h1 =Health&h2=Medicine&search=&height=&type=&scope=&order=&keyword= &lstPage=&num=&year=1996&month=08 (accessed December 5, 2010).

CHAPTER 13. THE RISKS OF PLANNING A CESAREAN

1. V. P. Ward et al., "Enhanced Surgical Site Infection Surveillance following Caesarean Section: Experience of a Multicentre Collaborative Post-Discharge System," *Journal of Hospital Infection* 70, no. 2 (October 2008): 166–73; L. Charrier et al., "Post-Partum Surgical Wound Infections: Incidence after Caesarean Section in an Italian Hospital," *Journal of Preventive Medicine and Hygiene* 50, no. 3 (September 2009): 159–63; Fiona M. Smaill and Gillian M. Gyte, "Antibiotic Prophylaxis versus No Prophylaxis for Preventing Infection after Cesarean Section," *Cochrane Database of Systematic Reviews (Online)*, no. 1 (2010): CD007482.

2. Margaret A. Olsen et al., "Risk Factors for Endometritis after Low Transverse Cesarean Delivery," *Infection Control and Hospital Epidemiology* 31, no. 1 (January 2010): 69–77.

3. Ibid.

4. David M. Haas, Sarah Morgan, Al Darei, and Karenrose Contreras, "Vaginal Preparation with Antiseptic Solution before Cesarean Section for Preventing Postoperative Infections," *Cochrane Database of Systematic Reviews* (Online) 3 (2010): CD007892.

5. Charrier et al., "Post-Partum Surgical Wound Infections."

6. Antonio De Vivo et al., "Wound Length and Corticosteroid Administration as Risk Factors for Surgical-Site Complications following Cesarean Section," *Acta Obstetricia et Gynecologica Scandinavica* 89, no. 3 (March 2010): 355–59.

7. Olsen et al., "Risk Factors for Endometritis"; Eran Hadar et al., "Timing

and Risk Factors of Maternal Complications of Cesarean Section," *Archives of Gynecology and Obstetrics* 283, no. 4 (March 31, 2010): 735–41.

8. Gokhan Yildirim et al., "When Should We Perform Prophylactic Antibiotics in Elective Cesarean Cases?" *Archives of Gynecology and Obstetrics* 280, no. 1 (July 2009): 13–18.

9. Mara J. Dinsmoor et al., "Perioperative Antibiotic Prophylaxis for Non-laboring Cesarean Delivery," *Obstetrics and Gynecology* 114, no. 4 (October 2009): 752–56; Smaill and Gyte, "Antibiotic Prophylaxis."

10. E. Boselli et al., "Antimicrobial Prophylaxis for Caesarean Delivery: before or after Cord Clamping? A Meta-Analysis" [in French], *Annales Françaises d'Anesthèsie et de Rèanimation* 28, no. 10 (October 2009): 855–67.

11. American College of Obstetricians and Gynecologists Office of Communications, "All Women Need Antibiotics One Hour before Cesarean Delivery," news release, August 23, 2010, http://www.acog.org/from_home/publications/press_releases/nr08-23-10-1.cfm (accessed February 24, 2011).

12. Gwyneth Lewis, ed., *Why Mothers Die 2000–2002* (London: RCOG, 2004), http://www.library.nhs.uk/womenshealth/ViewResource.aspx?resID=114586 (accessed February 24, 2011).

13. J. M. Morris, C. S. Algert, and C. L. Roberts, "Incidence and Risk Factors for Pulmonary Embolism in the Postpartum Period," *Journal of Thrombosis and Haemostasis: JTH* 8, no. 5 (May 2010): 998–1003; Winnie W. Sia et al., "The Incidence of Deep Vein Thrombosis in Women Undergoing Cesarean Delivery," *Thrombosis Research* 123, no. 3 (2009): 550–55.

14. Andra H. James, "Thromboembolism in Pregnancy: Recurrence Risks, Prevention, and Management," *Current Opinion in Obstetrics and Gynecology* 20, no. 6 (December 2008): 550–56.

15. Morris, Algert, and Roberts, "Incidence and Risk Factors."

16. Sia et al., "Incidence of Deep Vein Thrombosis."

17. Marc Blondon et al., "Thromboprophylaxis with Low-Molecular-Weight Heparin after Cesarean Delivery," *Thrombosis and Haemostasis* 103, no. 1 (January 2010): 129–37.

18. C. L. Roberts et al., "Amniotic Fluid Embolism in an Australian Population-Based Cohort," *BJOG: An International Journal of Obstetrics and Gynaecology* (July 7, 2010); Marian Knight et al., "Incidence and Risk Factors for Amniotic-Fluid Embolism," *Obstetrics and Gynecology* 115, no. 5 (May 2010): 910–17.

19. Nissar Shaikh and Firdous Ummunisa, "Acute Management of Vascular Air Embolism," *Journal of Emergencies, Trauma, and Shock* 2, no. 3 (September 2009): 180–85; T. W. Lew, D. H. Tay, and E. Thomas, "Venous Air Embolism during Cesarean Section: More Common than Previously Thought," *Anesthesia and Analgesia* 77, no. 3 (September 1993): 448–52.

20. Paolo Erba et al., "Fat Embolism Syndrome after Combined Aesthetic Surgery," *Scandinavian Journal of Plastic and Reconstructive Surgery and Hand Surgery* 45, no. 1 (February 17, 2010): 51–53; Drazen Cuculić et al., "Trauma Related Fat Embolism Syndrome in Forensic Practice," *Collegium Antropologicum* 34, no. 2 (June 2010): 723–26.

21. Knight et al., "Incidence and Risk Factors."

22. Chang Seok Kim et al., "Venous Air Embolism during Surgery, Especially Cesarean Delivery," *Journal of Korean Medical Science* 23, no. 5 (October 2008): 753–61.

23. Christina Larsson et al., "Estimation of Blood Loss after Cesarean Section and Vaginal Delivery Has Low Validity with a Tendency to Exaggeration," *Acta Obstetricia et Gynecologica Scandinavica* 85, no. 12 (2006): 1448–52.

24. O. Kor-Anantakul et al., "Comparing Complications in Intended Vaginal and Caesarean Deliveries," *Journal of Obstetrics and Gynaecology* 28, no. 1 (January 2008): 64–68; Catherine Deneux-Tharaux et al., "Postpartum Maternal Mortality and Cesarean Delivery," *Obstetrics and Gynecology* 108, no. 3 (September 2006): 541–48; Shiliang Liu et al., "Maternal Mortality and Severe Morbidity Associated with Low-Risk Planned Cesarean Delivery versus Planned Vaginal Delivery at Term," *CMAJ: Canadian Medical Association Journal* 176, no. 4 (February 13, 2007): 455–60.

25. M. E. Van Wolfswinkel et al., "Maternal Mortality and Serious Maternal Morbidity in Jehovah's Witnesses in the Netherlands," *BJOG: An International Journal of Obstetrics and Gynaecology* 116, no. 8 (July 2009): 1103–10.

26. Toril Kolås, Pål Øian, and Finn Egil Skjeldestad, "Risks for Peroperative Excessive Blood Loss in Cesarean Delivery," *Acta Obstetricia et Gynecologica Scandinavica* 89, no. 5 (May 2010): 658–63.

27. Ibid.

28. Gabriela Bencaiova, Tilo Burkhardt, and Ernst Beinder, "Abnormal Placental Invasion Experience at 1 Center," *Journal of Reproductive Medicine* 52, no. 8 (August 2007): 709–14; S. L. Clark, P. P. Koonings, and J. P. Phelan, "Placenta Previa/Accreta and Prior Cesarean Section," *Obstetrics and Gynecology* 66, no. 1 (July 1985): 89–92; Todd Rosen, "Placenta Accreta and Cesarean Scar Pregnancy: Overlooked Costs of the Rising Cesarean Section Rate," *Clinics in Perinatology* 35, no. 3 (September 2008): 519–29.

29. A. Cristina Rossi, Richard H. Lee, and Ramen H. Chmait, "Emergency Postpartum Hysterectomy for Uncontrolled Postpartum Bleeding: A Systematic Review," *Obstetrics and Gynecology* 115, no. 3 (March 2010): 637–44; Kolås, Øian, and Skjeldestad, "Risks for Peroperative."

30. Qiuying Yang et al., "Comparison of Maternal Risk Factors between Placental Abruption and Placenta Previa," *American Journal of Perinatology* 26, no. 4 (April 2009): 279–86.

31. M. S. Rahman et al., "Bladder Injuries during Cesarean Section in a University Hospital: A 25-Year Review," *Archives of Gynecology and Obstetrics* 279, no. 3 (March 2009): 349–52.

32. Ellika Andolf, Malin Thorsell, and Karin Källén, "Cesarean Delivery and Risk for Postoperative Adhesions and Intestinal Obstruction: A Nested Case-Control Study of the Swedish Medical Birth Registry," *American Journal of Obstetrics and Gynecology* 203, no. 4 (October 2010): 406.1–6.

33. S. Al-Took, R. Platt, and T. Tulandi, "Adhesion-Related Small-Bowel Obstruction after Gynecologic Operations," *American Journal of Obstetrics and Gynecology* 180, no. 2 (February 1999): 313–15.

34. Mette C. Tollånes et al., "Reduced Fertility after Cesarean Delivery: A Maternal Choice," *Obstetrics and Gynecology* 110, no. 6 (December 2007): 1256–63; Lucky Saraswat et al., "Caesarean Section and Tubal Infertility: Is There an Association?" *Reproductive Biomedicine Online* 17, no. 2 (August 2008): 259–64.

35. Dilek Uygur et al., "Multiple Repeat Caesarean Section: Is It Safe?" *European Journal of Obstetrics, Gynecology, and Reproductive Biology* 119, no. 2 (April 1, 2005): 171–75.

36. Antonio Malvasi et al., "Effects of Visceral Peritoneal Closure on Scar Formation at Cesarean Delivery," *International Journal of Gynaecology and Obstetrics* 105, no. 2 (May 2009): 131–35; Zhu Yiyang, Cai Qunxi, and Wu Weiling, "Closure versus Nonclosure of the Peritoneum at Cesarean Delivery," *International Journal of Gynaecology and Obstetrics* 94, no. 2 (August 2006): 103–07; Michael Sbarra, Marc Boyd, and Thomas S. Dardarian, "Complications due to Adhesion Formation following Cesarean Sections: A Review of Deliveries in Three Cases," *Fertility and Sterility* 92, no. 1 (July 2009): 394.13–16.

37. Khadeen Cheesman et al., "Epidemiology of Anesthesia-Related Complications in Labor and Delivery, New York State, 2002–2005," *Anesthesia and Analgesia* 109, no. 4 (October 2009): 1174–81.

38. C. Imarengiaye and I. Ekwere, "Postdural Puncture Headache: A Cross-Sectional Study of Incidence and Severity in a New Obstetric Anaesthesia Unit," *African Journal of Medicine and Medical Sciences* 35, no. 1 (March 2006): 47–51; A. W. Ross et al., "The Sprotte Needle and Post Dural Puncture Headache following Caesarean Section," *Anaesthesia and Intensive Care* 21, no. 3 (June 1993): 280–83.

39. A. Zeidan et al., "Does Postdural Puncture Headache Left Untreated Lead to Subdural Hematoma? Case Report and Review of the Literature," *Middle East Journal of Anesthesiology* 20, no. 4 (February 2010): 483–92.

40. Arzu Kaya and Salih Ozgocmen, "Thoracic Disc Herniation Causing Transient Paraplegia Coincident with Epidural Anesthesia: A Case Report," *Cases Journal* 2 (2009): 6228; Claude Lentschener et al., "Central Sensory-Motor Deficit after Uneventful Single-Dose Spinal Morphine Administration in a

Patient with Preexisting Migraine Headaches," *Anesthesia and Analgesia* 109, no. 5 (November 2009): 1688–90.

41. K. Schwabe and H. B. Hopf, "Persistent Back Pain after Spinal Anaesthesia in the Non-Obstetric Setting: Incidence and Predisposing Factors," *British Journal of Anaesthesia* 86, no. 4 (April 2001): 535–39.

42. T. W. Breen et al., "Factors Associated with Back Pain after Childbirth," *Anesthesiology* 81, no. 1 (July 1994): 29–34.

43. J. M. Price and R. L. Carpenter, "Anesthesia Safety, Outcomes, and Prospective Study Design," *Anesthesiology* 89, no. 3 (September 1998): 790–92.

44. Yves Auroy et al., "Major Complications of Regional Anesthesia in France: The SOS Regional Anesthesia Hotline Service," *Anesthesiology* 97, no. 5 (November 2002): 1274–80.

45. M. J. Paech, R. Godkin, and S. Webster, "Complications of Obstetric Epidural Analgesia and Anaesthesia: A Prospective Analysis of 10,995 Cases," *International Journal of Obstetric Anesthesia* 7, no. 1 (January 1998): 5–11.

46. Liu et al., "Maternal Mortality and Severe Morbidity Associated with Low-Risk Planned Cesarean Delivery versus Planned Vaginal Delivery at Term."

47. L. Guglielmo et al., "Conversion of Spinal Anesthesia into General Anesthesia: An Evaluation of More than 35,000 Spinal Anesthetics," *Minerva Anestesiologica* 76, no. 9 (July 1, 2010).

48. Pi-Ying Chang et al., "Butterfly-Like Knotting of a Lumbar Epidural Catheter," *Acta Anaesthesiologica Taiwanica: Official Journal of the Taiwan Society of Anesthesiologists* 48, no. 1 (March 2010): 45–48.

49. Paech, Godkin, and Webster, "Complications of Obstetric Epidural Analgesia."

50. Brendan Carvalho et al., "Patient Preferences for Anesthesia Outcomes Associated with Cesarean Delivery," *Anesthesia and Analgesia* 101, no. 4 (October 2005): 1182–87.

51. Eugene Declercq et al., "Maternal Outcomes Associated with Planned Primary Cesarean Births Compared with Planned Vaginal Births," *Obstetrics and Gynecology* 109, no. 3 (March 2007): 669–77.

52. Shiliang Liu et al., "Risk of Maternal Postpartum Readmission Associated with Mode of Delivery," *Obstetrics and Gynecology* 105, no. 4 (April 2005): 836–42.

53. Chuma J. Chike-Obi, Patrick D. Cole, and Anthony E. Brissett, "Keloids: Pathogenesis, Clinical Features, and Management," *Seminars in Plastic Surgery* 23, no. 3 (August 2009): 178–84.

54. Johanna M. F. W. Vermelis et al., "Prevalence and Predictors of Chronic Pain after Labor and Delivery," *Current Opinion in Anaesthesiology* 23, no. 3 (June 2010): 295–99.

55. Caroline Signore, Anusha Hemachandra, and Mark Klebanoff,

"Neonatal Mortality and Morbidity after Elective Cesarean Delivery versus Routine Expectant Management: A Decision Analysis," *Seminars in Perinatology* 30, no. 5 (October 2006): 288–95.

56. Zilgia Benoît et al., "The Effect of Increased FIO2 before Tracheal Extubation on Postoperative Atelectasis," *Anesthesia and Analgesia* 95, no. 6 (December 2002): 1777–81.

57. Lucky Jain and Golde G. Dudell, "Respiratory Transition in Infants Delivered by Cesarean Section," *Seminars in Perinatology* 30, no. 5 (October 2006): 296–304.

58. Anne Kirkeby Hansen et al., "Risk of Respiratory Morbidity in Term Infants Delivered by Elective Caesarean Section: Cohort Study," *British Medical Journal (Clinical Research Ed.)* 336, no. 7635 (January 12, 2008): 85–87.

59. P. M. Hull, "Rapid Responses to Risk of Respiratory Morbidity in Term Infants Delivered by Elective Caesarean Section: Cohort Study," *British Medical Journal*, March 3, 2008, http://www.bmj.com/content/336/7635/85.full/reply #bmj_el_191467 (accessed September 10, 2010).

60. Roberta De Luca et al., "Incidence of Early Neonatal Mortality and Morbidity after Late-Preterm and Term Cesarean Delivery," *Pediatrics* 123, no. 6 (June 2009): 1064–71.

61. Clarissa Bonanno and Ronald J. Wapner, "Antenatal Corticosteroid Treatment: What's Happened Since Drs. Liggins and Howie?" *American Journal of Obstetrics and Gynecology* 200, no. 4 (April 2009): 448–57.

62. James M. Alexander et al., "Fetal Injury Associated with Cesarean Delivery," *Obstetrics and Gynecology* 108, no. 4 (October 2006): 885–90; J. J. Wiener and J. Westwood, "Fetal Lacerations at Caesarean Section," *Journal of Obstetrics and Gynaecology* 22, no. 1 (January 2002): 23–24; National Health Service, "NHS Maternity Statistics, England 2004–05," NHS Information Centre for Health and Social Care, May 26, 2006, http://www.ic.nhs.uk/pubs/maternity eng2005 (accessed September 10, 2010).

63. Alan T. N. Tita et al., "Timing of Planned Repeat Cesarean Delivery at Term and Neonatal Outcomes," *New England Journal of Medicine* 360, no. 2 (January 8, 2009): 111–20.

64. "Anesthesia and Queen Victoria," Department of Epidemiology, UCLA School of Public Health, http://www.ph.ucla.edu/epi/snow/victoria.html (accessed September 10, 2010).

65. C. R. Davis, "Infection-Free Surgery: How to Improve Hand-Hygiene Compliance and Eradicate Methicillin-Resistant Staphylococcus Aureus from Surgical Wards," *Annals of the Royal College of Surgeons of England* 92, no. 4 (May 2010): 316–19.

66. Ian M. Gould, "Alexander Gordon, Puerperal Sepsis, and Modern The-

ories of Infection Control: Semmelweis in Perspective," *Lancet Infectious Diseases* 10, no. 4 (April 2010): 275–78.

67. Robert A. Yoho, Jeremy J. Romaine, and Deborah O'Neil, "Review of the Liposuction, Abdominoplasty, and Face-Lift Mortality and Morbidity Risk Literature," *Dermatologic Surgery* 31, no. 7 (July 2005): 733–43; D. N. Lucas et al., "Urgency of Caesarean Section: A New Classification," *Journal of the Royal Society of Medicine* 93, no. 7 (July 2000): 346–50.

68. Leanne S. Dahlgren et al., "Caesarean Section on Maternal Request: Risks and Benefits in Healthy Nulliparous Women and Their Infants," *Journal of Obstetrics and Gynaecology Canada* 31, no. 9 (September 2009): 808–17.

CHAPTER 14. THE DAY OF SURGERY: WHAT HAPPENS, STEP BY STEP

1. Emmanuel Bujold et al., "The Role of Uterine Closure in the Risk of Uterine Rupture," *Obstetrics and Gynecology* 116, no. 1 (July 2010): 43–50.

2. Colin A. Walsh, "Evidence-Based Cesarean Technique," *Current Opinion in Obstetrics and Gynecology* 22, no. 2 (April 2010): 110–15.

CHAPTER 17. INFORMED CHOICE: NECESSARY, COMPLEX, AND CHALLENGING

1. Gary D. V. Hankins, Shannon M. Clark, and Mary B. Munn, "Cesarean Section on Request at 39 Weeks: Impact on Shoulder Dystocia, Fetal Trauma, Neonatal Encephalopathy, and Intrauterine Fetal Demise," *Seminars in Perinatology* 30, no. 5 (October 2006): 276–87.

2. Scott A. Farrell, "Cesarean Section versus Forceps-Assisted Vaginal Birth: It's Time to Include Pelvic Injury in the Risk-Benefit Equation," *CMAJ: Canadian Medical Association Journal* 166, no. 3 (February 5, 2002): 337–38.

3. S. A. Johnson, "Ethical Dilemma: A Patient Refuses a Life-Saving Cesarean," *MCN. The American Journal of Maternal Child Nursing* 17, no. 3 (June 1992): 121–25; J. V. Pinkerton and J. J. Finnerty, "Resolving the Clinical and Ethical Dilemma Involved in Fetal-Maternal Conflicts," *American Journal of Obstetrics and Gynecology* 175, no. 2 (August 1996): 289–95; Elizabeth Butler-Sloss, "Legal Aspects of Medical Ethics," *Web Journal of Current Legal Issues*, 2006,

http://webjcli.ncl.ac.uk/2006/issue2/butlersloss2a.html; American College of Obstetricians and Gynecologists Office of Communications, "New ACOG Opinion Addresses Elective Cesarean Controversy," news release, October 31, 2003, http://www.acog.org/from_home/publications/press_releases/nr10-31-03 -1.cfm (accessed February 24, 2011).

4. Margaret Olivia Little et al., "Mode of Delivery: Toward Responsible Inclusion of Patient Preferences," *Obstetrics and Gynecology* 112, no. 4 (October 2008): 913–18.

5. American College of Obstetricians and Gynecologists, "ACOG Committee Opinion No. 394, December 2007. Cesarean Delivery on Maternal Request," *Obstetrics and Gynecology* 110, no. 6 (December 2007): 1501.

6. Barbara A. Bettes et al., "Cesarean Delivery on Maternal Request: Obstetrician-Gynecologists' Knowledge, Perception, and Practice Patterns," *Obstetrics and Gynecology* 109, no. 1 (January 2007): 57–66.

7. Jenny Gamble et al., "A Critique of the Literature on Women's Request for Cesarean Section," *Birth* 34, no. 4 (December 2007): 331–40; Annika Karlström et al., "Behind the Myth: Few Women Prefer Caesarean Section in the Absence of Medical or Obstetrical Factors," *Midwifery* 27, no. 5 (October 2011): 620–27; Eugene Declercq, "Myth of the Maternal Request Cesarean: Exploring Mothers' Attitudes toward Cesarean Birth," paper presented at the 134th Annual Meeting and Exposition of the American Public Health Association, Boston, MA, November 2006, http://apha.confex.com/apha/134am/techprogram/paper _144003 .htm (accessed February 24, 2011).

8. American College of Obstetricians and Gynecologists, "ACOG Committee Opinion No. 395: Surgery and Patient Choice," *Obstetrics and Gynecology* 111, no. 1 (January 2008): 243–47.

9. Robin B. Kalish, Laurence B. McCullough, and Frank A. Chervenak, "Patient Choice Cesarean Delivery: Ethical Issues," *Current Opinion in Obstetrics and Gynecology* 20, no. 2 (April 2008): 116–19.

10. Jill Milne et al., "Developing and Pre-Testing a Decision Board to Facilitate Informed Choice about Delivery Approach in Uncomplicated Pregnancy," *Biomed Central (BMC) Pregnancy and Childbirth* 9 (2009): 50.

11. Joanne Morrison and I. Z. MacKenzie, "Cesarean Section on Demand," *Seminars in Perinatology* 27, no. 1 (February 2003): 20–33.

CHAPTER 18. THE EVOLUTION OF NATURAL BIRTH AND THE FUTURE OF CESAREAN BIRTH

1. M. M. Abitbol, "Evolution of the Ischial Spine and of the Pelvic Floor in the Hominoidea," *American Journal of Physical Anthropology* 75, no. 1 (January 1988): 53–67.

2. Tom Hogervorst, Heinse W. Bouma, and John de Vos, "Evolution of the Hip and Pelvis," *Acta Orthopaedica. Supplementum* 80, no. 336 (2009): 1–39.

3. W. R. Trevathan, "The Evolution of Bipedalism and Assisted Birth," *Medical Anthropology Quarterly* 10, no. 2 (June 1996): 287–90; K. R. Rosenberg and W. R. Trevathan, "The Evolution of Human Birth," *Scientific American* 285, no. 5 (November 2001): 72–77; Karen Rosenberg and Wenda Trevathan, "Birth, Obstetrics, and Human Evolution," *BJOG: An International Journal of Obstetrics and Gynaecology* 109, no. 11 (November 2002): 1199–206.

4. Timothy D. Weaver and Jean-Jacques Hublin, "Neandertal Birth Canal Shape and the Evolution of Human Childbirth," *Proceedings of the National Academy of Sciences of the United States of America* 106, no. 20 (May 19, 2009): 8151–56; W. R. Trevathan and K. Rosenberg, "The Shoulders Follow the Head: Postcranial Constraints on Human Childbirth," *Journal of Human Evolution* 39, no. 6 (December 2000): 583–86.

5. Stuart Weiner, Janet Monge, and Alan Mann, "Bipedalism and Parturition: An Evolutionary Imperative for Cesarean Delivery?" *Clinics in Perinatology* 35, no. 3 (September 2008): 469–78, ix; Trevathan, "Evolution of Bipedalism"; Anna Blackburn Wittman and L. Lewis Wall, "The Evolutionary Origins of Obstructed Labor: Bipedalism, Encephalization, and the Human Obstetric Dilemma," *Obstetrical and Gynecological Survey* 62, no. 11 (November 2007): 739–48.

6. Herbert Oliver Elftman, "The Evolution of the Pelvic Floor of Primates," *American Journal of Anatomy* 51, no. 2 (1932): 307–46.

7. Rosenberg and Trevathan, "Birth, Obstetrics, and Human Evolution."

8. Weiner, Monge, and Mann, "Bipedalism and Parturition."

9. Ibid.

10. Rosenberg and Trevathan, "Birth, Obstetrics, and Human Evolution."

11. Jordan B. Peterson, *Maps of Meaning: The Architecture of Belief* (London: Routledge, 1999).

Index

delivery type, 29, 101, 171, 205–206, 228, 269
Denmark, 278
    cesarean rates in, 66, 161
developing world, as it relates to birth rate and delivery type, 21, 92, 100, 162–63, 176–77, 212
diabetes, 253, 255, 344. *See also* gestational diabetes
dilation and curettage (D&C), 259, 297
dilemma, of doctors, 100, 148, 346
disabled, children by birth, 323, 353
double incontinence, 162. *See also* incontinence
doula, 185, 190
dyspareunia, 237, 240. *See also* pain during sex

economics, 130
    health economics, 153
    See also under cost
Ecuador
    increased cesarean rates in, 124
    reduced deaths of mothers in, 124
edema (fluid swelling), 266, 288
education, 18, 110, 114, 118, 135, 144, 150, 157, 162, 163, 186
Egypt
    increased cesarean rates in, 124
    reduced deaths of mothers in, 124
electivecesarean.com, 324
elective cesarean
    debate over, 21, 139, 149, 151, 154, 163, 165, 178, 190–91, 198, 344–45, 348
    long-term risks of, 348
    preference for, 65, 160, 162, 250
    safety of, 41–55, 66, 185, 191, 199, 202, 220–21
electrocautery, 293, 300
embolism
    air embolism, 255–57, 298
    amniotic fluid embolism, 255–56
    embolization, 261
    fat embolism, 255–56

pulmonary embolism, 102, 254
thromboembolism, 143, 175, 253–55
    See also deep vein thrombosis (DVT); pulmonary embolism
emergency cesarean
    avoiding, 249
    cost of, 224, 226–27, 229–31
    increased risks of, 44, 142, 144, 150
    and love hormones, 63
    trauma of, 47. *See also* trauma
emotion, 19, 21, 35, 59, 91, 104, 111, 113, 132, 174, 198, 206, 208, 209, 219, 324, 330
empowerment, 21, 70, 74, 107, 164
endometritis, 250–52
England, 151, 154–55, 333
    research and surveys in, 59, 65, 67, 150, 153, 156, 279
epidemic. *See under* obesity, 143
epidural, 30, 92, 109, 122, 161, 174, 181, 185, 232, 265–71, 276, 281, 315, 335
episiotomy, 31, 87, 88, 90, 112, 114–17, 138, 160, 169, 237, 275, 320, 329, 335
Egypt
    cesarean rates in, 124
    mortality rate of mothers in, 124
Erb's palsy, 49, 323. *See also under* brachial plexus
ethics, 133, 163, 185, 348
ethnicity as factor in childbirth, 129, 169, 201, 249, 256
Europe
    European Perinatal Health Report, 135
    fertility rates in, 202
    healthcare in, 146, 148, 338
    hospitals in, 43
    perinatal mortality rates in, 134
evidence-based, 21, 44, 50, 157, 173, 274, 342
evolution, 177, 221, 282–83, 343, 353–58, 360
exercise, 104, 114, 117, 145, 170, 212, 230, 282, 285, 305, 308, 310, 311

430   INDEX